THE NURSE'S DICTIONARY

Twenty-eighth edition

THE
NURSE'S DICTIONARY

originally compiled by

HONNOR MORTEN

Twenty-eighth edition

revised by

P. JEAN CUNNINGHAM

B.A., S.R.N., S.C.M.
Health Visitor's Certificate

(Sixty-fifth printing)

FABER AND FABER LIMITED
3 Queen Square
London

Twenty-eighth edition 1976
Published by Faber and Faber Limited
3 Queen Square, London W.C.1
Printed in Great Britain by
Western Printing Services Ltd, Bristol
All rights reserved

ISBN 0 571 04896 X

PREFACE TO THE TWENTY-FIFTH EDITION

To mark the quarter of a century in editions of this dictionary the publishers have decided on a new format, so that once again this dictionary will fit into the pocket as it did in the earliest editions.

Many new entries appear in this edition, of words in current use, and with the emphasis on mental health today I have tried to add the psychological terms which the nurse is likely to meet. Some drugs have been added and others deleted, but as the number of new drugs is legion, no attempt has been made to list them all, which would only cause confusion. The section on diets has been revised. There is a new section on poisons and their antidotes, and I have described the mouth-to-mouth method of artificial respiration, which Mrs. Audrey Besterman has illustrated. Many have helped with this revision including: Dr. J. G. Bate, Mr. C. W. F. Burnett, F.R.C.S., F.R.C.O.G., Dr. J. Caradoc Evans, Dr. D. Knight Jones, Dr. D. Weitzman, Miss Gloria Gerson, Mrs. Shirley Gillis and Miss E. More O'Ferrall.

I very much hope that the student nurse coming from abroad may find the guide to pronunciation helpful; it is often more difficult for her to grasp where the stress comes in a word, than the correct pronunciation of each syllable.

Finally, I would like to say that the student nurse is in many ways faced with a greater problem than the medical student, who is not often obliged to turn so quickly from one subject to another as the student nurse, who may have a variety of patients in her ward, all suffering from diseases which belong to the various specialties.

1962   P.J.C.

PREFACE TO THE TWENTY-SIXTH EDITION

Many additions and alterations have been made to keep this dictionary in line with modern developments. There are also a number of new drawings by Audrey Besterman and a new Appendix on Blood explaining its constituents and blood chemistry.

It is hoped that the dictionary will continue to meet the needs of nurses, medical auxiliaries, and all those who need a concise dictionary to help them in their work, and I would like to thank the many people who have given me help with this new edition.

1966   P.J.C.

PREFACE TO THE TWENTY-SEVENTH EDITION

Many have helped to compile this new edition in which there are over three hundred new entries. New procedures are mentioned and a number of words, now out of fashion, have been deleted. There is a short alphabetical list of some common drugs in the Appendix.

I would like to thank all those who have helped with this new edition and am indebted to Mrs. Audrey Besterman for the new line drawings she has produced.

1972   P.J.C.

PREFACE TO THE TWENTY-EIGHTH EDITION

A number of additions have been made throughout the dictionary to keep it up to date, and some new drugs have been added to the list of some common drugs in Appendix IV.

My aim has been to keep the dictionary as concise as possible, and 'portmanteau' words such as acrocephalosyndactyly are usually omitted when the meaning is obvious.

I have to thank many for their help in revising the dictionary, and in particular Miss Heather Potter, B.Sc.

1974   P.J.C.

CONTENTS

ABBREVIATIONS OF LATIN TERMS AS USED IN PRESCRIPTIONS, &c.

Abbreviation	Latin	
a.c.	ante cibos	before meals
ad.	adde	up to
ad lib.	ad libitum	to the desired amount
alt. dieb.	alternis diebus	every other day
aq.	aqua	water
aq. dest.	aqua destillata	distilled water
aurist.	auristillae	ear drops
b.d.	bis die	twice a day
B.N.F.	—	British National Formulary
B.P.	—	British Pharmacopoeia
bal.	balneum	bath
c.	cum	with
comp.	compositus	compounded of
crem.	cremor	a cream
dil.	dilue	dilute
ext.	extractum	extract
gutt.	gutta or guttae	drop or drops
haust.	haustus	a draught
in d.	in dies	daily
inj.	injectio	an injection
lot.	lotio	lotion
mist.	mistura	mixture
mit.	mitte	send
noct.	nocte	at night
oc.	oculentum	eye ointment
o.m.	omni mane	every morning
o.n.	omni nocte	every night
p.c.	post cibos	after meals
pig.	pigmentum	paint
p.r.	per rectum	by the rectum
p.r.n.	pro re nata	as occasion arises
pulv.	pulvis	powder
p.v.	per vaginam	by the vagina
q.d. q.d.s. }	quarter in die	four times a day
q.s.	quantum sufficit	as much as is required
R.	recipe	take

Abbreviations   *Latin*

rep.	repetatur	let it be repeated
sig.	signetur	let it be labelled
s.o.s.	si opus sit	if necessary
stat.	statim	immediately
syr.	syrupus	syrup
t.d. t.d.s. }	ter in die	thrice a day
tinct. tr. }	tinctura	tincture
ung.	unguentum	ointment

COMPARATIVE WEIGHTS AND MEASURES

WEIGHT

Metric System

1 kilogram (kg)	=	1,000 grams
1 gram (G or g)	=	1,000 milligrams
1 milligram (mg)	=	1,000 micrograms
1 microgram (μg)	=	1,000,000 micromicrograms

Imperial System

(The standard is the pound Avoirdupois)

1 pound (lb.)	=	16 ounces	=	7,000 grains (gr.)
1 ounce (oz.)	=	437·5 grains		

Apothecaries Weight (Imperial and U.S.A.)

1 ounce (℥)	=	8 drachms	=	480 grains
1 drachm (ʒ)	=	3 scruples	=	60 grains
1 scruple (Ə)	=	20 grains		

Conversions

Imperial System		Metric System
1 pound (lb.)	=	453·59 grams
1 ounce (oz.)	=	28·34 grams
1 grain (gr.)	=	0·0648 gram or 64·8 milligrams (mg)

Metric System		Imperial System
1 kilogram (kg)	=	2·2046 pounds or 35·274 ounces or 15,432 grains
1 gram (G or g)	=	15·432 grains
1 milligram (mg)	=	0·015432 grain

SOME USEFUL EQUIVALENTS

Milligrams		Grains	Milligrams		Grains
1000	=	15	20	=	1/3
800	=	12	15	=	1/4
600	=	10	10	=	1/6
500	=	8	6	=	1/10
400	=	6	4	=	1/15
300	=	5	2·5	=	1/24
250	=	4	1·5	=	1/40
200	=	3	1·25	=	1/50
125	=	2	1	=	1/60
100	=	1½	0·8	=	1/75
60	=	1	0·6	=	1/100
50	=	3/4	0·25	=	1/240

VOLUME

Metric System

1 litre (l) = 1,000 millilitres
1 millilitre (ml) = 1·000028 cubic centimetres (cc)
(The millilitre and cubic centimetre are usually treated as identical.)

Imperial (Apothecaries) System

1 gallon (C) = 8 pints = 76,800 minims
1 pint (pt.) (O) = 20 fluid ounces = 9,600 minims
1 fluid ounce (fl.oz.) (℥) = 8 fluid drachms = 480 minims
1 fluid drachm (fl.dr.) (ℨ) = 60 minims (m.)

U.S.A. Apothecaries

1 gallon (C) = 8 pints = 61,440 minims
1 pint (O) = 16 fluid ounces = 7,680 minims
1 fluid ounce (f℥) = 8 fluid drachms = 480 minims
1 fluid drachm (fℨ) = 60 minims (m.)

Conversions

Imperial System		Metric System
1 pint (pt.)	=	568·25 millilitres
1 fluid ounce (fl.oz.)	=	28·412 millilitres
1 fluid drachm (fl.dr.)	=	3·5515 millilitres
1 minim (m.)	=	0·059192 millilitres

Metric System		Imperial System
1 litre (l)	=	1·7598 pints or 35·196 fluid ounces
1 millilitre (ml)	=	16·894 minims

Imperial System		U.S.A. Apothecaries
1 pint	=	1·25 pints
U.S.A. Apothecaries		Imperial System
1 pint	=	0·8 pints

(A 1 per cent w/v solution means:

10 grams dissolved in water and the volume diluted to 1 litre, or 1 ounce dissolved in water and the volume diluted to five pints.)

LENGTH

Metric System

1 metre (m)	=	10 decimetres
1 decimetre (dm)	=	10 centimetres
1 centimetre (cm)	=	10 millimetres
1 millimetre (mm)	=	1,000 microns
1 micron (μ)	=	1,000 millimicrons
1 millimicron (mμ)	=	1,000,000 micromicrons ($\mu\mu$)

British System

1 mile	=	1,760 yards
1 yard	=	3 feet
1 foot	=	12 inches

Conversions

Metric System		*British System*
1 metre (m)	=	39·370 inches
1 decimetre (dm)	=	3·9370 inches
1 centimetre (cm)	=	0·39370 inches
1 millimetre (mm)	=	0·039370 inches
1 micron (μ)	=	0·000039370 inches
1 millimicron (mμ)	=	0·000000039370 inches

British System		*Metric System*
1 mile	=	1609·344 metres
1 yard	=	91·44 centimetres
1 foot	=	30·48 centimetres
1 inch	=	2·540 centimetres

FLUID MEASURE

1 minim	= 1 drop (approx.)—Symbol (m)
60 minims	= 1 drachm— „ (℈)
8 drachms	= 1 ounce— „ (℥)
20 ounces	= 1 pint— „ (O)
8 pints	= 1 gallon— „ (C)

A teaspoonful is about a drachm. Two tablespoonfuls are about an ounce.

COMPARISON OF CENTIGRADE AND
FAHRENHEIT THERMOMETRIC SCALES

Boiling-point $= 212°$ F $= 100°$ C

Freezing-point $= 32°$ F $= 0°$ C

Normal temperature of the body $= 98.4°$ F
$= 37°$ C

To convert degrees F into degrees C deduct
32, multiply by 5, and divide by 9.
e.g. 104° F to centigrade,
$104 - 32 = 72 \times 5 = 360 \div 9 = 40$
$\therefore 104°$ F $= 40°$ C

To convert degrees C into degrees F multiply
by 9, divide by 5, and add 32 to the result.
e.g. 36.6° C to Fahrenheit,
$36.6 \times 9 = 330 \div 5 = 66 + 32 = 98$
$\therefore 36.6°$ C $= 98°$ F

C	F
100	212
95	203
90	194
85	185
80	176
75	167
70	158
65	149
60	140
55	131
50	122
45	113
40	104
35	95
30	86
25	77
20	68
15	59
10	50
5	41
0	32
-5	23
-10	14
-15	5
-18	0

SOME USEFUL EQUIVALENTS IN
CLINICAL THERMOMETER READINGS

Fahrenheit		Centigrade
107·5	←→	41·9
107	←→	41·7
106·5	←→	41·4
106	←→	41·1
105·5	←→	40·8
105	←→	40·6
104·5	←→	40·3
104	←→	40
103·5	←→	39·7
103	←→	39·4
102·5	←→	39·2
102	←→	38·9
101·5	←→	38·6
101	←→	38·3
100·5	←→	38·1
100	←→	37·8
99·5	←→	37·5
99	←→	37·2
98·4	←→	36·9
97·8	←→	36·6

A GUIDE TO PRONUNCIATION

The pronunciation for the twenty-fifth edition of the *Nurse's Dictionary* was completely revised and simplified, and I have tried to consider the special needs of student nurses from all parts of the world who by studying nursing in the English language have to use a foreign tongue.

After each entry in the dictionary the pronunciation is found in brackets. The stress mark ' shows where the emphasis should be made in a word of more than one syllable, and these are divided by hyphens. Where the emphasis or stress comes in a word is often one of the most difficult parts in learning to speak a language. For example, an-ti'-mo-ni (antimony) always has the emphasis on the second syllable, and the English ear is jarred if the stress is put anywhere else.

The basic vowel and consonant sounds are listed below with examples taken from the dictionary:

Vowel sound			Example
a	as in	bat	cataract (*kat'-a-rakt*)
ā	,, ,,	mate	flatus (*flā'-tus*)
ah	,, ,,	father	after (*ahf'-ter*)
ar	,, ,,	far	carbon (*kar'-bon*)
ā-r	,, ,,	air	aerosol (*ā'-rō-sol*)
aw	,, ,,	fall	audiometer (*aw-dē-om'-et-er*)
e	,, ,,	get	electric (*e-lek'-trik*)
ē	,, ,,	been	ether (*ē'-ther*)
ē-r	,, ,,	ear	sclera (*sklē'-ra*)
i	,, ,,	bit	nicotinic (*ni-kō-tin'-ik*)
ī	,, ,,	bite	eye (*ī*), hydro- (*hī-drō*)
o	,, ,,	hop	optics (*op'-tiks*)
ō	,, ,,	hope	isotopes (*ī-zō-tōps*)
oo	,, ,,	soon	croup (*kroop*)
or	,, ,,	for	orbit (*or'-bit*)
ow	,, ,,	how	sound (*sownd*)
oy	,, ,,	boy	boil (*boyl*)
u	,, ,,	cup	tongue (*tung*)
ū	,, ,,	mute	cubit (*kū-bit*)

Consonant sound							Example
f	the sound of	ph as in phobia (*fō'-bi-ah*)
j	,,	,, ,,	g	,,	,, dermalgia (*der-mal'-ji-a*)

21

Consonant sound   *Example*

k	the sound of	c	as in	catalyst	(*ka'-ta-list*)
ks	,,	,,	x	,,	X-ray (*eks'-rā*)
kw	,,	,,	qu	,,	quintan (*kwin'-tan*)
s	,,	,,	c	,,	lucid (*loo'-sid*)
shon	,,	,,	tion	,,	ablution (*ab-loo'-shon*)
zhon	,,	,,	sion	,,	invasion (*in-vā'-zhon*)

THE NURSE'S DICTIONARY

A

a- or **an** (*ā or an*). Prefix denoting 'lack of', *e.g.* achlorhydria, lack of hydrochloric acid; anuria, lack of urine, etc.

ab (*ab*). A prefix signifying from, away from, *e.g. Abenteric*, situated away from and not in the intestine, etc.

abalienation (*ab-ā-lē-en-ā-shon*). Mental derangement.

abasia (*ab-ā'-si-a*). Motor incoordination in walking.

abdomen (*ab-dō'-men*). The belly. The body cavity immediately below the thorax, bounded above by the diaphragm, below by the pelvis, behind by the lumbar vertebrae, and in front and at the sides by muscular walls. It contains many important organs, including the stomach, intestines, liver, kidneys, spleen, pancreas, bladder, uterus and ovaries. It is lined with a serous membrane called the peritoneum, which is reflected onto many of the organs in the abdomen (*see* illustration).

abdominal (*ab-dom-in-al*). Pertaining to the abdomen.

abdomino-perineal (*ab-do-mi-nō-pe-ri-nā-al*). Used to

AREAS OF THE ABDOMEN

describe operation utilizing approach from both abdominal and perineal incisions.

abducent nerves (*ab-dū'-sent nervs*). The sixth pair of cranial nerves, activating the external rectus muscle of the eye-ball, which rotates the eye-ball outwards.

abduct (*ab-dukt'*). To draw away from the mid-line.

abduction (*ab-duk-shon*). The act of moving a limb away from the middle line of the body.

abductor (*ab-duk'-ter*). A muscle which draws a limb from the median line of the body, *e.g.* deltoid.

aberration (*ab-er-ā'-shon*). Deviation from the normal. In optics, defect in focus of a lens. *Mental A.* Mental disturbance or peculiarity.

ablatio retinae (*ab-lah-tē-ō re-ti-nē*). Detachment of the retina.

ablation (*ab-lā'-shon*). Removal or detachment of a part.

ablution (*ab-loo'-shon*). Cleansing by washing.

abnormal (*ab-nor'-mal*). Irregular, unusual.

abort (*a-bort*). To terminate a process before the full course is run.

abortifacient (*a-bor-ti-fā'-si-ent*). A drug taken for the purpose of procuring abortion.

abortion (*a-bor'-shon*). Discharge of the gestation sac from the pregnant uterus before the fetus is viable, *q.v.* Abortion may be *complete* or *incomplete*; it may be *threatened* or *inevitable*, according to the cervical canal being closed or open. Finally it may be *missed*: that is, the fetus may be dead, but may not be discharged immediately. *Tubal A.* When an ovum developing in the Fallopian tube becomes detached, and is thrown off through the abdominal ostium of the tube into the Pouch of Douglas.

abortus fever (*ab-or'-tus fē-ver*). An undulant fever, also called brucellosis, caused by infected cow's milk.

abrasion (*ab-rā'-zhon*). A superficial injury to the skin or mucous membrane.

abreaction (*ab-rē-ak'-shon*). A state of mind brought about during the process of psychoanalysis. The patient lives again through past painful experiences which may unconsciously be causing the neurosis.

abscess (*ab'-ses*). A collection of pus in a cavity, the result of inflammation. *Alveolar A.* One which develops in the socket of a tooth. *Blind A.* One with no external opening. *Cold A.* One which develops slowly, without inflammation, as in tuberculosis. *Ischiorectal A.* One in the ischiorectal fossa. *Metastatic A.* Secondary to an abscess elsewhere; caused by an infected embolus. *Psoas A.* One due to disease of the vertebrae. The pus descends in the sheath of the psoas muscle, forming a fluctuating tumour above or below Poupart's ligament. It is usually tuberculous in origin. *Residual A.* One developing in old inflammatory products. *Stitch A.* One formed around a stitch or suture.

absolute values. In blood counts these are the actual numbers and not the percentage figures.

absorbent (*ab-sorb'-ent*). Taking up by suction. Gauze and wool are absorbent dressings. *A. drug.* One that causes absorption of diseased tissue, *e.g.* potassium iodide.

acanthosis (*ak-an-thō'-sis*). Any disease of the prickle-layer, the lowest stratum of the epidermis. *A. Nigricans.* General pigmentation of the skin with mole-like growths.

acapnia (*ā-kap'-ni-a*). A lessened amount of carbon dioxide in the blood.

acardia (*ā-kar'-di-ah*). Congenital absence of the heart.

Acarus (*ak'-a-rus*). The name of a group of animal parasites. *A. Scabiei* is the parasite causing scabies.

acatalepsy (*ā-ka-ta-lep'-si*). Uncertainty, lack of understanding.

acataphasia (*a-kat-a-fā'-zi-a*). Difficulty in expressing ideas in logical sequence.

accessory nerves (*ak-se-so-ri*). Eleventh pair of cranial nerves.

accidental haemorrhage (*ak-si-den'-tal hem-o-rāj*). Bleeding from the pregnant uterus in the later months of pregnancy due to premature separation of normally situated placenta. It may be *concealed*, when the bleeding remains internal; or *external*, when the blood escapes by the vagina. *See* ANTEPARTUM HAEMORRHAGE.

accommodation (*ak-om-o-dā'-shon*). In ophthalmology the power to adjust the eye to obtain clear vision at different distances.

accouchement (*ak-koosh-mor*). Childbirth.

accretion (*ak-krē-shon*). Accumulation of foreign matter.

acephalic (*ā-ke-fa-lik*). Headless.

acetabuloplasty (*a-se-tab-ū-lō-pla'-sti*). A plastic operation performed on the hip joint for osteo-arthritis.

acetabulum (*a-se-tab'-ū-lum*). The cuplike socket in the hip

Hip bone

Acetabulum

Femur

HIP JOINT
(Showing Acetabulum)

or innominate bone into which the head of the femur fits.

acetate (*as'-et-āt*). A salt of acetic acid.

acetazolamide (*a-sē-ta-zol-a-mīd*). A non-mercurial diuretic. Also used in glaucoma as it decreases intra-ocular pressure, and in epilepsy. Proprietary name, Diamox.

acetic acid (*a-sēt'-ik*). The acid of vinegar. It is used in testing urine for albumin.

aceto-acetic acid (*as-ē-tō-a-sē-tik*). Produced at an intermediate stage of fatty acid oxidation. If metabolism is disturbed, as in diabetes mellitus, it is found in excess in the blood and the urine. Syn. diacetic acid.

acetomenaphthone (*a-sē-tō-men-af'-thōn*). A chemical with activity similar to that of vitamin K.

acetonaemia (*as'-ē-tō-nē-me-ah*). The presence of acetone in the blood.

acetone (*ass'-e-tōn*). A colourless volatile solvent. This substance is formed in the body when metabolism is upset, as in starvation, excessive vomiting, diabetes mellitus. It is excreted in the urine and the breath.

acetonuria (*as'-ē-tōn-ū'-ri-a*). The presence of acetone in the urine. For test *see* Appendix, p. 383.

acetylcholine (*ass-ē-til-kō'-lēn*). A chemical substance liberated from parasympathetic nerve endings when they are stimulated. They are thus called cholinergic fibres.

acetylsalicylic acid (*ass-ē'-til-sa-li-sil'-ik as-id*). Aspirin, *q.v.*

achalasia (*ak-al-ā'-ze-ah*). Failure to relax. *Cardiac A.* Contraction of the sphincter at the cardiac orifice of the stomach, with dilatation of the lower end of the oesophagus.

Achilles tendon (*a-kil-lēz ten'-don*). The large tendon which attaches the calf muscles to the heel.

achillorrhaphy (*a-kil-o-ra-fi*). Surgery to rejoin the Achilles tendon after rupture.

achlorhydria (*ā-klor-hī'-dri-a*). Absence of hydrochloric acid in the gastric juice; may occur in pernicious anaemia and cancer of the stomach.

acholia (*ā-kō-li-a*). Absence of bile.

acholuria (*a-kol-ū'-ri-a*). The absence of bile pigment from the urine.

acholuric jaundice (*a-kol-ū'-rik*). *See* JAUNDICE.

achondroplasia (*a-kon'-drō-plā-zi-a*). A form of arrested development of the long bones, leading to dwarfism. The intellect is not affected.

achromasia (*a-krō-mā'-zi-a*). (1) Absence of colour. (2) Loss of staining reaction in a cell.

achromatopsia (*a-krō-mat-op'-si-a*). Colour blindness.

Achromycin (*a-kro-mī'-sin*). Proprietary drug. Tetracyclines, *q.v.*

achylia, achylosis (*a-kī'-li-a*). Absence of chyle. *A. gastrica*, dysfunction of gastric juice by atrophy of mucous membrane of the stomach.

acid (*as'-id*). A substance capable of uniting with alkalis to form salts. Acids turn blue litmus paper red and when in liquid form have a sour taste, *e.g.* vinegar and lemon juice both contain acids. (For individual acids *see under* special name.)

acidaemia (*a-sid-ē-mi-a*). The blood is abnormally acid and the pH below 7·3.

acid-base balance. The balance between the acidic and basic components which determine the pH of body fluids.

acid-fast. In bacteriology a term applied to certain bacteria which retain the red carbol-fuchsin stain after the application of an acid solution. Other organisms are decolorized. Tubercle bacilli are 'acid-fast'.

acidity (*as-id'-it-ē*). The proportion of acid in a given substance. Thus gastric juice contains normally 0·2 per cent of hydrochloric acid.

acidosis (*as-id-ō'-sis*) or ketosis. A condition believed to be due to diminished alkalinity of the blood. There is an abnormal production and faulty elimination of acids. The condition occurs in association with acetonuria and is due to the same causes. The acids found in the blood and urine are oxybutyric and diacetic.

acid phosphatase (*fos-fa-tāz*). Enzyme produced by the prostate gland and secreted in seminal fluid. Serum acid phosphatase is raised in carcinoma of the prostate when there is bone involvement.

acinus (*a-sē-nus*), pl. **acini** (*a-sē-nē*). A minute grape-like structure whose cells secrete; as in the breast. Acini are also found in the lungs and other racemose glands. Syn. alveolus, pl. alveoli.

acme (*ak'-mē*). The highest point attained: the crisis.

acne (*ak'-nē*). Inflammation of the glands of the skin, causing the formation of little pustules, and of blackheads. Often found among adolescents.

acousma (*a-kūs-ma*). The hearing of imaginary sounds.

acoustic (*a-koo'-stik*). Relating to sound or hearing.

acquired (*ak-wī-rd*). Contracted after birth, not congenital.

acrid (*ak'-rid*). Sharp, burning.

acriflavine (*ak'-ri-flā-vin*). An antiseptic acridine dye, used in the treatment of wounds in solution of 1 in 1,000. Similar compounds are euflavine and proflavine. All are yellow in colour.

acro- (*ak-rŏ*). Extremity of (prefix).

acrocephaly (*ak-ro-ke-fa-li*). Congenitally malformed, cone-shaped head.

acrocyanosis (*ak-rŏ-sī-a-nō-sis*). Blueness of the extremities.

acrodynia (*ak-rŏ-din'-i-a*). See PINK DISEASE.

acromegaly (*ak-rŏ-meg'-a-lē*). A disease marked by enlargement of the face, hands and feet, and due to a pathological condition of the pituitary gland. The commonest form of gigantism.

acromion (*ā-krō'-mi-on*). The outward extremity of the spine of the scapula. *See* SCAPULA.

acronyx (*ak'-rō-niks*). An ingrowing of the nail.

acroparaesthesia (*ak-rō-pa-res-thē-zi-a*). A tingling feeling in the hands with numbness.

acrophobia (*ak-rō-fō'-bi-a*). Morbid fear of being at a height.

acrylics (*a-kril-iks*). Plastic substances used for prostheses.

ACTH Adrenocorticotrophic hormone, of the anterior lobe of the pituitary body, controlling the function of the adrenal cortex and the release of cortisone. It may be given by intramuscular or slow intravenous injection. ACTH gel is a long-acting form for intramuscular injection only.

actinism (*ak'-tin-izm*). Chemical changes produced by radiant energy, *e.g.* light rays.

actinodermatitis (*ak-ti-nō-der-ma-ti'-tis*). Inflammation of the skin from ultra-violet or other rays.

Actinomyces (*ak-ti-nō-mī'-sez*). A genus of fungoid organisms; ray fungus.

actinomycin. Cytotoxic drugs used to treat malignant disease.

actinomycosis (*ak-tin-ō-mi-kō-sis*). Disease due to Actinomyces. There are usually chronic discharging abscesses.

actinotherapy (*ak-tin'-o-the-rapi*). Treatment by ultra-violet and infra-red radiations.

action potential (*ak-shon-po-ten-shal*). Electrical charges occurring when a nerve conducts an impulse.

action tremor. Tremor of the limbs or incoordination of movement as in ataxia.

activator (*ak-ti-vā'-tor*). A physical or chemical agent which initiates some reaction in which the activator itself does not take part.

active movements. A term used by physiotherapists to denote a movement done by the patient or with their help.

active principle. The substance in a drug which gives it a medicinal character.

acuity (*a-kū-it-i*). Sharpness and clearness.

acupuncture (*ak-ū-pungk-chur*). A treatment to relieve oedema. The oedematous tissue—usually of the legs—is stabbed all over with straight cutting needles, *see* illustration.

acute (*ak-yoot'*). Rapid; severe. *A. abdomen.* A surgical emergency resulting from disease or damage of abdominal viscera.

acute yellow atrophy (*at'-ro-fi*). Severe damage to liver due to toxic agents.

Section

ACUPUNCTURE NEEDLES

acystia (*a-sis'-ti-a*). Absence of bladder.

adactylia (*ā-dak-til'-i-a*). Absence of fingers or toes.

Adam's apple. The laryngeal prominence formed by the thyroid cartilage.

adamantinoma (*a-da-man-ti-nō'-ma*). Epithelial tumour of jaw.

Adams-Stokes disease. Syncope, due to bradycardia and associated with heart block.

adaptation (*a-dap-tā'-shon*). (1) Adjustment by structural or functional change to new circumstances. (2) The process whereby the eye adjusts to sudden changes from light to dark and vice versa.

addiction (*ad-dik'-shon*). State of physical and mental dependence on a drug, usually alcohol or narcotics.

Addis count (*ad-dis kownt*). Number of red blood cells in the urine, per 24 hours.

Addison's anaemia. Pernicious anaemia, *q.v.*

Addison's disease. A disease of the suprarenal gland causing anaemia, vomiting, wasting, low blood pressure and a bronzed skin.

adducent muscle of eye (*a-dū-sent*). Internal rectus muscle.

adduct (*ad-dukt*). To draw towards the midline.

adduction (*ad-duk'-shon*). The act of moving a limb towards the midline of the body.

adductor (*ad-duk'-ter*). A muscle which draws towards the midline of the body, *e.g.* A. *muscles* of the thigh draw the legs together.

adendritic (*ā-den-dri'-tik*). A nerve cell without dendrons.

adenectomy (*ad-en-ek'-to-mē*). Excision of a gland.

adenine (*a-de-nēn*). An amino purine base important for the synthesis of nucleic acids.

adenitis (*ad-en-i'-tis*). Inflammation of a gland.

adenocarcinoma (*ad-en-ō-kar-sin-ō'-ma*). A carcinomatous tumour of a gland.

adenoid (*ad'-en-oyd*). Lymphoid tissue, in the nasopharynx, which when swollen hinders breathing.

adenoidectomy (*ad-en-oyd-ek-to-mi*). Operation to remove adenoids.

adenoma (*ad-en-ō'-ma*). A benign tumour of glandular tissue.

adenomyoma (*ad-en-ō-mī-ō-ma*). A benign growth, esp. in uterus, of glandular and muscle tissue.

adenopathy (*ad-en-op'-ath-ē*). A disease of a gland, especially a lymphatic gland.

adenovirus (*a-de-nō-vīr'-us*). One group of the 'orphan' viruses. They do not cause specific clinical diseases and are said to be 'viruses in search of a disease'.

adeps (*a-deps*). Lard. Once used as a basis for ointments, now replaced by more satisfactory bases. *A. lanae hydrosus*, lanolin.

adermin (*ad-er-min*). Pyridoxin or vitamin B_6, concerned with the metabolism of amino-acids. Used as a drug in muscular dystrophy, nausea or vomiting of pregnancy, irradiation sickness and acute alcoholism.

adherent (*ad-hār'-ent*). Fixed firmly to.

adhesion (*ad-hē'-zhon*). A sticking together of two surfaces or parts. Bands of fibrous tissue, usually the result of inflammation.

adiaphoresis (*ā-dī-a-for-ē-sis*). Deficiency of perspiration.

adipose (*ad'-ip-ōz*). Fatty.

aditus (*ad'-it-us*). An entrance. A portal. *A. ad antrum* is the narrow passage between the mastoid antrum and the tympanic cavity of the ear.

adjustment (*ad-just-ment*). The change made by a person to adapt to circumstances.

adjuvant (*ad'-jū-vant*). A secondary ingredient in a prescription, aiding the chief drug, e.g. lead in *pilula plumbi c. opio* by inhibiting the secretion of the mucous

membrane aids the sedative action of the opium in checking diarrhoea.

Adler's theory. The theory that people develop neuroses to compensate for some inferiority.

adnexa (*ad-nek'-sa*). Appendages. Usually applied to the uterine appendages.

adolescence (*ad-ō-les'-sens*). The period between puberty and maturity.

adrenal (*ad-rē'-nal*). SUPRARENAL GLAND, *q.v.*

adrenalectomy (*ad-rē-nal-ek'-to-mi*). The removal of one or both adrenal glands.

adrenaline (*ad-re'-na-lin*). Secretion of the suprarenal medulla. Used locally as a styptic as it constricts small blood vessels. Injected hypodermically it raises the blood pressure and is used for anaphylactic reactions. It relieves asthma.

adrenergic (*a-dren-er-jik*). Applied to autonomic nerve fibres whose stimulation leads to the production of adrenaline and noradrenaline.

adrenocortical steroids (*ad-rē-nō-kor-ti-kal ste-royds*). Endocrine secretions of the adrenal cortex. See ALDOSTERONE, CORTISONE, DEOXYCORTICOSTERONE.

adrenocorticotrophic hormone (*ad-rē-nō-kor-ti-kō-tro-fik hor-mōn*). See ACTH.

adrenogenital syndrome (*ad-rē-nō-je-ni-tal sin-drōm*). Development of secondary male characteristics in the female or secondary female characteristics in the male. Usually due to hyperplasia or adenoma of the adrenal cortex.

adrenolytic (*ad-rē-no-li-tik*). A drug antagonistic to adrenaline.

adrenotropin (*a-drē-nō-trō-pin*). Also called adrenocorticotropic hormone. An anterior pituitary hormone acting upon the adrenal gland.

adsorbent. Substance causing adsorption.

adsorption (*ad-sorp'-shon*). The property possessed by certain porous substances, *e.g.* charcoal, of taking up other substances.

adulteration (*a-dul-te-rā'-shon*). Fraudulent addition of unnecessary substances to foods or medicines.

advancement (*ad-vans-ment*). An operation for the cure of squint. The procedure consists in dividing one of the eye muscles at its insertion into the eyeball and reattaching it farther forward.

adventitia (*ad-ven-tish'-a*). Outer coat of a blood vessel.

adventitious (*ad-ven-tish-us*). Accidental.

Aëdes aegypti (*a-ē-dās ā-jip'-tē*). Species of mosquito transmitting yellow fever, etc.

aeration (*ā-rā-shon*). Charging with air or gas.

aerobes (*ā-rōbs*). Term applied to bacteria needing oxygen for respiration, *cf.* anaerobes.

aerobic (*ā-rō'-bik*). Requiring free oxygen or air to support life.

aerocele (*ār-ō-sēl*). A diverticulum of larynx, trachea or bronchus.

aerogen (*ā-rō-jen*). Any gas-producing bacterium, *e.g.* clostridium Welchii, the cause of gas gangrene.

aerophagy (*ar-of'-a-ji*). Excessive air swallowing.

aerosol (*ā'-rō-sol*). Finely atomized solution used to sterilize the air, or may be used as an inhalation.

Aesculapius (*ē-skū-lā-pē-us*). A Greek god, the founder of the art of healing.

aesthesia (*es-thē'-zi-a*). Feeling.

aetas (*ā-tas*). Latin for age.

aetiology (*ē-tē-ol'-o-ji*). The science of the causation of disease.

afebrile (*ā-feb'-ril*). Without fever.

affect (*af-ekt*). Term used in psychology for an emotion associated with ideas.

affective disorders. Group of psychiatric illnesses primarily due to reaction to internal or external stress. They include anxiety states, depression, mania and hypomania.

afferent (*af'-er-ent*). Leading to the centre, applied to the lymphatic vessels and to sensory nerves.

affiliation (*a-fil-ē-ā'-shon*). The fixing of paternity of an illegitimate child on the putative father.

affinity (*af-fin'-it-ē*). Attraction. In chemistry the property of an element which prefers to combine with some other particular element.

after-birth (*ahf'-ter-berth*). The placenta, cord, and membranes as expelled after labour.

after-care (*ahf'-ter-kār*). Care of the convalescent, including rehabilitation.

after-image. A retinal impression persisting although the stimulus of light has eased.

after-pains (*ahf'-ter pānz*). Pains from uterine contractions following labour.

Ag. Chemical symbol for Silver.

agammaglobulinaemia (*ā-gam-a-glo-bū-lin-ē'-mi-a*). Absence or deficiency of gamma-globulin in plasma proteins, leading to inadequate response to infection.

agar-agar (*ā-ga-ā-ga*). A gelatinous substance prepared from seaweed and used by bacteriologists for the cultivation of micro-organisms. Also prescribed as a laxative, as it absorbs water and increases bulk in the colon.

agenesis (*ā-je'-ne-sis*). Defective development of a structure.

agglutination (*a-gloo-ti-nā-shon*). The sticking together of cells, *e.g.* red blood cells, bacteria, due to an alteration of surface charge. Usually brought about by the effect of antibodies.

agglutinins (*ag-gloo'-tin-ins*). Antibodies such as those found in the blood serum of persons suffering from typhoid or paratyphoid fever. They have the property of causing bacteria to clump together or 'agglutinate'. *See* WIDAL REACTION.

agglutinogen (*ag-gloo-ti-nō-jen*) A factor stimulating the production of specific antibodies in the blood.

aggregate (*ag-re-gāt*). To group together.

aggressin (*ag-gre-sin*). A product of certain bacteria increasing their action on the host.

aggression (*ag-gre-shon*). A hostile attitude born of a feeling of inferiority or frustration.

aglutition (*ā-glū-ti-shun*). Inability to swallow.

agnosia (*ag-nō-zia*). A disturbance in recognizing sensory impression.

agonist (*a-go-nist*). Muscle which shortens when in action.

agoraphobia (*a'-gor-af-ō'-bi-a*). Neurotic fear of open spaces.

agranulocytosis (*ā-gran-ū-lō-sī-tō'-sis*). Absence or marked reduction in the blood of the polymorphonuclear cells. May be caused by drugs such as the sulphonamides or irradiation of the bone marrow.

agraphia (*ā-graf'-i-a*). Loss of the power to express words and ideas in writing.

ague (*ā-gū*). *See* MALARIA.

A.I.D. Artificial insemination (donor other than husband).

A.I.H. Artificial insemination with semen from the husband.

air. *See* ATMOSPHERE. *A., tidal.* The air breathed in and out in ordinary breathing.

air embolism. Embolism caused by air entering the circulatory system.

air-encephalography (*ăr-en-ke-fal-o'-gra-fi*). Radiography of the brain after air has been introduced into the subarachnoid space.

air hunger. Respiratory distress caused by lack of oxygen.

akinesis (*ă-ki-nē'-sis*). Loss or imperfection of movement.

Al. Chemical symbol for aluminium.

ala (*ā-la*). A wing. *A. nasi.* The outer side of the external nostril.

alastrim (*a-la'-strim*). Variola minor, *q.v.*

Albee's (*al-bēz*) **operation.** (1) The hip joint is ankylosed by a plastic operation. (2) A bone grafting operation to the spine performed in tuberculous disease of the spine. The graft is taken from the tibia.

Albers-Schönberg's disease (*albers shern-bărgs*). Marble bone disease.

albino (*al-bē-nō*). A male with white hair, fair skin, and pink eyes, due to pigmentary deficiency. Female is albiness.

albumin (*al-bū'-min*). Serum protein with relatively low molecular weight (M.W. = 70,000) which is of great importance in controlling water exchanges between the blood and tissue fluids.

albuminuria (*al-bū-min-ū'-ri-a*). Albumin in the urine; occurs in diseases of the kidneys. *Test for albumin: see* URINE TESTING in Appendix, p. 381.

albumose (*al-bū-mōs*). Intermediate product formed in digestion of protein.

alcohol (*al-ko-hol'*). Chemically the hydroxides of a great number of organic radicles are known as alcohols: the term usually refers to ethyl alcohol, the alcohol present in intoxicating drinks. *Absolute A.* May contain up to 1 per cent by weight of water. Rectified spirit is 90 per cent alcohol.

alcoholism (*al'-kō-hol-izm*). A morbid state produced by excessive use of alcoholic drinks.

aldosterone (*al-dos'-ter-ōn*). One of the adreno-cortical hormones which regulates metabolism of electrolytes, *q.v.*

aleukaemia (*ā-lū-kē'-mi-a*). Deficiency of leucocytes in the blood.

alexia (*a-leks'-i-a*). Inability or difficulty in understanding the written or printed word, owing to a lesion of the brain.

Algae (*al-jē*). A group of plants including seaweed and some fresh-water plants. Used for purification of water by their filtering action.

algesia (*al-jē'-si-a*). Sensibility to pain. (-algia is a suffix meaning pain.)

alienation (*āl-yen-ā'-shon*). Insanity.

alignment (*a-līn'-ment*). Bringing into line.

alimentary (*al-i-men'-tar-ē*). Pertaining to the absorption of nourishment. The *alimentary canal* is the whole digestive tract, extending from the mouth to the anus.

alimentation (*a-lē-men-tā'-shon*). Nourishment.

aliquot (*a-li-qwot*). One of equal parts of a compound.

alkalaemia (*al-ka-lē-mi-a*). Abnormally alkaline blood with a pH above 7·5.

alkali (*al'-ka-lī*). A substance which combines with an acid to form a salt, and with a fat to form a soap. Turns red litmus paper to blue. Ammonia, soda and potash are examples of alkalis. *A. reserve.* The amount of buffer-alkalis available in the body to neutralize acids.

alkaline. Containing alkali. Blood, milk and saliva are normally slightly alkaline.

alkalinity (*al-ka-lin'-it-ē*). Proportion of alkali in a given substance.

alkaloid (*al'-ka-loyd*). An organic substance having some of the properties of an alkali, especially that of combining with an acid to form a salt.

Morphine and quinine are alkaloids. Salts of these are morphine tartrate, morphine hydrochloride, quinine sulphate, etc.

alkalosis (*al-kal-ō'-sis*). Alkalaemia. An increase in the alkalinity of the blood due to excessive intake of alkali or accumulation of it, or to loss of acids in the body caused by sweating, vomiting, diarrhoea or deep breathing.

alkapton (*al-kap'-ton*). A nitrogenous substance derived from the decomposition of proteins.

alkaptonuria (*al-kap-ton-ūr-i-a*). The presence of alkapton in the urine due to a chemical disorder of metabolism.

alkylating agents (*al-ki-lā-ting ā-jens*). Drugs such as nitrogen mustard interfering with the growth of malignant cells.

all or none law. Physiological law regarding irritable tissues, *e.g.* nerves, by which there are only two possible reactions to a stimulus, either no reaction or full response. There is no grading of response according to the strength of the stimulus.

allantois (*al-lan'-tō-is*). An embryonic structure contained in the umbilical cord. (*See* illustration.)

allelomorphs (*al-lē-lō-morfs*). Inborn characteristics determined by contrasting genes.

allergen (*al'-er-jen*). A substance that produces the allergic state.

uterine wall
umbilical cord
placenta
allantois
chorion
yolk sac
amnion
coelom
embryonic gut
embryo
amniotic cavity

DIAGRAM OF EARLY OVUM
SHOWING THE ALLANTOIS

allergic state (*al'-ler-jik*). The patient is sensitive to a particular foreign protein which acts as a poison, producing certain reactions. Some of these proteins are derived from animal emanations, from pollens, or are found in the diet. Asthma, urticaria, hay fever are often allergic conditions. Syn. allergy.

allocheiria (*al-lō-ki-ri-a*). A sensation felt on the opposite side to that which is touched.

allograft (*a-lō-grahft*). Graft with material obtained from a donor.

alloy (*al'-oy*). A mixture of two or more metals obtained by fusing them together.

aloes (*al'-ōz*). A vegetable laxative drug of bitter taste.

aloin (*al'-ō-in*). The active principle of aloes. Aloin purges mainly by stimulation of the lower bowel.

alopecia (*al-ō-pē'-si-a*). Absence of hair, baldness.

alpha rays (*al-fah rās*). Nuclear radiation consisting of two protons and two neutrons which is the helium nucleus. Will penetrate only a few mm into tissue.

alternating current (*orl'-ter-nā-ting ku-rent*). Electric current in which the direction periodically reverses.

alum. Ammonium or potassium aluminium sulphate. Astringent and haemostatic. Alum precipitated toxoid protects against diphtheria.

aluminium (*al-yū-min'-ium*). A white metal of low specific gravity. *A. hydroxide* used as an antacid for gastric ulcer. *A. silicate.* Kaolin used for poultices and also given by mouth as a gastric antacid.

alveoli (*al-vē'-ō-lī*). (Sing. is **alveolus.**) (1) The sockets of the teeth. (2) The air cells in the lungs. (3) The secreting units of the breasts.

alveolitis (*al-vē-ō-lī-tis*). Inflammation of an alveolus.

Alzheimer's disease (*alz'-hī-mer*). Degeneration of the brain cortex. Loss of memory, aphasia, and paralysis occur.

amalgam (*am-al-gam*). An alloy of mercury and other metals. *Dental A.* is of silver, tin and mercury. Used for filling teeth.

amastia (*ā-mas-ti-a*). Absence of breasts.

amaurosis (*am-aw-rō'-sis*). Blindness from disease or defect of the nervous system of the eye; occurs in uraemia.

amaurotic family idiocy (*a-maw-ro-tik*). This condition, also known as Tay-Sach's disease, occurs in infants. There is optic atrophy, rigidity of the limbs and coma.

ambidextrous (*am-bi-deks'-trus*). Equally skilful with each hand.

ambivalence (*am-bi-va-lens*). Contrary emotions, such as love and hate, are experienced towards the same object or person.

amblyopia (*am-bli-ō'-pi-a*). Indistinct vision; approaching blindness.

amblyoscope (*am-bli-o-skōp*). Instrument used in orthoptics for the correction of squint.

amboceptor (*am'-bo-sep'-tor*). A substance which has the specific power of binding 'complement', *q.v.*, to the cell or bacterium for which the amboceptor is specific. *See also* EHRLICH'S THEORY.

ambulance (*am-bū-lanz*). A vehicle for the conveyance of sick and wounded.

ambulant (*am-bū-lant*). Able to walk.

ambulatory (*am'-bū-lā-to-rē*). Relating to walking; moving about. *A. treatment of frac-*

tures. Enables the patient to remain up and about. The limb is immobilized in plaster of Paris.

amelioration (*a-mēl-i-or-ā'-shon*). General improvement in the condition of the patient.

amenorrhoea (*a-men-o-re'-a*). Absence of menstruation. In *primary A.*, menstruation has never been established. *Secondary A.* occurs after menstruation has commenced. There is amenorrhoea in pregnancy, and it may occur in certain endocrine disorders, anaemia, etc.

amentia (*a-men'-she-a*). Absence of intellect; idiocy.

amethocaine hydrochloride *a-mē-thō-kān hī-drō-klo'-rīd*). Syn. Anethaine, Decicain. A local anaesthetic used in a 1 per cent solution. Used specially in preparation for gastroscopy.

ametria (*a-mē-tri-a*). Absence of uterus.

ametropia (*am-e-trō'-pi-a*). Defective vision due to abnormal form or refractive power of the eye.

amidone hydrochloride (*a-mē-dōn*). Methadone hydrochloride. An analgesic. Proprietary name, Physeptone.

amidopyrine (*am-id-ō-pī'-rin*). Powerful analgesic. Has caused agranulocytosis and should be used with caution.

amino-acids (*am'-īn-ō*). Nitrogen containing organic acids of which proteins are built.

Ten are considered to be essential to health and must be present in the food. They are leucine, phenylalanine, lysine, arginine, histidine, valine, tryptophane, isoleucine, methionine and threonine.

aminophylline (*am'-in-ō-fil-ēn*). Theophylline derivative used in heart failure, asthma, cardiac and renal oedema. May be given orally, by intramuscular or intravenous injection, or by suppository.

aminopterin (*a-min-op'-ter-in*). A folic acid antagonist.

amiphenazole (*a-mē-fen-a-zōl*). Drug which stimulates the respiratory centre. Often used with bemegride for treatment of barbiturate poisoning. Is an antagonist of morphine. Proprietary name, Daptazole.

amitosis (*a-mit-ō'-sis*). Direct cell division.

ammonia (*am-mō'-ne-a*). A volatile alkali with a pungent odour. *Ammonium bicarbonate* is used as an expectorant. *Ammoniated mercury* ointment: unguentum Hydrargyri Ammoniati dilutum, usually known as ung. H.A.D., is an antiseptic ointment.

ammonium mandelate (*am-mō'nē-um-man'-de-lāt*). See MANDELIC ACID.

amnesia (*am-nē'-si-a*). Loss of memory. *Anterograde A.* Inability to remember recent events. *Retrograde A.* Symptom of concussion. The pa-

tient cannot remember what happened immediately before the accident.

amniocentesis (*am-ni-ō-sen-tē-sis*). Aspiration of liquor amnii from the uterus.

amniography (*am-ni-o-gra-fi*). Radiographic demonstration of amniotic sac by injection of radio-opaque dye.

amnion (*am'-nē-on*). The sac directly encircling the foetus in utero. (*See diagram of early ovum, p. 37.*)

amniotic fluid (*am-nē-o-tik floo-id*). See LIQUOR AMNII.

amoeba (*am-ē'-ba*). A microscopic unicellular animal, one variety of which causes amoebic dysentery.

amoebiasis (*am-ē-bī'-as-is*). Infection with pathogenic amoebae (plural of amoeba).

amoebicide (*am-ē-bi-sīd*). Substance lethal to amoeba.

amorphous (*ā-mor-fus*). Formless.

ampère (*ahm-pār*). Unit measure of electric current.

amphetamine (*am-fet-a-mēn'*). Drug which stimulates the central nervous system. Used in depressive states, narcolepsy, and to postpone fatigue.

amphiarthrosis (*am-fi-ar-thrō'-sis*). A slightly movable joint, *e.g.* the articulations of the spine.

amphoteric (*am-fo-ter'-ik*). Having the power of turning red litmus blue and blue litmus red.

ampicillin (*am-pi-si-lin*). Widespectrum antibiotics used in urinary tract infections due to Gram-negative organisms. Also given in cases of bronchitis, pneumonia and influenza.

ampoule (*am'-pūl*). A sealed phial containing some drug or solution sterilized ready for use.

ampulla (*am-pū-la*). Any flask-shaped dilatation. *A. of Vater.* See VATER'S AMPULLA.

amputation (*am-pū-tā'-shon*). The removal of a limb or organ. It is termed primary if performed immediately after the injury; secondary if performed later.

amyl nitrite (*am'-il nī'-trīt*). A remedy for angina pectoris. A few drops are contained in a glass capsule which is crushed in its cotton covering and the vapour inhaled. It dilates the coronary blood vessels, thus relieving the ischaemia.

amylase (*am'-il-āz*). An enzyme which has a digestive action on carbohydrates. It converts starch into maltose. It is found as ptyalin in the saliva and as amylopsin in the pancreas.

amylobarbitone (*a-mi-lō-bar-bi-tōn*). Barbiturate of intermediate action given to control insomnia.

amyloid disease (*am'-il-oyd*), also called fatty or lardaceous (*lar-dā-'she-us*) disease. Wax-like material is laid down in the liver, kidneys, spleen and blood vessels. It usually occurs as a result of long-standing infection.

amylopsin (*am-il-op'-sin*). Amylase, *q.v.*

amylum. Starch.

amyotonia (*ā-mī-o-tōn'-i-a*). A form of muscular feebleness or paralysis, often congenital.

amyotrophic (*ā-mī-o-trō'-fik*). Pertaining to muscular atrophy.

Amytal (*a'-mi-tal*). Official name, amylobarbitone. A barbituric hypnotic.

ana. Used in prescriptions to mean so much of each. Syn. aa.

anabolic compound (*a-na-bo-lik kom-pownd*). Chemical substance which helps to repair body tissue.

anabolism (*an-ab'-o-lizm*). See METABOLISM.

Anacardone (*a-na-kar-dōn*). Official name nikethamide, *q.v.*

anacrotism (*an-a'-krot-ism*). A small additional wave or notch found in the ascending limb of the tracing of the pulse curve.

anaemia (*a-nē-mi-a*). Diminished oxygen-carrying capacity of the blood, due to a reduction in the number of red cells or in their content of haemoglobin, or both. The cause may be inadequate production of red cells or excessive loss of blood. (For different types, *e.g.* Pernicious A., see under special name.) *See* BLOOD COUNT.

anaerobe (*an-ār-ōb*). Any micro-organism that can live and multiply in the absence of free oxygen, *e.g.* tetanus.

anaesthesia (*an-es-thē'-zi-a*). Absence of sensation; loss of feeling. *Basal A.* Partial general anaesthesia obtained by a drug such as morphine given before an inhalation anaesthesia. *Dissociated A.* Loss of sensation to pain and temperature, sense of touch being retained. *General A.* This gives loss of consciousness. *Glove A.* Hysterical loss of feeling in the area of the hand a glove covers. *Intravenous A.* A general anaesthesia produced by intravenous injection. *Local A.* Anaesthesia of a certain area only. *Nerve block A.* Local anaesthesia produced by injecting an anaesthetic into a sensory nerve. *Rectal A.* General anaesthesia by administering an anaesthetic rectally. *Refrigeration A.* Anaesthesia produced by intense cold. *Spinal A.* An anaesthetic is injected into the subarachnoid space of the spinal cord producing anaesthesia in the lower half of the body.

anaesthetic (*an-es-thet-ik*). An agent which produces insensibility. (As an adjective it means insensible to touch.)

anaesthetist (*an-ēs'-thet-ist*). The administrator of anaesthetics.

anal (*ā-nal*). Of the anus.

analeptic (*an-a-lep-tik*). A restorative. A drug which restores to consciousness, *e.g.* nikethamide.

analgesia (*an-al-jē'-zi-a*). Diminished sensibility to pain. A symptom in certain nervous diseases, *e.g.* syringomyelia.

analgesic (*an-al-jē-zik*). Relieving pain; remedy for pain.

analogous (*a-nal'-ō-jus*). Similar in certain respects.

analysis (*a-na'-li-sis*). In chemistry, the breaking down of a substance into its constituent parts. In psychiatric medicine, psycho-analysis, *q.v.*

analyst (*an'-al-ist*). The person who analyses.

anaphase (*an'-a-fāz*). A stage in mitosis when the daughter cells pass towards the poles.

anaphoresis (*an-a-for-ēs'-is*). Diminished activity of the sweat glands.

anaphylaxis (*a-na-fi-lak'-sis*). A state of shock induced by an antigen-antibody reaction occurring in cells which cause the release of substances acting on the vascular system.

anaplasia (*an-a-plā'-si-a*). The reversion of a special tissue or cells to a less differentiated type.

anastomosis (*an'-as-to-mō'-sis*). In anatomy the intercommunication of the terminal branches of two or

more blood vessels. In surgery the establishment of
some artificial connection,
as, for instance, between two
parts of the intestine.

anatomy (*an-at'-o-mē*). The
science of organic structure.
A., applied. As applied to
diagnosis and treatment.

anconeus (*an-kō'-nē-us*). A
small extensor muscle of the
forearm.

androgen (*an-drō-jen*). A hormone producing male sex
characteristics.

android pelvis (*an-droyd pelvis*). Shaped like a male
pelvis. The narrow fore-
pelvis, shallow posterior segment and straight lateral
walls make child-bearing
difficult.

androsterone (*an-dro-ste-rōn*).
A breakdown product of
testosterone, *q.v.*

anencephalous (*an-en-kef'-al-
us*). Having no brain; occurs
in monsters; incompatible
with life.

anergic (*an-er'-jik*). Inactive.
Slack.

aneroid (*a-nār'-oyd*). Without
liquid. *A. barometer.* One
that measures air pressure
by its action on elastic lid
of box exhausted of air, not
by height of fluid column.

aneurine hydrochloride (*a-nū-
rin hī-drō-klo-rīd*). Vitamin
B₁. *See* VITAMINS.

aneurysm (*an'-ū-rizm*). A
permanent dilatation of an
artery usually with rupture
of the internal and middle

coats. It may be *fusiform* or
sacculated (*see diagrams*).
The thoracic aorta and the
innominate artery are those
usually affected, more rarely
the abdominal aorta. *Arteriovenous A.* is a communi-
cation between an artery and
a vein, usually the result of
injury.

FUSIFORM SACCULATED DISSECTING
ANEURYSM ANEURYSM ANEURYSM

aneurysm needle (*an'-yu-rizm*).
A blunt instrument which
can be passed under a vessel;
the eye is then threaded and
the needle withdrawn, leaving
the ligature beneath the
vessel ready to tie.

ANEURYSM NEEDLE

angiectasis (*an-ji-ek'-ta-sis*).
Dilatation of blood-vessel.

angiitis (*an-ji-ī-tis*). Inflammation of blood-vessels.

angina (*an-jī'-na*). Suffocating
pain; thus any severe sore
throat associated with swel-

ling of the walls of the air passages may be termed angina. Ludwig's angina, Vincent's angina, are examples; but the commonest use of the term is in angina pectoris.

angina pectoris (*an-jī'-na pek'-tor-is*). A disease characterized by sense of suffocation, with pain in the chest due to insufficient blood supply to the heart, the arteries being diseased. It occurs on effort. Inhalation of amyl nitrite (*q.v.*) is helpful.

angiocardiogram (*an-jē-ō-kar'-dē-o-gram*). The X-ray film taken in angiocardiography, *q.v.*

angiocardiography (*an-jē-ō-kar-dē-o'-graf-ē*). An opaque liquid is injected into a vein and X-ray photographs are taken when the liquid circulates through the heart.

angiogram (*an-jē-ō-gram*). X-ray film showing blood-vessels.

angiography (*an-jē-og'-raf-ē*). An opaque liquid is injected to show the blood-vessels on X-ray

angioma (*an-jē-ō'-ma*). A tumour composed of blood-vessels, often called a naevus.

angioneurotic (*an'-ji-ō-nū-rot'-ik*). Having to do with the nervous control of the blood-vessels. Thus *angioneurotic oedema* is a persistent or intermittent swelling of parts such as the eyelid or lip. It may be an allergic symptom.

angioparalysis (*an-jē-ō-pa-ra'-li-sis*). Vasomotor paralysis.

angioplacentography (*an-ji-ō-pla-sen-to'-gra-fi*). Radiography of placental blood vessels by injection of radio-opaque dye.

angioplasty (*an-jē-ō-plas'-ti*). Plastic surgery of the blood-vessels.

angiosarcoma (*an-jē-ō-sar-kō'-ma*). A sarcoma composed of vascular tissue.

angiospasm (*an-jē-ō-spazm*). The blood-vessels contract in spasms.

angiotensin (*an-ji-ō-ten-sin*). A polypeptide raising blood pressure and formed by the action of renin, *q.v.* on plasma globulins.

Angström unit (*ang-strer-m*). Unit of measurement of wavelengths of light, equal to one ten thousand millionth of a metre.

anhidrosis (*an-hī-drō'-sis*). Deficiency of perspiration.

anhidrotics (*an-hīd-rot'-iks*). Drugs which reduce the amount of perspiration, *e.g.* belladonna, hyoscyamus.

anhydrous (*an-hī'-drus*). Without water.

aniline (*a-nil-īn*). Phenylamine. Used in preparing dye-stuffs.

animalcule (*an-im-al'-kūl*). Microscopic animal.

anion (*an'-ī-on*). An ion which holds a negative charge of electricity and is repelled from the negative pole, or cathode, of a battery.

aniridia (*a-ni-ri-di-a*). Absence or defect of iris.

anisocoria (*an-is-o-ko'-ri-a*). Inequality of the pupils.

anisocytosis (*an-i-so-sī-tō'-sis*). Inequality of size of the red blood corpuscles.

anisomelia (*an-is-o-me'-li-a*). Unequal limbs which should be a pair.

anisometropia (*a-ni-sō-me-trō-pi-a*). Refraction of the two eyes is different.

ankle (*ang'-kl*). The joint between the leg and the foot. The bones which articulate are the tibia and fibula above and the astragalus below.

Tibia — Fibula
Talus —
Calcaneum

ANKLE JOINT

ankyloblepharon (*an-ki-lō-blef'-a-ron*). Adhesion of the edges of the eyelids.

ankyloglossia (*an-ki-lō-glo'-si-a*). Inability to protrude the tongue fully and tendency for it to deviate to one side, usually the result of damage to the tongue muscles.

ankylosing spondylitis (*an-ki-lō-sing spon-di-lī-tis*). Disease of joints, of unknown aetiology, in which destruction of the joint space occurs and is followed by sclerosis and calcification. The sacroiliac joints are predominantly affected.

ankylosis (*an-kil-ō'-sis*). Immobility in a joint, following inflammation or prolonged immobilization. *False A.* Fixation or stiffness produced by conditions around the joint, such as contraction of skin, *e.g.* after burns, or of tendons, by ossification of muscles, or by outgrowths of bone. *True A.* Fixation or stiffness produced by conditions in the joint such as injury or arthritis. *Fibrous A.* Fixation by fibrous tissue. *Bony A.* The articular surfaces of the bones are fused together.

Ankylostoma duodenale (*an-ki-lo-stō'-ma du-ō-den-ar'-li*). A minute parasitic hookworm which may inhabit the duodenum in large numbers and cause profound anaemia.

ankylostomiasis (*an-ki-lō-stō-mī'-a-sis*). Hook-worm disease. Infection with the Ankylostoma duodenale.

annular (*an'-ū-lar*). Ring-shaped. *A. ligament.* The ligament around the wrist or ankle.

anode (*an'-ōd*). Electrode with positive charge.

anodyne (*an'-o-dīn*). A pain-relieving drug.

anomalous (*an-om'-al-us*). Irregular. Out of the ordinary.

anomia (*a-nō-mi-a*). Inability to name objects and recall names.

anonychia (*ā-nō-ni'-ki-a*). Without nail formation.

anoperineal (*ā-nō-pe-rin-ē-al*). Relating to anus and perineum.

Anopheles (*an-of'-el-ēz*). A genus of mosquitoes. They are carriers of the malarial parasite, their bite being the means of transmitting the disease to human beings.

anorchous (*an-or'-kus*). Having no testes, or the condition in which the testes have not descended into the scrotum.

anorectal (*ā-nō-rek-tal*). Of the anus and rectum.

anorexia (*an-o-rek'-sē-a*). Lack of appetite, abhorrence of food. *A. nervosa*. Patients may imagine that certain articles of diet are harmful to them. Their diet becomes progressively limited resulting in extreme emaciation. Psychological treatment is indicated.

anosmia (*an-os'-mi-a*). Loss of sense of smell.

anovular (*a-no-vū-la*). Without ovulation, esp. of menstrual bleeding when ovulation has not occurred.

anovulation (*an-ov-ū-lā'-shon*). Cessation of ovulation.

anoxaemia (*an-ok-sē'-mi-a*). Insufficient oxygen in the blood.

anoxia (*a-nok-si-a*). Absence of oxygen. Often implies insufficient oxygen available for normal respiratory metabolism, *e.g.* hypoxia.

Antabuse (*an-ta-būs*). *See* TETRAETHYLTHIURAM DISULPHIDE.

antacid (*ant-as'-id*). Any substance neutralizing an acid, *e.g.* sodium bicarbonate.

antagonist (*an-tag'-on-ist*). An organ such as a muscle that acts in opposition to another, or a drug neutralizing another drug.

antaphrodisiac (*ant'-af-ro-diz'-i-ak*). An agent which diminishes sexual desire.

ante (*an-tē*). Before.

anteflexion (*an-tē-flek'-shon*). A bending forward, as of the normal position of the uterus.

ante mortem (*an-tē maw-tem*). Before death.

antenatal (*an-tē-nā-tal*). Before birth.

Antepar (*an-ti-par*). *See* PIPERAZINE.

antepartum (*an-tē-par'-tum*). Before birth. *Antepartum haemorrhage* may be inevitable or accidental when it is due to partial separation of the placenta; incidental when it is due to diseases of the cervix.

anterior (*an-te'-ri-or*). In front of.

anterior chamber of eye. The space between cornea in front and the iris and lens behind, which contains the aqueous humour.

anterior commissure (*kom'-mis-sūr*). A bundle of nerve fibres crossing the mid-line in front of the third ventricle and serving to connect certain parts of the two cerebral hemispheres.

anterior fontanelle. *See* FONT-ANELLE.

anterior poliomyelitis (*pol-i-ō'-mi-el-ī'-tis*). Inflammation of the anterior horns of the grey matter in the spinal cord. Infantile paralysis.

anterior root. Motor root, *syn.* ventral root. Nerve root emerging from the spinal cord carrying motor fibres.

anterograde (*an-ter-ō-grād*), Going forwards.

antero-inferior (*an-te-rō-in-fār'-i-or*). Lying in front and below.

antero-interior (*an-te-rō-in-tār'-i-or*). Lying to the front and internally.

anterolateral (*an-te-rō-la'-ter-al*). In front and to the side.

anteromedian (*an-te-rō-mē'-di-an*). Lying in front and near the mid-line.

anteroposterior (*an-te-rō-pō-stā'-ri-or*). From front to back.

anterosuperior (*an-te-rō-soo-pā'-ri-or*). In front and above.

anteversion (*an'-tē-ver'-shon*). The state of being inclined forward. It is the normal position of the uterus.

anthelmintic (*an-thel-min'-tik*). A remedy for intestinal worms, *e.g.* santonin, extract of filix mas, etc.

Anthisan (*an-ti-zan*). Antihistamine drug.

anthracosis (*an-thra-kō'-sis*). Disease caused by inhaling coal dust or soot into the lungs. Seen in miners.

anthrax (*an'-thrax*). An acute, infectious disease produced by the Anthrax bacillus. *Skin A.* and *Pulmonary A.* are the two main forms.

anthropoid (*an'-thro-poyd*). Manlike. *A. apes* include animals most closely related to man. *A. pelvis* has a narrowed transverse inlet which is long antero-posteriorly.

anthropology (*an-throp-ol'-o-ji*). The natural history of mankind.

anti (*an-ti*) Prefix meaning against.

antibiotic (*an-ti-bī-o'-tik*). Opposed to life; drugs, derived from living cells, especially fungi, which prevent micro-organisms from multiplying, *e.g.* penicillin.

antibodies (*an-ti-bo-dis*). Protein substances, usually circulating in the blood, which neutralize corresponding antigens.

anticholinergic (*an-ti-kō-li-ner-jik*). Term applied to drugs inhibiting the action of acetylcholine, *q.v.*

anticoagulant (*an-ti-kō-ag-ū-lant*). Substance which delays the clotting of blood.

anticonvulsant (*an-ti-kon-vul'-sant*). A drug used to prevent a convulsion.

antidepressants (*an-ti-de-pre-sant*). Drugs used to treat depression. They may be mono-amine oxidase inhibitors, the imipramine group of drugs or stimulants.

antidiuretic hormone (*an-ti-dī-ū-re-tik hor-mōn*). Posterior pituitary hormone regulating the amount of water passing from the uriniferous tubules into the renal substance.

antidote (*an'-ti-dōt*). The corrective to a poison. *See* POISONS in Appendix, p. 385.

antigen (*an'-ti-jen*). Substance capable of stimulating the formation of antibodies.

antihistamine (*an-ti-his'-ta-mēn*). Drug counteracting the effects of the liberation of histamine in the tissues, *e.g.* Anthisan, Benadryl, Dramamine, Phenergan, etc.

anti-infective factor (*an-ti-in-fek-tif fak-tor*). Found in vitamin A.

antimetabolites (*an-ti-me-ta-bo-līts*). Chemical substances used to prevent cell division in malignant disease.

antimitotic (*an-ti-mī-to-tik*). Substance which prevents mitosis.

antimonii et potassii tartras. Tartar emetic. Dose 30 to 60 mg as an emetic; vomiting occurs in twenty to thirty minutes. It increases bronchial and sweat secretion. In small doses acts as an expectorant. Now administered intravenously in cases of parasitic infections such as

kala-azar and bilharzia with excellent results. Poison.

antimony (*an-ti'-mo-ni*). A metallic poison, like arsenic in its properties.

antimycotic (*an-ti-mī-ko-tik*). Substance used to treat fungus diseases.

antiperistalsis (*an-ti-pe-ri-stal'-sis*). Reverse peristalsis, *i.e.* from below upward. *See* PERISTALSIS.

antiphlogistic (*an-ti-flo-jis'-tik*). Relieving inflammation.

Antiphlogistine (*an-ti-flo-jis'-tēn*). *See* POULTICE, KAOLIN.

antipruritic (*an-ti-proo-rit-ik*). Substance relieving itching.

antipyretic (*an-ti-pī-ret'-ik*). A drug which reduces the high temperatures of feverish conditions.

antipyrin (*an-ti-pī'-rin*). Syn. PHENAZONE, *q.v.*

antirachitic factor (*an-ti-rak-it-ik fak-tor*). *Syn.* Vitamin D. Prevents rickets.

antiscorbutic (*an-ti-skor-bū'-tik*). *Syn.* Vitamin C or ascorbic acid. Prevents scurvy.

antiseptic (*an-ti-sep'-tik*). A substance opposing sepsis by arresting the growth and multiplication of micro-organisms. Iodine, phenol, biniodide of mercury, chlorine, formalin, lysol, quaternary ammonium compounds, chloroxylenols, hypochlorites are common antiseptics.

antiserum (*an-ti-sā-rum*). Serum, usually prepared from horses containing a high titre, *q.v.*, of antibody to a specific organism or toxin.

anti-siphonage (*an-ti-sī'-fon-āj*). Preventing siphonage. *A. pipe*. Small pipes leading from the soil pipe which contain air. They are necessary when lavatories are placed one above another on different floors. They prevent the suction of water from the traps of the lavatories as the water from the upper floors rushes down.

antisocial (*an-ti-sō-shal*). Against the normally accepted behaviour in society.

antispasmodic (*an-ti-spaz-mo'-dik*). An agent relieving spasm.

antistatic (*an-ti-sta-tik*). Applied to ways of preventing a build-up of static electricity.

antithrombin (*an-ti-throm'-bin*). A substance in the blood having the power of retarding or preventing coagulation.

antithyroid drugs (*an-ti-thī-royd*). Substances which restrict the secretion of thyroid hormones by interference in the intermediary metabolism of the gland.

antitoxin (*an-ti-tok'-sin*). A specific antibody produced in the blood in response to a toxin or poison. The antibody is capable of neutralizing that particular toxin.

antitragus (*an-ti-trā'-gus*). The prominence of the lower portion of the external ear.

antivenin (*an-ti-ven'-in*). An antidote injected in cases of poisoning by snake bite.

antrostomy (*an-trost'-o-mi*). Incision of an antrum.

antrum (*an'-trum*). A cave; applied to the auxiliary sinus, called the antrum of Highmore, and the cavity in the mastoid bone communicating with the middle ear. *See* SINUS, MAXILLARY.

Antuitrin (*an-tū-it-rin*). Official name Gonadotrophinum Chorionicum. Anterior lobe pituitary extract.

anuria (*an-ū'-ri-a*). Cessation of the production of urine; to be distinguished from retention of urine, due to inability to empty the bladder.

anus (*ā'-nus*). The rectal exit. *Imperforate A.* A congenital malformation where a child is born with no anal opening, or an anus is present but does not communicate with the bowel above. Treatment is operative and success depends on degree of development of lower bowel.

anxiety neurosis (*ang-zī-e-ti nū-rō'-sis*). A neurosis in which fear and apprehension mainly control the patient's behaviour and ideas.

aorta (*ā-or'-ta*). The large artery arising from the left ventricle of the heart and supplying blood to the whole body.

aortic incompetence (*ā-or'-tik in-kom'-pe-tens*). Blood from the aorta regurgitates back into the left ventricle, due to inefficiency of the valve.

aortic stenosis (*ā-or-tik ste-nō-sis*). Narrowing of the aortic valve due to malformation or disease.

aortic valves. Three semi-lunar valves guarding the entrance from the left ventricle to the aorta and preventing the backward flow of the blood.

aortitis (*ā-or-tī'-tis*). Inflammation of the aorta.

aortography (*ā-or-to-gra-fi*). Radiography of the aorta visualized by the injection of radio-opaque dye.

apathy (*ap'-a-thi*). Absence of emotion or feeling.

apepsia (*ā-pep'-si-a*). Failure of digestion due to deficiency of gastric juice.

aperient (*a-pār-i-ent*). A purgative medicine, e.g. cascara.

aperistalsis (*ā-per-i-stal'-sis*). Cessation of peristalsis.

apex (*ā-peks*). Top, extreme point, summit. *A. of the heart*. Narrow end of heart enclosing left ventricle. *A. beat*. The heart beat as felt at its most forcible point on the chest wall. This corresponds approximately with the position of the apex of the left ventricle.

Apgar score (*ap-gu-skaw*). System for assessing vitality of new-born infant, esp. heart rate and respiratory effort.

aphagia (*a-fā'-ji-a*). Inability to swallow.

aphakia (*a-fā-ki-a*). Absence of lens of the eye.

aphasia (*a-fā'-zi-a*). Speechlessness; due to disease or injury of brain.

aphonia (*a-fō'-ni-a*). Loss of voice.

aphrodisiac (*af-rō-diz'-i-ak*). An agent which increases sexual power.

aphthae (*af'-thē*). Small white ulcers in the mouth.

aphthous stomatitis (*af-thus sto-ma-tī'-tis*). Inflammation of the mucous membrane of the mouth due to herpes simplex virus, *cf.* thrush.

apical (*ā'-pik-al*). Pertaining to the apex.

apicectomy (*ā-pi-sek-to-mi*). Excision of the root-end of a tooth.

apicolysis (*ā-pi-ko-lī'-sis*). Stripping of the parietal pleura from the chest wall to collapse a tuberculous apex of lung.

aplasia (*ā-plā'-si-a*). Non-development of an organ or tissue.

aplastic anaemia (*ā-plas-tik a-nē-mi-a*). Anaemia resulting from destruction of bone marrow cells.

apnoea (*ap-nē'-a*). Suspended respiration.

apocrine glands (*a-po-krin glans*). Specialized sweat glands found in the axillae and genital regions.

apomorphine (*ap-o-mor'-fēn*). A synthetic alkaloid derived from morphine. A prompt emetic: acts by stimulating the vomiting centre in the medulla; used also in small doses as an expectorant. For emesis, dose, 2 to 8 mg subcutaneously.

aponeurosis (*ap-o-nū-rŏ′-sis*). A tendon-like fibrous tissue, which invests the muscles and transmits their movements to the structures upon which they act.

apophysis (*ap-off′-is-is*). A bony protuberance or outgrowth.

apoplexy (*ap′-o-plek-si*). A stroke. The effects of a cerebrovascular accident, *q.v.*

apothecary (*ap-oth′-e-ka-ri*). A druggist or pharmacist.

appendicectomy (*ap-pen-di-sek′-to-mi*). Removal of the vermiform appendix.

appendices epiploicae (*ep-pi-plŏ′-i-sē*). Small peritoneal bags of fat projecting from the peritoneal coat of the large intestine.

appendicitis (*ap-pen-di-sī′-tis*). Inflammation of the appendix.

appendix vermiformis (*ap-en-diks ver-mi-for′-mis*). A worm-like offshoot from the caecum, ending blindly, and 1 to 5 in. long.

apperception (*ap-er-sep-shon*). The conscious reception of a sensory impression.

applicator (*ap′-li-kā-tor*). An instrument for applying local remedies, *e.g.* radium.

apposition (*a-po-zi′-shon*). The lying together or the fitting together of two structures.

Ascending Colon

Appendix

Caecum

APPENDIX VERMIFORMIS

apraxia (*a-prak′-si-a*). Motor aphasia and inability to perform certain purposive movements. The lesion is in the cerebral cortex.

Apresoline. Proprietary form of hydrallazine hydrochloride. Used to lower blood pressure.

A.P.T. Alum precipitated toxoid. A diphtheria prophylactic.

aptitude (*ap′-ti-tūd*). A facility or a particular bent for certain work or actions.

aptyalism (*ap-tī-a-lism*). Absence of salivation.

apyrexia (*ā-pī-rek′-si-a*). Without fever.

aqua (*a′-kwa*). Water: abbreviation is *aq.*, see p. 13.

aqueduct (*ak′-wē-dukt*). Certain canals of the body, such as the A. of Sylvius which leads from the third to the fourth ventricle of the brain.

aqueous humour (*ā'-kwē-us hū'-mor*). Fluid in the eye between the cornea and the iris and the lens.

arachnodactyly (*a-rak-nō-dak-ti-li*). Abnormally long and slender bones of the extremities.

arachnoid (*a-rak'-noyd*). Resembling a web. *A. membrane*, surrounds the brain and spinal cord. It is between the dura and pia mater.

Aran-Duchenne's disease (*a-ran-dū-shenz*). The commonest myopathy occurring in children. Also known as pseudo-hypertrophic muscular dystrophy.

arbor vitae (*ah-bor vē-tī*). Tree-like appearance seen in a section of the cerebellum and also applied to that seen in the interior folds of the cervix of the uterus.

arborization (*ah-bor-ī-zā-shon*). Branching of processes of nerve cells.

arboviruses (*ah-bo-vī'-ru-sez*). Insect-borne viruses causing diseases such as yellow fever.

arcus. An arch or ring. *A. Senilis.* An opaque circle round the edge of the cornea, occurring in the aged.

areola (*ā-re'-ō-la*). The pigmented skin round the nipple of the breast.

areolar tissue (*a-rē'-ō-la ti-shoo*). Filmy connective tissue of the body.

AREOLA

(*a*) Nipple; (*b*) Montgomery's follicles; (*c*) primary areola; (*d*) secondary areola, develops in the early weeks of pregnancy.

Arfonad (*ah-fon-ad*). Proprietary form of trimetaphan camphorsulphonate used to lower blood pressure rapidly. It is short acting.

argentaffinoma (*ar-jen-ta-fi-nō-ma*). Also known as carcinoid tumour. Arises from so-called argentaffin cells in the gastrointestinal tract.

argenti nitras (*ar-jen'-ti nī'-tras*). *See* NITRATE OF SILVER.

argentum. Silver

arginine (*ah-ji-nēn*). An essential amino-acid which helps to form urea.

argon (*ar'-gon*). An inert gaseous element in the atmosphere in very small quantities.

Argyll-Robertson (*ar-gil-ro'-bert-son*) **pupil.** Pupil of eye which is small, reacting to accommodation but not to light. Seen in diseases of the nervous system, *e.g.* tabes dorsalis.

argyria (*ar-ji'-ri-a*). Discoloration of the skin from the continued use of preparations of silver.

Argyrol (*ar'-jir-ol*). Official name Argentoproteinum mite. A dark brown organic silver compound. Used for eyedrops.

arrector pili (*a-rek-tor pē-lē*). Muscle fibres around the hair follicles which on contraction produce 'goose-flesh'.

arrhenoblastoma (*a-rā-nō-blas-tō-ma*). A neoplasm of the ovary associated with masculinization.

arrhythmia (*a-rith'-mi-a*). Disturbance of rhythm (usually the heart's rhythm). *Sinus A.* Increased pulse rate during inspiration, decreased during expiration; common in infants.

arsenic (*ar'-sen-ik*). a poison: used sometimes as Liq. arsenicalis in the treatment of skin diseases. Report at once if the tongue is furred, or diarrhoea or gastric pains commence. Treatment for overdose, *see* Appendix, p. 386.

Artane (*ar'-tān*). Benzhexol.

artefact (*ar'-te-fakt*). A lesion produced by artificial means.

arterial (*ar-tār-i-al*). Pertaining to an artery. Thus *arterial tension* means the pressure of the blood circulating in a given artery.

arteriectomy (*ar-tār-i-ek-to-mi*). Excision of part of an artery.

arteriography (*ar-tār-i-og'-raf-i*). The photographing of blood-vessels by special technique after they have been injected with a substance opaque to X-rays.

arterioles (*ar-te-ri-ōls*). Small arteries with contractile muscular walls which control the supply of blood to the capillaries.

arteriopathy (*ar-tār-i-o-pa-thi*). Disease of the arteries.

arterioplasty (*ar-tār-i-ō-pla-sti*). Surgery to reform an artery, especially for aneurysm.

arteriorrhaphy (*ar-tār-i-ōr'-raf-i*). Suture of an artery.

arterio-sclerosis (*ar-tār'-i-ō-skler-ō'-sis*). Degeneration of an artery with hardening of its walls, seen chiefly in old age. The condition is accompanied by high blood pressure.

arteriotomy (*ar-tār-i-o-to-mi*). Incising an artery.

arteriovenous aneurysm (*ar-tār-i-ō-vē'-nus an'-ūr-ism*). *See* ANEURYSM.

arteritis (*ar-ter-ī'-tis*). Inflammation of the arteries.

artery (*ar'-te-ri*). A vessel carrying blood from the heart.

arthralgia (*ar-thral'-ji-a*). Pain in the joints.

arthrectomy (*ar-threk'-to-mi*). The removal by operation of the whole or part of a joint.

arthritis (*ar-thrī'-tis*). Inflammation of a joint. *See* RHEUMATOID A.

arthro (*ar-thrō*). Prefix referring to a joint.

arthroclasia (*ar-thrō-klā-si-a*). An operation for breaking up an ankylosed joint to produce free movement.

arthrodesis (*ar-thrō-dē'-sis*). Fixation of a joint by means of a surgical operation.

arthrodial (*ar-thrō'-di-al*). Term applied to a joint which glides.

arthrodynia (*ar-thrō-din'-i-a*). Pain in the joints.

arthrography (*ar-thro'-gra-fi*). Radiography of joint after the injection of radio-opaque fluid to outline the joint space.

arthropathy (*ar-thro-pa-thi*). Disease of the joints. Commonly used to imply secondary damage to joints as a result of other disease processes.

arthroplasty (*ar-thrō-plas'-ti*). The making of an artificial joint.

arthrotomy (*ar-throt'-o-mi*). Incision into a joint.

articular (*ar-tik'-ū-lar*). Relating to the joints; the articulation of a skeleton is the manner in which the bones are joined together.

articulation (*ar-tik-ū-lā-shon*). (1) A joint between two or more bones. (2) The enunciation of words.

artificial feeding (*ar-ti-fi-shal*). Feeding of an infant with food other than its mother's milk.

artificial insemination. Artificial introduction of spermatozoa into the vagina.

artificial kidney. Dialysing apparatus through which blood from the patient is pumped so that excretory products such as urea may be extracted in the event of the patient's own kidneys not functioning.

artificial pneumothorax. *See* PNEUMOTHORAX.

artificial respiration. *See* Appendix, p. 430.

arytenoid (*ar-i-tē-noyd*). The term applied to two funnel-shaped cartilages of the larynx.

asbestos (*as-bes'-tos*). A mineral substance which is incombustible and which does not conduct heat.

asbestosis (*as-bes-tō-sis*). Disease of the lung caused by inhalation of asbestos dust.

ascariasis (*as-kar-ī-a-sis*). Infestation of the bowel by roundworms (ascarides).

ascaricide (*a-ska-ri-sīd*). Lethal to roundworms.

Ascaris (*as'-kar-is*). A genus of parasitic roundworm. *A. lumbricoides*, long roundworm.

Aschheim-Zondek test. *See* ZONDEK-ASCHHEIM TEST.

Aschoff nodules (*ash-off no-dūls*). The focal lesions of acute rheumatism consisting of perivascular necrosis of collagen. These nodules tend to occur in the heart, muscles and connective tissues.

ascites (*as-sī'-tēz*). Fluid collection in the abdominal cavity.

ascitic fluid (*a-si-tik floo-id*). Fluid of ascites which can be aspirated.

ascorbic acid (*a-scaw-bik*). Vitamin C. *See* VITAMINS.

asepsis (*ā-sep'-sis*). The state of being free from living pathogenic micro-organisms.

aseptic (*ā-sep'-tik*). Free from bacteria. In aseptic surgery all instruments, dressings, etc., are sterilized before use.

asexual (*ā-sek-shal*). Having no sex. A method of reproduction as opposed to sexual.

Aspergillus (*as-per-gil-us*). The name of a group of fungi, some species of which are pathogenic, causing aspergillosis which may infect the ear, eye or lungs.

aspermia (*ā-sper-mi-a*). Inability to produce semen.

asphyxia (*as-fik'-si-a*). Suffocation.

aspiration (*as-pi-rā'-shon*). The operation of drawing off fluids from the body, for example, in a case of pleural effusion or an abscess. Suction is usually applied by means of a syringe or aspirator. One type is Potain's aspirator which consists of a trocar and cannula fitted to a rubber tube connected to a bottle from which the air is exhausted with a pump. The trocar and cannula are inserted into the chest, the trocar withdrawn, and the fluid from the chest runs into the bottle. (*See illustration.*) Fluid may be removed from the pleural cavity by *siphonage*, or a two-way aspirating syringe is used.

aspirator (*as'-pi-rā-tor*). The apparatus used for aspiration.

POTAIN'S ASPIRATOR

aspirin. Syn. acetylsalicylic acid. It relieves pain and is antipyretic. Dose 0·3 to 1 g.

assimilation (*as-im-il-ā'-shon*). The absorption and utilization of nourishment by the living tissues. *A. pelvis.* One in which the fifth lumbar vertebra is incorporated in the sacral body.

TWO-WAY ASPIRATING SYRINGE

association (*as-sō-si-ā'-shon*). Co-ordination. 'Association of ideas,' *i.e.* a phrase used to denote the secondary thoughts that arise on the receipt of any individual mental impression.

asteatosis (*ā-ste-a-tō'-sis*). Deficient action of sebaceous glands.

astereognosis (*a-ster-e-og-nō'-sis*). Loss of power to recognize the shape of objects by touch.

asthenia (*as-the'-nē-a*). Failure of strength; debility.

asthenopia (*as-then-o'-pi-a*). Weakness of sight.

asthma (*as'-ma*). Paroxysms of difficult breathing, with sense of suffocation. There is difficulty in expiration. *Bronchial A.* is generally an allergic state, *q.v.* The attacks are relieved by injections of adrenaline. *Cardiac A.* occurs later in life and is due to failure of left ventricle.

astigmatism (*as-tig'-ma-tizm*). Inequality in the curvature of the cornea or lens, with consequent blurring and distortion of the images thrown upon the retina.

astragalus (*as-trag'-a-lus*). The ankle bone. See ANKLE.

astringent (*as-trinj'-ent*). A substance applied to produce local contraction of blood-vessels and inhibit secretion, *e.g.* tannin, adrenaline.

astrocytoma (*as-tro-sī-tō-ma*). A tumour occurring in the central nervous system.

asymmetry (*ā-sim'-me-tri*). Lack of symmetry.

asymptomatic (*ā-simp-tō-ma-tik*). Without any symptoms.

asynclitism (*a-sin'-clit-ism*). Engagement in the pelvis of a diameter of the foetal head other than the biparietal. It may occur with a contracted pelvis.

ataxia, ataxy (*at-ak'-si*). Literally, disorder; applied to any defective control of muscles and consequent irregularity of movements. *See also* LOCOMOTOR ATAXIA and FRIEDREICH'S ATAXIA.

atebrin (*a-te-brin*). *See* MEPACRINE HYDROCHLORIDE.

atelectasis (*at-e-lek'-ta-sis*). Imperfect expansion of the lungs of the new-born. Term also used for collapse of part of the lung from some other cause.

atherogenic (*a-the-rō-je-nik*). Applied to factors which may cause atheroma.

atheroma (*ath-e-rō'-ma*). A degeneration of the walls of the arteries.

atherosclerosis (*a-the-rō-skle-rō-sis*). Fatty degeneration and hardening and narrowing of the arteries.

athetosis (*ath-e-tō'-sis*). A condition marked by continuous and purposeless movements, especially of the hands and fingers.

athlete's heart. Aortic incompetence from strain. *A. foot.* Infectious disease of the skin, between and behind the toes, due to parasitic fungi.

atlas (*at'-las*). First cervical vertebra.

ATLAS

atmosphere (*at'-mōs-fē-er*). The air surrounding the earth. Atmospheric pressure is 15 lb. per sq. in. As it is equal in all directions it is not felt. It is measured by means of a barometer and is sufficient to support a column of mercury 760 mm high at sea level. The higher the altitude, the lower the pressure. Moist air is lighter than dry air, and so the barometer falls in damp weather.

atom (*a'-tom*). The structural unit of an element.

atomic weight (*ā-tom'-ik wāt*). The weight of an atom as compared with that of an atom of hydrogen.

atomizer (*at'-om-ī-zer*). A spray for providing a shower of very minute droplets.

atony (*at'-o-ni*). Wanting in muscular tone or vigour; weakness.

atresia (*at-trē'-si-a*). Absence of a natural passage. Closure of a duct.

atria (*ā-tri-a*) (sing., **atrium**). The two thin-walled chambers of the heart into which the veins drain.

atrial fibrillation (*ā-tri-al fī-bri-lā-shon*). Cardiac arryhthmia caused by the independent contraction of muscle bundles in the atrial walls. There is no co-ordinated atrial contraction and the ventricular contractions are stimulated irregularly.

atrial septal defect (*ā-tri-al sep-tal dē-fekt*). Defect in the development of the heart leaving a hole in the wall separating the right and left atrium.

atrio-ventricular bundle (bundle of His) (*ā-tri-ō ven-tri-kū-la*). A neuromuscular bundle of fibres connecting the atria with the ventricles of the heart, by means of which the impulse to contract is conducted. Degeneration of this bundle produces heart-block, a condition in which the ventricle contracts independently of the atrium. *See* STOKES-ADAMS' SYNDROME.

atrophy (*at'-ro-fi*). Wasting of a part, from disuse or lack of nutrition.

atropine (*at'-ro-pin*). The active principle of belladonna. It paralyses para-sympathetic nerve endings, therefore inhibits glandular secretions, and peristalsis, increases the rate of the heart beat and dilates the pupil of the eye. It is used to inhibit bronchial secretion before an anaesthetic and 0·6 mg atropine sulphate may be given subcutaneously together with 15 mg morphine sulphate. To dilate the pupil of the eye, drops are instilled in a 1 per cent solution.

atropine methyl nitrate. Eumydrin, *q.v.*

atropinism (*at'-rō-pin-ism*), **atropism** (*at'-rō-pism*). Poisoning by atropine. *Symptoms*: Dryness of throat and mouth, restlessness and delirium, red erythematous rash. *Treatment: see* Appendix, p. 388.

attenuation (*at-ten-ū-ā-shon*). A weakening or dilution.

atypical (*ā-ti-pi-kal*). Not typical, *e.g. A. Pneumonia* which does not follow the usual pattern.

audiogram (*aw-di-ō-gram*). Chart showing how the ear responds to sounds of differing pitch.

audiometer (*aw-dē-om'-et-er*). An instrument for measuring the acuteness of hearing.

audiometry (*aw-di-o'-me-tri*). Measurement of hearing ability. The results are usually plotted as an audiogram.

auditory (*aw-di-to-ri*). Pertaining to the sense of hearing.

Auerbach's plexus (*ow'-er-bax*). The collection of nerve fibres (terminations of vagus and sympathetic nerves) and ganglia situated in the intestinal wall. Function: regulates peristalsis.

aura (*aw-ra*). A sensation arising indigenously in the percipient. May precede epileptic fits.

aural (*aw'-ral*). Pertaining to the ear.

Aureomycin (*aw'-re-ō-mī'-sin*). Chlortetracycline hydrochloride. Antibiotic produced by the growth of streptomyces aureofaciens. Is active orally, and has a wide range of action.

auricle (*aw'-ri-kl*). (1) The external ear. (2) One of the upper cavities of the heart now usually termed atrium. *See* HEART.

auricular (*aw-rik'-ū-lar*). Pertaining to the ear or to the auricles of the heart.

auricular fibrillation (*aw-rik-ū-lar fi-bri-lā-shon*). *See* ATRIAL FIBRILLATION.

auriculo-ventricular bundle (bundle of His) (*aw-rik'-ū-lō ven-trik'-ū-lar. See* ATRIO-VENTRICULAR BUNDLE.

auriscope (*aw-ri-skōp*). An instrument for examining the drum of the ear. An otoscope.

aurist (*aw-rist*). A specialist in diseases of the ear.

auscultation (*aws'-kul-tā-shon*). Listening to sounds of the body for the purpose of diagnosis. Usually a tube is employed, *e.g.* stethoscope.

autistic (*aw-tis-tik*). Self-absorbed.

auto (*aw'-tō*). A prefix meaning self, of itself.

autoclave (*aw'-tō-klāv*). An apparatus for sterilizing by steam.

autodigestion (*aw-tō-di-jest'-chon*). Process of self-digestion of tissues.

auto-eroticism (*aw-tō-e-ro-ti-sism*). Sexual gratification obtained by a person stimulating himself.

autogenous (*aw-toj'-en-us*). Self-produced.

autograft (*aw-tō-grahft*). Graft taken from the patient's own body. *See* GRAFT.

autographism (*aw-tog'-raf-ism*). Same as dermographism, *q.v.*

auto-hypnosis (*aw-tō-hip'-nō-sis*). Self-induced hypnotism.

auto-immunity (*aw-tō-im-mū'-ni-ti*). State of sensitization to products of one's own organs, *e.g.* as in Hashimoto's disease, *q.v.*

auto-infection (*aw'-tō-in-fek-shon*). Self-infection.

auto-intoxication (*aw-tō-in-toks-i-kā'-shon*). Poisoning by toxins generated within the body.

autolysis (*aw-tol'-is-is*). The process of self-digestion occurring in tissues under pathological conditions and in the uterus during the puerperium.

automatism (*aw-tom'-at-ism*). A condition in which actions are performed without consciousness or regulated purpose; sometimes follows a major or minor epileptic fit.

autonomic nervous system (*aw-to-no-mik ner-vus sis-tem*). Motor supply to smooth muscle and glands. Divided into sympathetic and para-sympathetic systems and characterized by synapsing in ganglia after fibres leave the central nervous system. Not directly under conscious control but there is considerable cortical representation.

autoplasty (*aw'-tō-plas-ti*). *See* AUTOGRAFT.

autopsy (*aw-top'-si*). A post-mortem examination.

auto-radiography (*aw-tō-rā-di-o-gra-fi*). Photography showing localization of radioactive substance in a tissue section.

auto-suggestion (*su-jes-chon*). Self-suggestion: used in the treatment of functional nervous disorders.

auto-transfusion (*aw-tō-trans-fū-zhon*). Transfusion of blood to a patient taken from another part of his body.

Auvard's (*ō-var'z*) **speculum.** *See under* SPECULUM.

avascular (*ā-vas-kū-la*). Bloodless.

aversion (*a-ver-shon*). An intensive dislike. *A. therapy.* The patient is made to dislike the desired object, such as alcohol, by associating something unpleasant with it.

Avertin. Official name bromethol. A basal anaesthetic for rectal administration. Dose 0·07 to 0·1 ml per kilogram body weight. Rapidly decomposed by moisture. It must be tested by the addition of two drops of 1 in 1000 solution of

Congo red to 5 ml of Avertin solution immediately before use. The resulting colour must be pure orange-red. It should not be heated above 40° C.

avian tuberculosis (*ā-vē-an*). Tuberculosis in birds. This is rarely transmitted to man.

avirulent (*ā-vi-rū-lent*). Not virulent.

avitaminosis (*ā-vi-tā-mi-nō'-sis*). Lacking in vitamins. Usually the particular vitamin deficiency is specified, *e.g.* avitaminosis A.

Avomine. Anti-emetic drug used in travel and irradiation sickness.

avulsion (*a-vul'-shon*). A tearing apart.

axilla (*aks-il'-la*). The arm-pit.

axillary artery (*ak-sil'-a-ri ar-te-ri*). The artery of the arm-pit, connecting the subclavian and brachial arteries.

axis (*ak'-sis*). The second cervical vertebra. Also a straight line through the centre of a body. The *axis of the pelvis* is a curved line which is everywhere at right angles to the planes of the pelvic cavity. *Axis traction* is force so

Odontoid process

groove for transverse ligament

(side view)

AXIS VERTEBRA

AXIS TRACTION FORCEPS

applied to the fetus by forceps that its effect is always exerted along the axis of the pelvis. *Axis traction forceps* is a special pattern of forceps, invented originally by Tarnier, to allow an axis traction to be secured. *A. cylinder*, AXON, *q.v.*

axon (*aks-ōn*). The long process of a nerve cell conducting impulses away from the cell body.

axonotmesis (*ak-son-ō-tmē-sis*). Damage causing the break-up of nerve fibres but the supporting tissue remains intact.

azoospermia (*ā'-zo-o-sper'-mi-a*). Absence of viable sperms in the semen causing male sterility.

azotaemia (*az-o-tē'-mi-a*). Excess urea in the blood.

azoturia (*az-o-tū'-ri-a*). An increase of urea in the urine.

azygos (*ā-zi'-gos*). Not paired but single.

B

Ba. Chemical symbol for barium.

Babinski's reflex (*bab-in-skēz rē-fleks*). Extensor plantar reflex. Extension instead of flexion of the great toe on stroking the sole of the foot. The sign is normal in infants and abnormal after about two years.

bacillaemia (*ba-si-lē-mi-a*). Bacilli in the blood.

bacillary dysentery (*ba-si-la-ri di-sen-te-ri*). Infection of the gut with Shigella bacilli.

bacilluria (*ba-sil-ū'-ri-a*). Bacilli in the urine.

bacillus (*ba-sil'-us*). See BACTERIA.

bacitracin (*ba-si-trā-sin*). Antibiotic from the Bacillus subtilis group. Sometimes used externally to treat skin infections.

bacteraemia (*bak-ter-ē-mi-a*). Bacteria in the blood.

bacteria (*bak-tār'-i-a*). Microscopic unicellular living organisms; some cause disease and are called pathogenic. The principal forms are: (1) *Cocci*, those which are rounded in shape. When these are disposed in pairs they are called *Diplococci*—these occur in pneumonia, some forms of meningitis, and gonorrhoea. When these occur in chains they are called *Streptococci*, when in clusters *Staphylococci*. (2) *Bacilli* are rod-shaped bacteria which include the Gram-positive organisms causing anthrax, tetanus and diphtheria; Gram-negative causing dysentery, typhoid and plague and the acid-fast organisms of tuberculosis and leprosy. (3) *Spirilla* are cork-

diplococci

streptococci

bacilli

staphylococci

spirilla

screw-like germs, or spiral rods with several twists, occurring in relapsing fever, and syphilis. The majority of bacteria are stationary, but some have power of movement. Bacteria have power of multiplying by splitting across their centre, this is known as binary fission: others form spores, which are small, round, glistening bodies able to withstand great extremes of heat and cold.

bacterial (*bak-tār'-i-al*). Pertaining to bacteria.

bactericidal (*bak-tār-i-sī'-dal*). Capable of killing bacteria.

bacteriologist (*bak-tār-ē-ol'-ō-jist*). One who specializes in the study of bacteria.

bacteriology (*bak-tār-ē-ol'-o-ji*). The study of bacteria.

bacteriolysin (*bak-tār-ē-ō-lī'-sin*). A specific antibody developed in the blood to destroy bacteria.

bacteriolytic (*bak-tā-ri-ō-lit'-ik*). Capable of dissolving bacteria.

bacteriophage (*bak-tār-i-ō-fāj'*). Micro-organism, resembling a virus, capable of attacking other larger micro-organisms and destroying them by lysis.

bacteriostatic (*bak-tār-ē-o-sta-tik*). Preventing the growth of bacteria.

bacteriuria (*bak-tā-ri-ū-ri-a*). Bacteria in the urine.

Bainbridge reflex (*bān-brij rē-fleks*). Inhibition of vagal impulses caused by raised right atrial pressure.

Baker's cysts (*sists*). Cysts originating from synovial pouches connected with joints.

baker's itch. An eczematous disease occurring on the hands of bakers from constant irritation.

B.A.L. British anti-Lewisite or dimercaprol. Antidote for poisoning by arsenic and heavy metals.

balanitis (*bal-an-ī'-tis*). Inflammation of the glans penis.

Balkan beam (*bawl-kan-bēm*). Frame, usually of wood, fitted over a bed to carry a sling for an injured limb.

ballooning (*ba-lū-ning*). The distension of a cavity by air, or by its natural contents.

ballottement (*bal-lot'-mo*). The sensation of a return tap against the fingers when the hand is suddenly pressed on the pregnant uterus and temporarily displaces the con-tained fetus as it floats in the liquor amnii. Ballottement may be elicited externally, or per vaginam.

balneotherapy (*bal'-ne-ō-ther'-a-pi*). The amelioration of disease or pain by baths.

balsam of Peru (*bawl'-sum of pe-rū*). Antiseptic constituent of Tulle Gras.

balsam of tolu (*tō-lū*). Used as an expectorant in cough mixtures.

bandages (*ban'-dā-jez*). Roller, made of muslin, domette, linen, crêpe of various widths. Triangular, made by cutting a piece of material, approximately 36 inches (90 cm) square diagonally in half. T, made by taking two strips of roller bandage and joining them to make a T, used for keeping dressings on the perineum (*see illustration*, p. 340). Manytail, made with five strips of 5 inch domette bandage long enough to encircle the abdomen. The strips overlap ⅜ of their width and are fastened together. Elastic bandages are used for varicose veins. A rubber bandage is sometimes applied before an operation on a limb.

Bandl's ring. *See* RETRACTION RING.

Bankhart's operation (*ban-kartz*). Operation to repair the glenoid cavity after repeated dislocation of the shoulder joint.

Banti's syndrome (*ban-tiz sin-drōm*). Characterized by anaemia with recurrent bleeding from the alimentary tract, leucopaenia and splenomegaly due to portal hypertension.

Banting's diet. Taken to reduce superfluous fat. It has a high protein and low carbohydrate content.

Barbados leg (*bar-bā-dos*). Elephantiasis, *q.v.*

barber's rash. A pustular eczema occurring in the area of the moustache and whiskers. Sycosis Barbae.

barbitone. A hypnotic drug. Mainly used to promote sleep. Its soluble form is barbitone sodium of which there are a number of proprietary preparations.

barbiturate drugs (*bar-bit-ū-rāt*). Derivatives of barbituric acid, *e.g.* Nembutal, Evipan, Pentothal, *q.v.*

barium (*bār'-i-um*). A metal, of which all the soluble salts are very poisonous. Barium sulphate is insoluble hence non-toxic. Being opaque to X-rays it is used extensively for examination, etc.

Barlow's disease (*bar-lōs di-sēz*). Infantile scurvy due to lack of vitamin C in the diet.

Barlow's sign (*bar-lōs-sīn*). Testing the newborn infant's legs for congenital dislocation of hip. Many hips become stable within a week or two after birth and the sign can then not be elicited. Early splintage may occasionally be necessary to overcome potential dislocation of the hip.

baroreceptor nerves (*ba-rō-re-sep-tor nervs*). Found in the carotids and arch of the aorta. They stem from the vagus and glossopharyngeal nerves.

barrier nursing (*ba'-ri-er*). The nursing of a patient with an infectious disease in a general ward, or a ward with patients having a variety of infectious diseases. Adequate precautions are taken so that cross infection does not occur.

Bartholin's glands (*bah-tō-lins*). Two small glands, one each side of the vulva, may develop into an abscess or its duct may distend into a cyst.

bartholinitis (*bah-tō-lin-ī'-tis*). Inflammation of Bartholin's glands.

basal ganglia (*bā-zal gan'-gli-a*). Four deeply-placed masses of grey matter within the cerebral hemisphere, known as the caudate, lentiform and amygdaloid nuclei, and the claustrum. Disease of the basal ganglia gives rise to athetosis and Parkinsonism.

basal metabolism (*met-ab'-o-lizm*). The heat given out per unit of time by the individual under standard conditions, at absolute rest, at least twelve hours after a meal. It indicates the rate of combustion of the foodstuffs and of the tissues of the body. In cases of exophthalmic goitre the metabolic rate is high, while in cases of myxoedema it is lower than normal. For clinical purposes it is determined indirectly by the amount of oxygen taken in and carbon dioxide given out.

basal narcosis (*nar-kō'-sis*). Sleep produced by drugs given before an anaesthetic. *See* ANAESTHESIA.

base (*bāss*). (1) The bottom. (2) The chief substance of a mixture. (3) In chemistry, the substance which combines with an acid to form its salt.

Basedow's disease (*ba-zā-dofs*). Exophthalmic goitre.

basement membrane. A very fine membrane separating the epithelium from the underlying structures.

basic (*bā-sik*). 1. Basal. 2. Alkaline.

basilar (*ba-si-lah*). Pertaining to the base.

basilic (*ba-zil'-ik*). The name of a vein on the inner side of the arm. *Median B. Vein.* Short trunk opening into the B. Vein, and usually the one chosen for intravenous injection or for withdrawing blood from the arm.

basophil(e) (*bās'-ō-fil*). Readily stained with basic dyes in which the cation is the active part. Nucleic acids are basophilic.

basophilia (*bās-ō-fi-li-a*). Abnormality of red blood cells found in lead poisoning in which there is punctate basophilic staining of the cytoplasm.

bath. Any liquid or gas used

to bathe the body. A *Water B.* may be cold, 32–70° F (0–21° C) used to stimulate body tissues; a warm bath is 90–104° F (32–40° C) and a hot bath is 98–108° F (37–42° C) and may be analgesic, sedative and diaphoretic. *Medicated Bs.* These may contain sodium bicarbonate, saline, wax, etc. Starch, oatmeal and bran were formerly much used for emollient purposes.

Bassini's herniorrhaphy (*ba-sī'-nis her-ni-or'-ra-fi*). Method of reconstruction of the inguinal canal in repair of hernia.

battered baby (*ba-terd-bā-bī*). A young child physically injured by his parent or his guardian *B.b.* syndrome. A recognized pattern of physical maltreatment of a young child by his parents. The parents are themselves psychologically disordered.

Battle's incision (*in-si-zhon*). Same as Lennander's, *q.v.*

battledore placenta (*pla-sen'-ta*). A placenta in which the umbilical cord is inserted into the edge instead of the centre.

Bazin's (*bā-zinz*) **disease.** Erythema induratum of tuberculous origin. Reddish or purple nodules appear on the legs which may ulcerate.

B.C.G. Bacille Calmette-Guérin. A vaccine used for inoculation against tuberculosis.

bearing down. Popular term

for the expulsive contractions during the second stage of labour when the cervix uteri is fully dilated.

beat (*bēt*). Applied to the beating of the heart and the pulsation of the blood.

Beaver breather. Type of respirator used in paralysis of respiratory muscles. It ventilates the lungs by positive pressure.

bed bug. Insect, Cimex lectularius, living in furniture.

bedsore. A sore on the buttocks, heels, ankles, shoulders or elbows, caused by constant pressure on these points when lying. This arises in long illnesses if the nurse is not very careful, and is specially likely to occur in cases of spinal injury if the patient is not frequently turned. Now usually called pressure sore.

Beer's knife. A knife with a triangular blade used in operations on the eye.

BEER'S KNIFE

behaviour (*bē-hā-via*). Conduct; or response to certain stimuli.

behaviourism (*bē-hā-vūr-ism*). A psychological approach made through the study of the individual's behaviour pattern.

bejel (*be-jel*). Skin disease caused by a treponema.

Belcroy feeder. Small feeding bottle with teat and rubber bulb to help the flow of milk. Used for premature and weak infants.

Bell's paralysis. Peripheral paralysis or palsy of facial nerve.

belladonna (*bel-la-don'-na*). Deadly nightshade, from which atropine is obtained. Used as tincture of belladonna as an antispasmodic in treatment of gastric ulcer.

belle indifference (*bel-in-dif-er-enz*). An hysterical manifestation. Lack of emotional response in an obviously distressing situation.

Bellocq's cannula or sound. Hollow sound with curved spring used to draw in a plug in acute nose bleeding.

bemegride (*be-me-grīd*). Drug used in treatment of barbiturate poisoning. (*See* p. 387.)

Bence-Jones protein. A protein found in the urine in disease of the bone marrow, *e.g.* myelomatosis.

bends. Decompression sickness. *See* CAISSON DISEASE.

Benedict's solution. Used in testing urine for sugar. (*See* Appendix, p. 383.)

benign (*be-nīn*). Non-malignant. Not cancerous.

Bennett's fracture (*ben-netz frak-tūr*). Fracture of the base of the first metacarpal due to a blow on the base of the thumb.

Benzedrine. Amphetamine, *q.v.*

benzene (*ben-zēn*). Hydrocarbon from coal tar.

benzhexol hydrochloride. Antispasmodic drug specially used in extrapyramidal parkinsonism.

benzocaine. Local anaesthetic used mainly as an ointment or in suppositories.

benzoic acid (*ben-zō'-ik as-id*). An antimycotic, antiseptic and preservative.

benzyl benzoate (*ben-zō-āt*). Used in the treatment of scabies.

benzylpenicillin (*ben-zil-pe-ni-si-lin*). One of the penicillins used in the treatment of a variety of infections.

beriberi (*ber-i-ber'-i*). An acute neuritis, due to lack of vitamin B₁ (thiamine). Common in some parts of the tropics, associated with anaemia and dropsy. *See* VITAMINS.

Berkefeld filter (*berk-felt fil-ter*). A tubular filter, made of diatomaceous earth, which can be fitted to a tap.

beryllium window (*be-ri'-li-um win'-dō*). Apparatus designed to allow minimum penetration of the beam in X-ray therapy.

Besnier's prurigo (*bes-nē-ās proo-ri'-go*). Eczema affecting nape of neck, behind the heels, etc. Occurs in children.

beta cells (*bē-ta sels*). The type of cell making up the major part of an island of Langerhans and producing insulin.

beta rays (*bē-ta-rās*). Electrons emitted by radio-active substances. They will penetrate to about 1 cm. in tissue.

Betz cells (*bets sels*). Large cells in the deeper layers of the cerebral cortex.

bezoars (*be-zō-ars*). Masses of foreign material present in the gastro-intestinal tract.

Bi. Symbol for bismuth.

bi. Prefix meaning two or twice.

bicarbonate (*bī-kar-bon-āt*). Any salt containing two equivalents of carbonic acid and one of a base. Sodium bicarbonate is much used in medicine as an antacid.

bicephalus (*bī-kef'-al-us*). A monster with two heads.

biceps (*bī'-seps*). The two-headed muscles in front of the humerus, *see* below, and behind the femur. The latter is known as biceps femoris.

Scapula
Supraglenoid tubercle (long head)
Biceps
Humerus
Radial tuberosity
Coracoid process (short head)
Bicipital aponeurosis Ulna

BICEPS OF ARM

biconcave (*bī-kon-kāv*). Hollow or concave on both sides, usually of a lens.

biconvex (*bī-kon-veks*). Bulging or convex on both sides, usually of a lens.

bicornuate (*bī-korn-ū-āt*). Having two horns. *B. Uterus* A congenital abnormality due to incomplete development—the uterus may be double or a single organ possessing two horns. Pregnancy may take place in one half and be normal. Very rarely twins may develop—one in each horn.

bicuspid (*bī-kus'-pid*). Having two points or cusps. The two teeth immediately behind the canines in each jaw are bicuspids. Bicuspid or mitral valve, the valve between the left atrium and left ventricle of the heart.

Bielchowski's disease (*bĕl-chow-skis di-sēz*). Early juvenile cerebro-macular degeneration, characterized by mental deterioration and blindness.

bifid. (*bī-fid*). Cleft.

bifocal (*bī-fō'-kal*). With a double focus. *B. spectacles* can be used for near and distant vision.

bifurcate (*bī-fer'-kāt*). Forked.

bigeminal (*bī-je-mi-nal*). Occurring in two pairs.

biguanides (*bī-gwa-nīds*). *See* DIGUANIDES.

bilateral (*bī-lat'-er-al*). Two sided. Pertaining to both sides.

bile (*bīl*). Gall. The secretion of the liver; greenish, bitter, and viscid. Alkaline. Specific gravity 1010 to 1040. It consists of water, inorganic salts, bile salts, bile pigments. It emulsifies fats and stimulates peristalsis.

bile pigments (*pig-ments*). Bilirubin, red, and biliverdin, green. These pigments are derived from haemoglobin and appear in the faeces as stercobilin, and in the urine as urobilin. In cases of jaundice the unaltered pigments bilirubin and biliverdin appear in the urine. *See* BILIURIA.

Bilharzia (*bil-har'-zi-a*). The same as Schistosoma. A parasitic worm infesting the portal vein and lymph spaces. The worm's eggs are the main cause of the symptoms in those affected; they are spiny, and therefore cause bleeding wherever they lodge. They are found in enormous numbers in the bladder and rectum.

biliary ducts (*bil'-ya-rē dukts*). Canals in the liver which convey the bile to the duodenum. (*See illustration,* p. 67.)

biligraphin (*bi-li-gra-fin*). Radio-opaque material used to visualize the gall bladder, etc., in cholangiography.

bilious (*bil'-yus*). Connected with bile. Term often used to denote nausea.

bilirubin (*bil-i-rū'-bin*). *See* BILE PIGMENTS.

biliuria (*bil-i-ūr'-i-a*). Presence of bile in the urine. Choluria.

To test for bile pigments, *see* URINE TESTING, p. 384.

Labels on diagram: Cystic duct, Common hepatic duct, Gall bladder, Bile duct, Pancreas, Pancreatic duct, Ampulla of Vater, Duodenum

DIAGRAM SHOWING BILE DUCTS

biliverdin (*bil-i-ver'-din*). See BILE PIGMENTS.

Billroth's operation. Partial gastrectomy.

bimanual (*bī-man'-ū-al*). With two hands. By the use of both hands.

binary fission (*bi-na-ri fish-on*). Division of a cell into two equal parts.

binaural (*bi-naw'-ral*). Pertaining to both ears.

Binet-Simon test (*Bi-nā Sē-mon'*). A test of intelligence. *See* INTELLIGENCE TEST.

biniodide of mercury (*bin-i'-ō-dīd*). A very poisonous antiseptic, similar in composition and properties to perchloride of mercury, but less irritating and less potent. *See* CORROSIVE SUBLIMATE.

binocular (*bi-nok'-ū-la*). Relating to both eyes.

binovular (*bi-nov-ū-la*). Produced by two ova. Binovular twins develop from two separate ova fertilized at the same time.

bio-assay (*bi-ō-a-sā*). Quantitative estimation of biologically active substances such as hormones.

biochemistry (*bi'-ō-kem-is-tri*). The chemistry of cell life.

biogenesis (*bi-ō-jen'-es-is*). The birth of living matter from living matter.

biology (*bi-ol-o-ji*). The science of life and living organisms.

biopsy (*bi-op'-si*). Examination of tissue from the living body.

bios. The Greek word for life; hence the derivation of such words as 'biology', 'biogenesis'.

biotin (*bi-o-tin*). Vitamin H.

Biot's respiration (*bē'ō*). Seen most commonly in meningitis. There are pauses in the respiration, but no waxing or waning as in Cheyne-Stokes respiration.

biparous (*bip-ar-us*). Bearing twins.

bipolar version. *See* VERSION.

B.I.P.P. Bismuth, iodoform, paraffin paste: used for packing septic cavities.

birth (*berth*). The act of being born. *B. mark*, congenital naevus. *B. paralysis*, paralysis due to injury at birth.

bisacodyl (*bi-sa-kō-dil*). Laxative acting on the large intestine.

bisexual (*bī-sek-shal*). Being of both sexes. Hermaphrodite.

bismuth (*biz'-muth*). A metal, the salts of which are used in medicine as a stomachic, sedative and tonic. Causes black stools. Is opaque to X-rays. When applied externally, soothing and astringent.

bistoury (*bis-tō-ri*). A surgical knife.

bitemporal hemianopia (*bī-tem-po-ral he-mi-a-nō-pi-a*). Loss of vision in the outer part of the visual field of each eye.

Bitot's spots (*bi-toz*). Shiny spots on the conjunctiva associated with vitamin A deficiency.

bitters. A group of drugs given to stimulate the appetite, *e.g.* gentian, strychnine.

biurate crystals (*bī-ū'-rāt*). Found in the articular cartilage of joints in gout.

bivalve. Having two valves.

blackhead. See COMEDONES.

black stools (*blak stools*). Sign of bleeding from the intestine. May also occur in patients taking large quantities of iron tablets.

blackwater fever. A form of malaria in which there is rapid haemolysis of red blood corpuscles so that the blood supply to vital organs such as the brain is impaired. There is high fever, haemoglobinuria and jaundice.

bladder. A hollow organ for the reception of fluid. *Urinary B.* receives the urine from the kidneys. See GALL BLADDER.

Blalock's operation (*blā-lok*). The subclavian artery is anastomosed to the pulmonary artery. Performed in cases of congenital pulmonary stenosis. See FALLOT'S TETRALOGY.

bland. Mild, non-irritating.

blastoderm (*blas-tō-derm*). Germinal membrane of ovum.

blastoma (*blas-tō'-ma*). A granular growth due to a microorganism.

blastomycosis (*blas-tō-mī-kō'-sis*). A skin disease caused by the invasion of a yeast-like organism.

blastula (*bla-stū-la*). The fertilized ovum after the morula stage. It is hollow and surrounded by epithelium.

Blaud's pills (*blawd*, properly *blō*). The original iron preparation for anaemia. Now largely replaced by ferrous sulphate.

B.L.B. mask. Designed by Boothby, Lovelace and Bulbulian of the Mayo Clinic. See OXYGEN ADMINISTRATION.

bleaching powder (*blē-ching*). Chlorinated lime. A disinfectant and decolorizer.

bleb (*bleb*). See BLISTER.

bleeder. See HAEMOPHILIA.

bleeding time. The duration of bleeding following puncture of the skin as of the ear lobe.

blennophthalmia (*blen-of-thal'-mi-a*). Catarrh of the conjunctiva.

blennorrhoea (*blen-nor-re'-a*). (1) Discharge of mucus from the urethra or vagina. (2) Purulent conjunctivitis.

blepharadenitis (*blef-ar-ad-en-i'-tis*). Inflammation of the Meibomian glands. Terms commencing 'blephar' refer to the eyelids.

blepharitis (*blef-a-rī'-tis*). Inflammation of the eyelids.

blepharoptosis (*blef-ar-op-tō'-sis*). *See* PTOSIS.

blepharospasm (*blef-a-rō-spa-zm*). Spasmodic closure of the eye. Commonly due to the presence of a foreign body in the eye or to ulceration of the cornea.

blindness (*blīnd*). Lack of sight. *Colour B.*, an inability to distinguish certain colours. *Cortical B.*, blindness due to a lesion of the visual centre in the brain. *Night B.*, or nyctalopia, vision subnormal at night, thought to be due to a deficiency of Vitamin A in the diet. *Snow B.*, dimness of vision with pain and lacrimation due to the glare of sunlight upon snow. *Word B.*, inability to recognize familiar written words owing to a lesion of the brain.

blind spot. Point where the optic nerve enters the retina.

blister. A collection of serum between the layers of the skin. A bleb, a vesicle.

blood (*blŭd*). The red fluid which circulates through the heart, arteries, capillaries and veins. Blood consists of a pale yellowish albuminous fluid, called plasma, in which are carried numerous minute

cells or corpuscles. There are the red blood corpuscles, or erythrocytes, which hold the haemoglobin, carry oxygen and give to blood its red colour; and the white blood corpuscles or leucocytes. The leucocytes are of various kinds, named as follows: polymorphonuclears: lymphocytes, small and large: monocytes, eosinophils and basophils. In blood diseases abnormal forms appear, and the total number and the ratio to each other of these various kinds differ. The blood also contains minute discs called platelets.

WHITE AND RED
BLOOD CELLS

The functions of the blood are to carry to the tissues the water and nourishment which they require, to take off the waste products of their growth and activities, and to distribute heat equally through the body. In addition, the blood carries the antitoxins and other substances which defend the system against bacterial invasion, and certain ferments and chemical compounds which are necessary for the general functions of the body or the individual functions of the various organs.

When blood is shed fibrinogen, a soluble protein in the plasma, is converted to an insoluble thread-like form, fibrin, which constitutes the clot. The change is affected by an enzyme, thrombin, which is not active in circulating blood, in which it exists as prothrombin. Prothrombin is converted to thrombin at the time of shedding blood by the action of a second enzyme, thrombokinase which is set free by the breaking-up of platelets. The process also requires the presence of calcium ions for its completion. (*See also* BLOOD COUNT.)

blood-brain barrier. Hypothetical barrier separating the blood from the parenchyma of the central nervous system.

blood casts (*karsts*). Small shreds of coagulated blood found in the urine in certain cases of disease or injury of the kidney.

blood count (*kownt*). Examination and enumeration microscopically of the various corpuscles in the blood. A normal blood count would be, in an average healthy man between 20 and 40 years: *Red cells*—4,000,000 to 5,000,000 per cubic millimetre; *White cells*—7,000 to 10,000. If the different forms of white cells are estimated, it is called a *differential white blood count* and the percentages are as follows: *polymorphonuclears* —60 to 70 per cent; *eosinophils*—2 to 3 per cent; *large and small lymphocytes*—20 to 25 per cent; *other rarer forms*—4 to 8 per cent. *See* HAEMOGLOBIN, COLOUR INDEX, EOSINOPHILIA, LEUCOCYTOSIS.

blood grouping. For a blood transfusion it is essential that the blood of the donor be compatible with that of the patient. Blood grouping is decided according to the presence or absence of certain agglutinogens in the corpuscles, two in number, A and B. The international nomenclature of the different groups is as follows: AB, A, B, O. Group AB are those who may receive blood from any other group, and are called universal recipients. Group A may receive blood from Groups A and O. Group B may receive blood from Groups B and O. Group O may receive only from Group O. From the above it will be seen that Group O can give blood to all other groups, and therefore is a universal donor. Before transfusion a direct match is always made between the red cells of the donor and the serum of the recipient. Any clumping together or agglutination of the corpuscles which can be seen even with the naked eye means incompatibility. *The Rhesus (Rh.) Factor.* It has been recently shown that 85 per cent of human beings of most races possess this agglutinogen in their red cells, and so are termed 'Rh. positive'. The remaining 15 per cent, 'Rh. negative', are liable to form an anti-body (agglutinin) against the agglutinogen, if it is introduced into their circulation. It may occur in an 'Rh. negative' woman if she becomes pregnant with a fetus whose blood cells are 'Rh. positive' or if an 'Rh. negative' person is transfused with 'Rh. positive' blood.

blood-letting. Bleeding, phlebotomy, venesection. The withdrawal of blood for therapeutic purposes from a vein.

blood plasma (*plaz-ma*). The fluid part of blood.

blood pressure (*pre'-sher*). The pressure exerted by the blood in the vessels in which it is contained. It is taken in the brachial artery and estimated in terms of the number of millimetres pressure of mercury required, on the upper arm, just to obliterate the pulse at the wrist. This figure is the *Systolic B. Pressure*. The average systolic pressure in a young adult is 100–120. The *Diastolic B. Pressure* is the pressure in the artery during the resting phase of the cardiac cycle, *i.e.* the lowest pressure. The average diastolic pressure is 70 to 90 in a young adult. It rises with age. High blood pressure is present in arteriosclerosis,

and some kinds of kidney and heart disease.

blood-sedimentation rate (*sed-i-men-tā-shon rāt*). 0·4 ml of a 3·8 per cent sol. of sodium citrate is drawn into a syringe. Blood is then taken into the syringe from a vein until the total quantity reaches 2 ml mark. The blood and citrate are thoroughly mixed and then sucked into a standard pipette to make a column 200 mm high. The pipette is placed vertically and the column of fluid examined exactly one hour later. It is found that the red cells have sedimented leaving a clear supernatant fluid. In health the length of clear fluid on top varies from 1 to 5 mm. In active tuberculosis or other toxaemic states it may be 20 to 100 or more mm.

blood serum (*sā-rum*). See SERUM.

blood sugar (*shoo'-ga*). The amount of sugar normally in the blood is about 0·08 to 0·12 per cent or 80 to 120 mg per 100 ml of blood. This figure rises slightly after a meal, but not to more than about 180 mg. Above this figure, sugar leaks through into the urine. The amount in the blood can be raised artificially by a meal of glucose; and the blood sugar is raised in diabetes mellitus.

blood transfusion (*tranz-fū-zhon*). The transference of blood from a healthy individual to one suffering from a grave degree of anaemia due to either haemorrhage or disease. The donor must be free from syphilis, and his blood must belong to the same or to a compatible group. *See* BLOOD GROUPING. Clotting is prevented by the addition of 3·8 per cent sodium citrate solution. The blood is taken from the median basilic or other suit-

GIVING SET
For Blood Transfusion

able vein of the arm; the quantity is usually 1 pint. This is allowed to flow from

the needle in the arm, along a piece of short tubing into a vacuum bottle containing citrate solution; all needles and tubing have previously been run through with citrate solution. The blood is injected into the patient by (1) the closed method, through a thick hollow needle into the vein. (2) The vein of the patient is cut down upon, isolated and lifted; an incision is made into it, a small cannula slipped into the opening and tied there. The blood is then slowly run in from a giving set through a drip cannula. After the cannula in the arm is withdrawn, the vein is tied above and below and the skin incision closed.

blood urea (*ū-re-a*). Normally about 30 mg per 100 ml of blood, or 0·03 per cent, rising to a higher figure with increasing age. An abnormal amount of urea present usually shows deficient kidney action.

blood volume (*blud vo-lūm*). The calculated amount of blood in the whole body. About 5 litres in the normal adult.

bloodless operation. An operation unaccompanied by loss of blood. In the case of operation on a limb the blood is expelled from the part operated upon by raising the limb and applying a tourniquet or by applying an elastic bandage.

blue baby. A cyanosed infant, due to congenital cardiac

defects called the tetralogy of Fallot.

blue line on gums. This is seen near the margin in cases of lead poisoning and aids diagnosis. The line is interrupted where there are no teeth.

blue paint. An antiseptic paint for the skin, containing methyl violet and brilliant green. Stains on linen, etc., can be reduced by spirit, those on hands by sal volatile.

blue stone. Copper sulphate.

B.M.R. Abbreviation for basal metabolic rate. *See* BASAL METABOLISM.

B.N.A. Abbreviation for *Basle Nomina Anatomica.* Naming of anatomical terms agreed in Switzerland in 1895.

Bodecker index (*bŏ'-dek-er in-deks*). The ratio between the number of tooth surfaces (five to a tooth) which are carious and the total number of surfaces of the teeth which could be affected.

Boeck's disease (*berks*). *See* SARCOIDOSIS.

Böhler's iron (*ber-lerz-ī-on*). An iron heel incorporated in plaster of Paris when applied to the leg, to permit walking.

boil (*boyl*). Furuncle. A staphylococcal infection of the skin, causing inflammation round a hair follicle.

bolus (*bŏ'-lus*). A large round mass such as that of food before it is swallowed.

bomb. An apparatus containing radium so that its rays

may be applied to any desired part of the body.

bone. Hard material forming the skeleton. It is made of cartilaginous and fibrous tissue, impregnated with mineral substance, chiefly phosphate and carbonate of lime. The hard, outer part is compact tissue and the inner is cancellous tissue.

bone graft. A portion of bone is transplanted to remedy a defect.

BONE

bone marrow. Fatty substance contained within the marrow cavity of bones. In the flat bones, and with children in the long bones as well, the fat is replaced by active blood-forming tissue, which is responsible for production of the granular leucocytes, the red cells and platelets.

boracic acid (*bo-ras'-ik as-id*). Boric acid. A mild antiseptic used for irrigation of eyes, usual strength, half saturated solution.

borax (*bor'-aks*). Sodium biborate. A weak antiseptic. With glycerin and honey it is used as a soothing drug in inflammation of the mouth.

borborygmus (*bor-bo-rig'-mus*). Rumbling of intestinal flatus.

boric acid. Boracic acid, *q.v.*

Bornholm disease (*bawn-hōm*). Epidemic diaphragmatic pleurodynia.

boss (*bos*). A projection.

Botallo's foramen (*bot-al-ōs faw-rā-men*). The foramen ovale in the interauricular septum of the foetal heart.

Both respirator. A cabinet respirator used for respiratory muscle paralysis in patients with acute anterior poliomyelitis. The cabinet is connected to a pump driven by an electric motor and air is driven in and out of the cabinet, and the varying pressure causes expansion and contraction of the thorax.

botulism (*bot-ū-lizm'*). Food poisoning by Bacillus botulinus. Usually fatal.

bougie (*boo'-jē*). (1) A slender solid instrument for dilating contracted passages, made of metal, elastic-gum, whalebone or catgut. (2) Small solid cylinders of oil of theobroma containing a drug for introduction into a small orifice as the urethra.

bouillon (*bū-i-yo*). (1) A broth or soup. (2) A liquid nutritive medium for culture purposes.

bovine (*bō-vīn*). Pertaining to or derived from the ox or cow.

bowel (*bow'-el*). The intestine. The gut. It consists of the small and large intestine. The small intestine is about 20 ft. long and is divided into: (1) *Duodenum*, 12 in. long; (2) *Jejunum*, about 8 ft. long; (3) *Ileum*, about 12 ft. long. The large intestine is about 5 ft. long and consists of (1) the *Caecum* (*sē'-kum*) with

BOWEL

the *Vermiform Appendix*; (2) *Ascending Colon*, running up the right side; (3) *Transverse Colon*, running from right to left; (4) *Descending Colon*, running down left side; (5) *Sigmoid* or *Pelvic Colon*, passing to (6) *Rectum* which opens externally via (7) the *Anal Canal*.

bow-leg (*bō*). Genu varum.

Bowman's capsules (*bō-manz cap-sŭlz*). *See* MALPIGHIAN CORPUSCLES.

Boyle's law. At any given temperature, the volume of a given mass of gas varies inversely to the pressure it bears.

Bozeman's catheter (*Bō'-z-mans kath'-e-ter*). An intrauterine catheter grooved for ensuring the unobstructed return of fluid.

B.P. British Pharmacopoeia. *See* FORMULARY.

B.P.C. British Pharmaceutical Codex.

brachial (*brā'-ke-al*). Pertaining to the arm. *B. artery*, the main artery of the arm; it is a continuation of the axillary artery. *B. neuralgia.* Syn. B. neuritis. Pain in arm due to pressure on the brachial plexus. *B. plexus*, the plexus of nerves supplying the arm, forearm, and hand.

brachium (*brā'-ki-um*). The arm.

brachytherapy (*bra-ki-the'-ra-pi*). Treatment by ionizing radiation at short range.

bradycardia (*brad-i-kar'-di-a*). Abnormally slow pulse. Occurs in heart block and head injuries.

Bragg-Paul respirator. Machine assisting respiration with compression of chest and upper abdomen by inflatable pneumatic jacket and motor-operated bellows.

brain (*brān*). The main integrating mass of nervous tissue situated in the skull.

THE BRAIN SEEN FROM THE SIDE

It may be divided into cerebral hemispheres, cerebellum and brain stem.

THE BRAIN SEEN FROM ABOVE

branchial (*bran'-ki-al*). Pertaining to the gills. Thus *branchial cysts* are sometimes found in certain regions of the neck as vestiges of the gill stage of fetal development.

Braun's splint. A combined splint and extension apparatus for the lower limb.

BRAUN'S SPLINT

breast (*brest*). (1) The milk-secreting gland. (2) The anterior surface of the thorax. *See* MAMMAE.

breath (*breth*). Air taken into and expelled from the lungs. *B. holding.* A behaviour disorder of infants and children. *B. of life.* Kiss of life. *See* MOUTH TO MOUTH RESPIRATION, p. 430. *B. sounds,* the sounds heard by auscultation of the chest during respiration.

breech (*brēch*). The buttocks. *B. Presentation,* presentation of buttocks of fetus.

bregma. *See* FONTANELLE.

Bright's disease (*brītz*). Disease of the kidney, characterized by albuminuria, casts, and oedema.

brilliant green (*bril'-yant grēn*). Antiseptic dye used as a lotion, 1 in 1000, and as ointment 2 per cent.

broad ligaments (*brawd*). The folds of peritoneum with the contained ligaments, blood-vessels, Fallopian tubes, etc., which pass outwards on each side of the uterus.

Broadbent's sign. Retraction of the lower left part of the chest wall when the pericardium is adherent.

Broca's area (*brō'-ka*). On left side of brain, exercising control of movements of lips, tongue and vocal cords, and therefore the motor speech area. *See* APHASIA.

Brodie's abscess. Chronic abscess of bone. The tibia is most commonly affected.

bromethol (*brō'-meth-ol*). Official name for Avertin, *q.v.*

bromides. Salts of Bromine. They consist of a combination of bromine with potassium, sodium, or ammonium. In large doses are valuable sedatives; in small doses they lessen cerebral excitement.

bromidrosis (*bro-mi-drō'-sis*). Offensive sweating, most common in the feet.

bromism (*brō'-mizm*). Poisoning by bromides. Symptoms: red, papular rash, conjunctivitis.

bronchi (*bron'-ki*). The two tubes into which the trachea divides, opposite the upper border of the fifth dorsal vertebra.

bronchial tubes (*bron'-ki-al*). The smaller tubes into which the bronchi divide in the lung.

bronchiectasis (*bron'-ki-ek'-tas-sis*). A disease of the bronchial tubes in which they become dilated and usually secrete offensive pus in large quantities. Treatment, postural drainage, antibiotics, lobectomy, pneumonectomy.

TRACHEA AND BRONCHI

bronchiole (*bron'-ki-ōl*). A minute bronchial tube.

bronchiolitis (*bron-kē-o-li'-tis*). Inflammation of the bronchioles.

bronchitis (*bron-kī'-tis*). Inflammation of the bronchial tubes.

bronchocele (*bron'-kō-sēl*). A diverticulum of a bronchus.

bronchogenic (*bron-kō-jen-ik*). Originating from a bronchus.

bronchography (*bron-ko-gra-fi*). Instillation of radio-opaque dye in the bronchi, so that they are apparent on X-ray.

broncholith (*bron-kō-lith*). A bronchial calculus.

bronchomycosis (*bron-kō-mī-kō-sis*). Infection of the bronchi by fungus infection of lungs.

bronchophony (*bron-kof'-o-ni*). Resonance of patient's voice as heard on auscultating the bronchi.

broncho-pleural fistula (*bron-kō-plor-al fis-tū-la*). An opening between a bronchus and the pleural cavity found in disease.

broncho-pneumonia (*bron-kō-nū-mō'-ni-a*). Pneumonia, beginning in the bronchioles, affecting scattered lobules of the lung and also the finest or capillary bronchioles.

bronchoscope (*bron'-ko-skōp*). An instrument for seeing into the main bronchi.

bronchoscopy (*bron-kos'-kō-pi*). Examination of the bronchi with a bronchoscope.

bronchospirometry (*bron-kō-spī-ro-me-tri*). The measurement of the capacity of a lung or one of its lobes.

brow. The forehead. *B. presentation.* An unfavourable but unusual presentation in labour at the uterine orifice. The mento-vertical diameter, which is 13·0 cm, presents.

Brownian movement (*brow'-nian*). Oscillatory movement seen under the microscope in fine particles suspended in a liquid.

Brucella abortus bovinus (*broo-sel-la ab-or-tus bō-vē-nus*). The bacterium from an infected cow causing undulant fever.

Brucella melitensis (*broo-sel-la me-li-ten'-sis*). Bacterium from an infected goat whose milk causes Malta fever in man.

brucellosis (*broo-sel-ō-sis*). Infection with an organism of the Brucella group.

bruise (*brooz*). A contusion. The skin is not broken but is discoloured due to bleeding in the underlying tissues.

bruit (*broo-ē'*). The French for 'sound', used with regard to sounds heard in auscultation.

Brunhilde virus (*broon-hil-de vī-rus*). A strain of poliomyelitis virus.

Brunner's glands (*broo'-ner*). Glands of the duodenum.

bubo (*bū'-bō*). Inflammatory swelling of glands, particularly of groin.

bubonic plague (*bū-bon'-ik plāg*). Oriental plague, which in some forms is characterized by the development of buboes.

buccal (*buk-kal*). Pertaining to the mouth.

buccinator (*buk'-sin-ā-tor*). The muscle of the cheek; one of the muscles of mastication.

Buerger's disease (*ber-gerz-di-sēz*). Thromboangiitis obliterans. Rare disease of blood vessels resulting in reduction of blood supply to extremities.

buffer. A substance preventing changes in the pH of a solution.

bulb. A rounded expansion of an organ.

bulbar palsy (*bul'-ba pawl'-zi*). Paralysis due to disease of medulla oblongata.

bulimia (*bū-lim'-i-a*). Morbid hunger.

bullae (*bul'-lē*). Large blisters.

Buller's shield. Used to protect the sound eye from discharge poured from the infected one in contagious ophthalmia. It consists of sticking plaster and a watch glass. The shield is made as follows: two pieces of plaster are taken, the one measuring 4¼ in. square, the other 4¾ in. square, and a circular hole cut in the middle. The larger piece is fixed to the bulging side of the watch glass, and is then turned over and the smaller piece fastened to the concave side. To apply shield, the overlapping margins are carefully fastened to nose, forehead, temple, and cheek, but the lower and outer sides are left open to admit air.

bundle of His. *See* ATRIOVENTRICULAR BUNDLE.

bunion (*bun'-yon*). Inflammation of a bursa situated over the metatarsophalangeal joint of the great toe.

burette (*būr'-ret*). A graduated tube for measuring a reagent.

burns. Burns are of different degrees according to the depth of tissue involved. Those of the first degree show redness, of the second degree, blistering; third-degree burns involve the entire thickness of the skin, fourth-degree burns show charring of muscle and bone. The first-aid treatment is to exclude air by applying a dressing soaked in a solution of soda bicarb. or saline, and to treat the shock. In hospital, the burn is cleansed under an anaesthetic and then treated by: (1) Closed method with application of sulphonamide, antibiotic, or quaternary cream. (2) Early excision of dead tissue and then grafting. (3) Application of Tulle Gras and thick dressings. (4) 'Envelope', *q.v.*, treatment.

burr hole (*ber hōl*). Circular hole cut in the cranium to allow access to the brain.

bursa (*ber'-sa*). A small sac interposed between movable parts. *B. mucosa.* A sac lined with synovial membrane secreting synovial fluid.

bursitis (*ber-sī'-tis*). Inflammation of a bursa.

butacaine sulphate (*bū-ta-kān sul-fāt*). A local anaesthetic with action of rapid onset. Used especially in ophthalmic work as it does not cause dryness of tissues and does not dilate the pupil.

Butazolidin (*bū-ta-zo-li-din*). Phenylbutazone.

butobarbitone A medium-acting barbiturate. Proprietary name Soneryl.

buttock (*bu-tok*). Breech. Nates.

byssinosis (*bis-sin-ō'-sis*). A type of pneumokoniosis caused by inhalation of cotton dust.

C

C. (1) Chemical symbol for carbon. (2) Centigrade. (3) Calorie.

Ca. Chemical symbol for calcium.

cacao butter (*kak-a'-o*). Cocoa butter. Syn. theobroma, *q.v.*

cachet (*kash'-ā*). Capsule in which powders of disagreeable taste are enclosed.

cachexia (*ka-chek'-si-a*). A chronic state of malnutrition and debility produced by absorption of toxins.

cadaver (*kad-av-er*). A corpse.

caeco-sigmoidostomy (*sē'-kō-sig-mōy-dos'-to-mi*). Operation for establishing direct communication between the caecum and sigmoid colon.

caecostomy (*sē-kos'-to-mi*). Operation to provide an opening into the caecum through the abdominal wall.

caecum (*sē'-kum*). The blind intestine, a cul-de-sac at the commencement of the large intestine. *See* BOWEL and APPENDIX VERMIFORMIS.

Caesarean section (*se-za'-rē-an sek'-shon*). Delivery of the fetus through an incision in the abdominal and uterine walls. Julius Caesar is supposed to have been thus born after the death of his mother.

Caesium 137 (*sē-si-um*). Radioactive isotope used in radiotherapy in place of radium.

caffeine (*kaf'-fēn*). The alkaloid of coffee and tea; a cerebral stimulant and diuretic.

caisson disease (*kā'-son*). Also known as 'the bends'. The effect on those working under a heavier atmospheric pressure than normal, *e.g.* in deep mines or under water. Return to normal pressure should be effected gradually or nitrogen bubbles form in the blood and tissues.

calamine (*kal'-a-mīn*). Zinc carbonate an astringent.

calcaneus (*kal-kă'-ne-us*). The os calcis or heel bone.

calcareous (*kal-kă'-re-us*). Containing lime.

calciferol (*kal-sif'-er-ol*). The official name for vitamin D.

calcification (*kal-si-fi-kă'-shon*). The deposit of lime-salts: occurs normally in bone tissue, and may occur in other tissues, if diseased, *e.g.* calcified fibroid of uterus.

calcitonin (*kal-si-tō-nin*). Hormone lowering plasma content of phosphorus and calcium.

calcium carbonate, C. lactate, C. gluconate. Salts of calcium. The carbonate is used as an antacid in gastric conditions. The other salts are prescribed in cases of calcium deficiency, *e.g.* rickets, tetany and for chilblains.

calculus (*kal'-kū-lus*). A concretion found in the various reservoirs of the body, *e.g.* pelvis of the kidney, bladder, gall bladder. Operations for the removal or crushing of the stone are lithotomy, lithotrity, and litholapaxy, *q.v.*

Caldwell-Luc operation (*kawl-dwel-look*). Operation to drain the maxillary sinus.

calibrate (*kal-ē-brāt*). To graduate an instrument for measuring by a given standard.

calipers or **callipers** (*kăl'-i-perz*). (1) Surgical instruments for measuring the chest, the pelvis, etc. (2) *Ice-tong caliper*, a two-pointed instrument used for fixing a bone by actual penetration of some part of it, as in the treatment of fractures. (3) *Walking caliper*, an instrument fixed at the lower end

WALKING CALIPER

to a boot. At the upper end is a padded ring which fits round the groin and under the ischial tuberosity. This takes the weight off an injured leg on walking.

callosity (*ka-lo'-sit-i*). A thickened horny layer of epidermis formed on palmar and plantar surfaces subject to much friction.

callous (*kal'-lus*). Hard, insensible, thickened.

callus (*kal'-lus*). A new bony deposit around a fracture.

Some of this is absorbed, the remainder develops into new bone which repairs the fracture.

calomel (*kal'-o-mel*). Subchloride of mercury. Mainly used as a purgative. Should not be given to infants as it may cause pink disease.

calor. Heat.

calorie (*kal'-or-ē*). Scientific term for the standard unit of heat. 1 Calorie is the amount of heat required to raise 1 litre of water through 1 degree Centigrade. The amount of heat produced in the body by the combustion of food can be estimated. 1 gram carbohydrate, 1 gram protein each yield 4·1 C. 1 gram fat yields 9·3 C. It is essential that a diet should yield an adequate number of calories per day, and that the three types of foodstuffs should be proportionately distributed. A man weighing 11 stone doing an average day's work requires about 3,300 Calories per day. *Small c.*, the amount of heat necessary to raise 1 gram of water through 1° Centigrade.

calorific (*kal-or-if-ik*). Producing heat.

calorimeter (*kal-or-im'-e-ter*). An apparatus for determining the amount of heat yielded by a substance.

calvarium (*kal-va'-ri-um*). The upper half of the skull. The cranial vault.

calyx (*kā-liks*). A cup-shaped organ or cavity such as those of the recesses of the pelvis of the kidney.

camphor (*kam'-for*). Substance with aromatic odour, given internally as a carminative, with syrup as an expectorant and applied externally as an analgesic in liniments.

canal of Nuck. A narrow passage along which the round ligament passes to the region of the pubes, it is sometimes the seat of inguinal hernia and occasionally of cysts.

canaliculus (*kan-al'-ik-ū-lus*). A small canal or groove, *e.g.* the hairlike passage leading from the edge of the eyelid to the lacrimal sac.

cancelli (*kan-sel'-i*). The minute spaces in a cancellous bone. See BONE.

cancer (*kan'-ser*). A malignant growth.

cancerophobia (*kan-ser-o-fō'-bi-a*). Excessive fear of cancer.

cancroid (*kan'-kroyd*). Like a cancer.

cancrum oris (*kan'-krum o'-ris*). Ulceration of the mouth. Has nothing to do with cancer.

Candida (*kan'-di-da*). A genus of fungi which may cause thrush.

canine teeth (*kā'-nīn*). The four eye-teeth, next to the incisors. See TEETH.

canker (*kang'-ker*). Ulceration.

cannabis indica (*kan'-na-bis in'-dik-a*). Indian hemp, hashish; a soporific and cerebral stimulant. One of the drugs controlled by the Misuse of Drugs Act.

cannula (*kan'-nū-la*). Surgical name for a metal tube used to withdraw fluid from a cavity. *See* TROCAR.

cantharides (*kan-thar'-i-dēz*). The Spanish fly. The active principle is Cantharidin and is contained in Liquor Epispasticus and Emplastrum Cantharidin. They are counter-irritants and produce a blister.

canthus (*kan'-thus*). The angle of the eyelids, outer or inner.

capelline (*kap'-e-lin*). Bandage for the head.

CAPELLINE BANDAGE

capillaries (*kap-il'-ar-ēz*). The network of microscopic vessels which communicate with the arterioles and the venules. The walls are formed of a single layer of endothelium.

capillarity (*ka-pi-la-ri-ti*). Effect of surface tension causing liquid to rise up inside a small tube.

capillurgy (*kap'-il-er-ji*). The art of destroying superfluous hair

capitate (*ka'-pi-tāt*). Like a head. One of the carpal or wrist bones.

capitellum (*kap-it'-el-um*). The round eminence on the lower end of the humerus which articulates with the radius.

capsular ligament (*kap'-sū-la lig'-a-ment*). A ligament surrounding a movable joint.

capsule (*kap'-sūl*). A sheath enclosing a part or organism.

capsulotomy (*cap-sūl-ot'-o-mi*). An incision of the capsule of the lens of the eye.

caput succedaneum (*suk-sē-dā-ne-um*). Swelling on infant's scalp, due to pressure during labour.

carbachol (*kar-bak'-ol*) A drug which contracts plain muscle and relaxes the sphincter. It is given to relieve post-operative distension of the bowel, and post-operative retention of urine.

carbogen (*kah'-bō-jen*). Carbon dioxide, 6 per cent in oxygen, given to stimulate respiration.

carbohydrate (*kar-bō-hī'-drāt*). Substances composed of carbon, oxygen, and hydrogen only. Sugar and starch are examples of carbohydrate foods that produce energy.

carbolfuchsin (*kar-bol-fūk'-sin*). A solution of fuchsin and carbolic acid in alcohol and water, used as a stain in pathological and bacteriological work.

carbolic acid (*kar-bol'-ik as-id*). Phenol. A powerful antiseptic obtained from coal tar.

Highly poisonous. Used in a solution of 2·5% to 5% as a disinfectant.

carbon (*kar'-bon*). Non-metallic element occurring as diamond, graphite, and charcoal, the latter only being used in medicine.

carbonaemia (*kar-bon-ēm'-ia*). An accumulation of carbon dioxide in the blood.

carbonate (*kar'-bon-āt*). Compound of carbonic acid and a base.

carbon dioxide (*dī-oks'-īd*). CO_2. A gas which is a product of combustion. It is formed in the system by the metabolic process of the body, and excreted through the lungs. It is a respiratory stimulant and is administered diluted with oxygen when respiration is depressed. At extremely low temperatures this gas forms a liquid, and lower still a substance resembling snow. The latter is often used for destroying naevi and similar superficial growths on the skin.

carbon monoxide poisoning. Poisoning by inhalation of carbon monoxide, *e.g.* from coal gas or motor vehicle exhaust. *Symptoms* begin as giddiness and singing of ears, then lividity of face and body; later, owing to combination of the gas with the blood, the patient may have a rosy tinge; loss of muscular power; violent action of heart and lungs; fixed dilated pupils, convulsions, coma or asphy-

xia. *Treatment:* fresh air, oxygen and artificial respiration if necessary. See p. 388 and p. 430.

carboxyhaemoglobin (*kar-boks-i-hēm-o-glō'-bin*). A compound of carbon monoxide and haemoglobin formed in coal-gas poisoning.

carbromal (*kar-brō-mal*). A mild sedative and hypnotic.

carbuncle (*kar'-bunk-l*). Severe staphylococcal inflammation of an area of skin and subcutaneous tissue. There is necrosis and liquefaction of the subcutaneous tissue and several points of discharge.

carcinogenic (*kar-sin-ō-jen-ik*). Term applied to substances producing or predisposing to cancer.

carcinoma (*kar-si-nō'-ma*). A type of cancer growing from epithelial tissue. Spread is by way of the lymph channels, and therefore glands near, and at a distance, are involved.

carcinomatosis (*kar-sin-ō-ma-tō-sis*). The spread of carcinomatous metastases.

cardamom (*kard'-a-mum*). A carminative and stomachic vegetable drug.

cardia (*kar'-dē-a*). (1) The heart. (2) The aperture between the oesophagus and the stomach.

cardiac (*kar'dē-ak*). Relating to the heart. *C. catheterization.* Investigation to diagnose certain heart conditions. A catheter is introduced through a vein in the arm into the chambers of the heart from which pressure recordings can be obtained. *C. massage.* Squeezing the heart rhythmically to stimulate the normal heart beat in an attempt to restart the circulation, having first gained access to the heart through an incision in the chest. *External C. massage.* Pressure on the chest with patient lying flat on back. The heart is rythmically pressed between the front and back of the thoracic cage.

cardiac cycle. The changes in the heart to produce one heart beat.

Cardiazol. Official name, Leptazol, *q.v.* A powerful respiratory and vaso-motor stimulant.

cardinal (*kar'-din-al*). Chief or principal. *C. ligaments.* Fan-shaped muscular expansions from the cervix and vagina to the pelvic wall.

cardiogram (*kar'-di-ō-gram*). The tracing obtained by the use of the cardiograph.

cardiograph (*kar'-di-ō-graf*). An instrument which records the movements of the heart.

cardiology (*kar-dē-ol'-o-ji*). The study of the heart and circulatory disorders.

cardiomyotomy (*kar-dē-ō-mī-ot'-om-i*). Operation to relieve muscular spasm at the lower end of the oesophagus.

cardio-omentopexy (*kar-dē-ō-o-men-tō-pek'-si*). An operation consisting of grafting part of the omentum on to the surface of the heart. The omentum is taken through the diaphragm. The object is to provide a better blood supply in cases where the coronary circulation is deficient.

cardiopathy (*kar-dē-o-pa-thi*). Disease of the heart.

cardiospasm (*kar'-dē-ō-spazm*). Cardiac achalasia. *See* ACHALASIA.

cardiovascular (*vas-kū'-la*). Pertaining to the heart and circulating system.

carditis (*kar-dī'-tis*). Inflammation of the heart muscle.

caries (*kā-rēz*). Decay of teeth.

carina (*ka-rē-na*). A keel-shaped structure, esp. the base of the trachea where it is joined by the bronchi.

carminative (*kar'-min-a-tiv*). A remedy for flatulence, *e.g.* oil of peppermint.

carneous (*kar'-nē-us*). Flesh-like.

carneous mole (*mōl*). *See* MOLE.

carotene (*kar-o-tēn'*). A yellow pigment occurring in some plants. It is a precursor of vitamin A.

carotid (*ka-rot'-id*). Name given to the two great arteries of the neck, and to structures connected with them.

carpal tunnel syndrome (*kar-pal tu-nel sin-drōm*). Numbness and tingling in the hand as a result of compression of the median nerve at the wrist.

carpometacarpal (*kar-pō-me-ta-kar-pal*). Relating to a carpus and metacarpus.

carpopedal spasm (*kar-pō-pe-dal*). Cramp in hands and feet, due to deficiency of ionized calcium in the blood.

carpus (*kar'-pus*). The wrist.

carrier (*ka'-ri-er*). An individual who harbours in his body the micro-organisms of disease, and thus acts as a carrier of infection, *e.g.* typhoid carrier, diphtheria carrier. The typhoid bacillus can be harboured for years.

cartilage (*kar'-ti-lāj*). Gristle; a transparent substance of the body, very elastic and softer than bone.

caruncle (*ka-run-kl*). Small pedunculated granulomatous mass. *Lacrimal C.* The small red globe at inner corner of the eye.

cascara sagrada (*kas-kar'a sa-gra'-da*). A bark with laxative effects. It may be given as a tablet or in the form of an elixir.

caseation (*kā-sē-ā'-shon*). Conversion into cheesy material, as in breaking down of tuberculous glands.

casein (*kā-sēn*). An albuminous component of milk.

caseinogen (*kā-zin-ō-jen*). When acted upon by rennin this protein of milk yields casein.

Casilan (*ka-si-lan*). A proprietary protein powder containing all the essential amino-acids.

Castle's factors. Two factors, one in gastric juice, the other in certain foods, providing the anti-anaemic factor.

castor oil (*kas'-ter oyl*). *Oleum Ricini.* A purge of unpleasant taste which can be mitigated by adding lemon. In the duodenum in the presence of bile, it is converted into glycerol and ricinoleic acid; the latter is an irritant.

castration (*kas-trā'-shon*). Removal of the testicles or ovaries.

casts. Pieces of material taking shape of cavity from which they have been expelled, *e.g.* blood or epithelial debris found in the urine in kidney disease, membranous casts from large bowel in mucous colitis.

catabolism (*kat-ab'-ol-izm*). Syn. KATABOLISM.

cataclysm (*kat'-a-klizm*). Sudden shock; a deluge.

catacrotic (*kat'-a-krot'-ik*). Waverings in the downward mark of the sphygmograph.

catalepsy (*kat'-a-lep-si*). A period of trance, during which the limbs remain in any position in which they are placed.

catalyst (*ka'-ta-list*). Substance which facilitates a chemical reaction without itself being altered, *e.g.* enzyme.

catamenia (*ka-ta-mē-ni-a*). The menses.

cataphoresis (*kat-a-for-ē'-sis*). Introduction of drugs through the unbroken skin, especially by means of an electric current.

cataplasm (*kat'-a-plazm*). A poultice.

cataplexy (*ka'-ta-plek-si*). A rigid muscular condition produced by fear or shock.

cataract (*kat'-a-rakt*). Opacity of the lens of the eye, causing blindness. The commonest cause is old age. *Treatment*, extraction of the lens.

catarrh (*ka-tar'*). Inflammation of the mucous membrane, generally applied to the nose and throat, but also to internal organs, *e.g.* the bile ducts.

catatonia (*ka-ta-tō-ni-a*). A schizophrenic condition.

catechu (*kat'-e-kū* or *kat'-e-choo*). A vegetable astringent, may be given in diarrhoea and dysentery.

catgut. Material prepared from sheep's intestine and used for absorbable ligatures. For sterilization, *see* Appendix, p. 457.

catharsis (*ka-thar'-sis*). Emotional relief brought about by the conscious realization of suppressed desires.

cathartic (*ka-thar'-tik*). A drastic purge, such as jalap, elaterium, colocynth.

catheter (*ka-the-ter*). Instrument used for the passage of fluids; usually from the bladder where there is urethral obstruction. *Nasal c.* (Ryle's tube). Used for the administration of fluid feeds. The tube passes through the nose down the throat into the stomach. *Eustachian c.* A special tube used to inflate the pharyngo-tympanic tube (Eustachian tube). *See also* CARDIAC.

cathode (*kath'-ōd*). The negative pole in an electric circuit.

cation (*kat-ī-on*). An ion which holds a positive charge of

straight plain

semi-coudé

coudé

bi-coudé

self-retaining

bulbous (olivary)

de Pezzer's

Foley's

TYPES OF CATHETERS

electricity and is attracted to the cathode when a current is passed through a solution which contains it.

cauda equina (*kaw'-da ek-wī'-na*). The bundle of sacral and lumbar nerves at the base of the spine.

caudal analgesia (*kaw-dal an-al-jē'-si-a*). Regional anaesthesia of the rectum and perineum produced by injecting local anaesthetics into the sacral canal through the sacral hiatus.

caul (*kawl*). Foetal membranes about the face and head of some infants at birth.

cauliflower growth (*ko-li-flah'*). Term applied to the shape of a tumour growing from a surface.

causalgia (*kaw-sal-ji-a*). Pain referred to in the distribution of a cutaneous nerve which persists long after an injury to that nerve. Often follows herpes zoster (shingles). The cause is not known.

caustic (*kaws'-tik*). A substance, usually a strong alkali or acid, which destroys cells and causes chemical burns. Silver nitrate, fused into a pointed cone and trichloroacetic acid, used as crystals, are common examples.

cautery (*kaw'-ter-i*). Application of heated metal to living tissue in order to destroy it or to arrest haemorrhage. Diathermy is used during operations to arrest bleeding and to destroy tissue when excising malignant growths.

cavernous respiration (*ka'-vernus res-pī-rā'-shon*). A hollow sound, heard on auscultation, when there is a cavity in the lung.

cavernous sinus (*sī'-nus*). A blood sinus on the body of the sphenoid bone.

cavernous tumour. An angioma, *q.v.*

cavitation (*ka-vi-tā-shon*). Process whereby cavities are formed.

cavity of pelvis. The space between the pelvic inlet and outlet.

cell (*sell*). (1) A minute mass of protoplasm. The structural unit of any living organism. An animal cell is usually of microscopic dimensions. It contains a nucleus which appears essential (*a*) for the chemical changes that go on in the cell; (*b*) for multiplication of cells by division of the

DIAGRAM OF A CELL

nucleus and cell substance into two parts (fission). (2) A small jar containing chemicals which can generate electricity when the two terminals are connected by a conducting material such as a wire.

cellulitis (*sel-lū-lī′-tis*). Inflammation of cellular tissue. *Pelvic C.*, see PARAMETRITIS.

cellulose (*sel-ū-lōz′*). The woody, fibrous part of plants. It has no food value but forms bulk in the colon and so stimulates peristalsis. In the form of wood wool, cellulose is used as an absorbent dressing.

censorship (*sen-so-ship*). Freudian term for the barrier preventing repressed memories, ideas and impulses from easily coming into consciousness.

Centigrade (*sen′-ti-grād*). The scale of thermometers for scientific purposes; the freezing-point is 0 deg., normal body temp. 37 deg., boiling-point 100 deg. *See* p. 19 for conversion of Fahrenheit into Centigrade, etc.

centimetre (*sen′-ti-mē-ter*). Metric unit of length, one hundredth part of a metre, about two-fifths of an inch.

Central Midwives Board. The statutory authority which controls and regulates the practice of obstetrics by those who are not qualified medical practitioners.

central nervous system (*sentral ner′-vus sis-tem*). Abbreviation C.N.S. Generally term incorporating the brain and spinal cord, as opposed to the *peripheral nervous system*, which includes the

nerves and sensory receptors outside the brain and spinal cord.

centrifugal nerve fibres (*sentri-fū-gal*). Those which conduct impulses leaving the central nervous system—otherwise called efferent.

centrifuge (*sen′-trif-ūj*). An instrument for separating substances of different specific gravity by rotation.

centriole (*sen-tri-ōl*). Small granule situated just outside the nuclear membrane and found in many resting cells. Just before mitosis this granule divides and at mitosis the two resulting centrioles move apart and form the poles of the spindle.

centripetal nerve fibres (*sentri′-pē-tal*). Usually called *afferent* nerves; those which conduct impulses entering the central nervous system.

centromere (*sen-tro-mār*). Spindle-attachment. The region of the chromosome which attaches it to the spindle which is composed of long protein molecules passing between chromosomes and the centriole when the cell is dividing.

centrosome (*sen-trō-sōm*). Region of differentiated cytoplasm in which the centriole is situated. (*See* diagram of a cell, p. 87.)

cephalhaematoma (*kef-al-hē-ma-tō′-ma*). A subperiosteal haemorrhage on head of an infant, usually due to pressure during a long labour. It is gradually absorbed.

cephalic version (*kef-al'-ik ver'-shon*). The production artificially of a cephalic presentation, from a breech presentation or transverse lie. *See also* VERSION.

cephalocele (*kef'-al-ō-sēl*). Hernia of the brain.

cephalometry (*ke-fa-lō-me-tri*). Estimation of the size of the head of a foetus, usually by radiographic means.

cerebellum (*ser-ē-bel'-lum*). Outgrowth from the hindbrain overlying the medulla oblongata. Concerned with the co-ordination of movement. *See* BRAIN.

cerebral haemorrhage (*se'-rebral hem'-o-rāj*). Rupture of an artery of the brain, due to either high blood pressure or disease of artery. Escape of blood causes destruction of brain tissue, and paralyses occur of that side of the body which is opposite to the injured side of the brain. If the haemorrhage has occurred on the left side of the brain, the speech is affected.

cerebral palsy (*pawl'-zē*). A condition in which the control of the motor system is affected due to a lesion in the brain resulting from a birth injury or pre-natal defect. The popular term is 'spastic'.

cerebral thrombosis (*se-re-bral throm-bō-sis*). Thrombus formation in vessels supplying the brain.

cerebration (*ser'-e-brā-shon*). Activity of the brain. Thinking.

cerebrospinal fever. Epidemic meningitis of the brain and spinal cord, caused by the meningococcus. The fever is often accompanied by a rash; hence the popular name 'spotted fever'.

cerebrospinal fluid. The clear watery fluid which lies in the subarachnoid space, surrounding the brain and spinal cord. It also fills the cavities or ventricles of the brain. Its function is to protect the brain and spinal cord.

cerebrovascular accident (*se-rē-brō-vas'-kū-ler ak'-si-dent*). General term referring to cerebral embolism, thrombosis or haemorrhage.

cerebrum (*ser'-e-brum*). The larger part of the brain occupying the cranium. *See* BRAIN.

cerumen (*se-rū'-men*). Waxy secretion of the external auditory meatus.

cervical (*ser-vi'-kal*). Pertaining to the neck or cervix of the uterus. *C. rib*. Outgrowth from the seventh cervical vertebra, passing out and down to join rib below. It may press on nerve trunks of the arm giving rise to tingling and pins and needles in hands and fingers. *C. spondylosis*. Degenerative changes in the intervertebral discs of the cervical spine with associated secondary osteo-arthritic changes in the intervertebral joints of the neck.

cervicectomy (*ser-vi-sek'-to-mi*). Excision of the cervix uteri.

cervicitis (*ser'-vi-sī-tis*). Inflammation of the cervix of the uterus.

cervix (*ser'-viks*). The neck. *C. uteri*. The neck of the uterus. The lowest third of the uterus, about one inch in length. It is traversed by a canal which opens into the vagina.

Cestoda (*ses-tōd'-er*). Tapeworms. See TAENIA.

Cetavlon (*set-av'-lon*). Official name Cetrimide, B.P., abbreviation, C.T.A.B., a detergent with antiseptic action, used as a 1% solution.

cetrimide (*set-ri-mīd*). Quaternary ammonium compound used to cleanse skin, etc.

chalazion (*kal-ā-zi-on*). Meibomian cyst. A small retention cyst in the eyelid, due to blocking of a meibomian follicle.

chancre (*shang'-ker*). Syphilitic ulcer of the first stage; occurs at the site of infection. Contagious.

chancroid (*shang-kroyd'*). See SOFT SORE.

change of life. Popular term for the menopause, *q.v.*

character (*ka-rak-ter*). Applied to a person's mental features and according to which his actions are made relatively stable and predictable.

charcoal (*tshar'-kōl*). Prescribed as a powder, lozenges or biscuits to absorb gases in the gastro-intestinal tract and thus relieve flatulence. *C. Poultice.* See POULTICES.

Charcot-Marie-Tooth disease (*shar-kō-ma-rē-tooth di-sēz*). Peroneal muscular atrophy. A familial condition of unknown cause in which there is atrophy of the spinal nerves and neuritis affecting the peroneal nerves with resultant wasting of the muscles of the feet and lower legs. The hands may also be affected.

Charcot's joint (*shar-kō'*). Painless destructive changes in a joint due to loss of sensation.

cheilitis (*kī-lī'-tis*). Inflammation of the lip.

cheiloplasty (*kī'-lo-plas-ti*). Plastic operation on the lips.

cheilorrhaphy (*kī-lo-ra-fi*). Operation to repair a hare lip.

cheiloschisis (*kī'-lō-ski-sis*). Hare lip.

cheilosis (*kī-lō-sis*). Condition affecting the lips and angles of the mouth which can be caused by riboflavin deficiency.

cheiropompholyx (*kī'-rō-pom'-fo-liks*). A disease characterized by the appearance of small vesicles on the hands.

chelating agents (*kē-lā-ting ā-jents*). Substances which inactivate certain metals and are thus used in the treatment of poisoning by them.

chemoreceptor (*ke-mō-rē-sep'-tor*). Nerve ending capable of

reacting to chemical stimuli,
e.g. taste and smell.

chemosis *kē-mō'-sis*). Oedema
of the conjunctiva.

chemotaxis (*kem-o-tak'-sis*).
The attraction or repulsion
of living cells for various
chemical substances.

chemotherapy (*ke-mō-the-ra-pi*). Healing by chemical
means, administration of
drugs.

Cheyne-Stokes breathing. Irregular respiration, at first
shallow, then increasing in
depth till a maximum is
reached, when it decreases
again until imperceptible and
a pause ensues, during which
breathing is absent. Usually
a bad sign, and due to a poor
supply of oxygen to that part
of the brain containing the
respiratory centre.

chiasm (*kī'-asm*). A crossing.

chiasma opticum (*kī'-as-ma op'-ti-kum*). The meeting and
crossing of the optic nerves.

chicken-pox (*chi'-ken poks*).
A virus disease. Varicella.
Rash appears on the chest on
the first day; the disease runs
its course in a fortnight.
Incubation period ten to
sixteen days. Quarantine
period for contacts, twenty
days.

chilblain (*chil-blān*). Pernio.
Inflammation of the skin due
to cellular damage as a
result of local deficiency in
the circulation.

chiniofon (*kin-i-o-fon*). Drug
used in the treatment of
amoebiasis.

chiropodist (*ki-rop'-ō-dist*). One
skilled in the treatment of
the feet.

chirurgical (*ki-rur'-ji-kal*). Surgical.

chloasma (*klō-az'-ma*). Pigmentation of the skin. *C.
gravidarum*, the brown discoloration of pregnancy.

chloral hydrate (*klo'-ral*). Hypnotic and sedative. Full doses
depress respiration and blood
pressure. Antidote for overdose, fresh air, nikethamide,
artificial respiration.

chlorambucil (*klor-am-bū-sil*).
Drug used to retard malignant growth.

chloramine. An antiseptic
which is non-irritant.

chloramphenicol (*klor-am-fen-i-kol*). Antibiotic given orally
and of particular value in
typhoid and paratyphoid
fever.

chlorate (*klo'-rāt*). Compound
of chloric acid and a base,
such as chlorate of potash.

chlorbutol. Official name for
Chloretone. A hypnotic and
remedy for seasickness.

chlorcyclizine (*klor-sī-kli-zēn*).
An antihistamine drug.

chlordiazepoxide (*klor-dī-āz-pok-sīd*). Drug used to relieve
anxiety and tension.

chlorhexidine (*klor-hex-i-dēn*).
Antiseptic derived from coal
tar.

chlorinated lime. A compound
of lime and chlorine much
used as a disinfectant.

chlorine (*klo'-rēn*). A yellow
gaseous element. A disinfect-

ant used in swimming baths and in minute quantities to disinfect drinking water. Poisonous.

chlorocresol (klo-rō-krē-sol). A powerful bactericide.

Chlorodyne (klo'-ro-din). A sedative and astringent; given to stop diarrhoea.

chloroform (klo'-ro-form). A colourless liquid which produces anaesthesia when inhaled. Chloroform must always be kept in the dark. Antidote for an overdose, oxygen, fresh air, artificial respiration, stimulants and injection of leptazol.

chloroma (klo-rō'-ma). A green-coloured sarcoma especially affecting the bones of the skull.

Chloromycetin (klo'-ro-mī-sē-tin). Chloramphenicol, q.v.

chlorophyll (klo'-ro-fil). The green colouring matter in the leaves of plants by which photosynthesis takes place. This is the assimilation of carbon dioxide under the influence of light.

chloroquine (klo-rō-kwin). Synthetic drug widely used in the prevention and treatment of malaria; also given in amoebic hepatitis.

chlortetracycline (klor-te-tra-sī'-klin). Broad spectrum antibiotic similar to tetracycline. See AUREOMYCIN.

chlorothiazide (klo-rō-thī-a-zīd). Diuretic given orally.

chloroxylenol (klo-rō-zi-le-nol). A non-irritant antiseptic.

chlorpheniramine maleate (klor-fen-i-ra-mēn ma-lē-āt). Antihistamine drug used to prevent allergic reactions. Proprietary name, Piriton.

chlorpromazine. Proprietary name, Largactil. Drug with wide range of activity on the nervous system. Used as a sedative in psychiatry, also to intensify the action of pain-killing drugs.

chlorpropamide (klor-prō-pa-mīd). Oral drug which reduces blood sugar level. Used in cases of mild diabetes.

cholaemia (ko-lē'-mi-a). The presence of bile pigment in the blood.

cholagogue (kol'-ag-og). A medicine which increases the flow of bile into the intestine, e.g. directly, bile salts; indirectly, calomel.

cholangiogram (kō-lan-jē-o-gram). X-ray showing the biliary system.

cholangitis (kōl-an-jī'-tis). Inflammation of the biliary system.

cholecystectomy (ko'-lē-sis-tek'-to-mi). Removal of the gall bladder.

cholecystenterostomy (ko'-lē-sis-ten-ter-os'-to-mi). Operation for forming an artificial communication between the gall bladder and the intestine.

cholecystitis (ko'-lē-sis-tī'-tis). Inflammation of the gall bladder.

cholecystogastrostomy (ko'-lē-sis-tō'-gas-tros'-to-mi). An operation for forming an artificial communication between the gall bladder and the stomach.

cholecystography (*ko'-lē-sistog'-ra-fi*). X-ray examination of the gall bladder, after it has been rendered opaque to X-rays by drugs such as pheniodol. No food allowed, but water as desired. The first skiagram taken is twelve hours later, and two further ones at intervals of 2½ to 3 hours. Sometimes a meal rich in fat is ordered before taking the later pictures, in order that the emptying power of the gall bladder may be observed.

cholecystolithiasis (*kō-lē-sistō-li-thī-a-sis*). A stone or stones in the gall bladder.

cholecystostomy (*ko'-lē-sistos'-to-mi*). Operation for making the gall bladder open to the exterior.

choledocholithotomy (*kol-ēdok-o-li-thot'-o-mi*). Incision of the common bile duct for the removal of gall-stone.

choledochotomy (*ko'-lē-dokot'-om-i*). Incision of the common bile duct.

cholelithiasis (*ko-lē-li-thī'-a-sis*). Formation of gall-stones.

cholemesis (*kō-lem'-e-sis*)· Vomiting of bile.

cholera (*kol'-e-ra*). An epidemic tropical disease spread by infected water. *Symptoms*: Cramp, vomiting, and rice-water stools caused by cholera vibrio.

cholesteatoma (*kol-es-tē-a-tō'-ma*). Small tumour containing fat-like material which occasionally is found in the external auditory meatus.

cholesterol (*ko-les'-ter-ol*). A sterol widespread in animal tissues, first isolated from bile. One of the substances which on precipitation gives rise to gall-stones.

choline (*kō-lēn*). An organic base which is a constituent of some important substances, *e.g.* phospholipids, acetylcholine. It is used in fat metabolism.

cholinergic (*ko-lin-er-jik*). *See* ACETYLCHOLINE.

cholinesterase (*kō-li-nes-te-rāz*). Specific for acetylcholinesterase: an enzyme found at motor end plates and other sites, which breaks down and inactivates acetylcholine. Non-specific or pseudocholinesterases are found in the blood.

choluria (*ko-lū'-ri-a*). Bile in the urine.

chondralgia (*kon-dral'-ji-a*). Pain in a cartilage.

chondrin (*kon'-drin*). Cartilaginous tissue.

chondritis (*kon-drī'-tis*). Inflammation of cartilage.

chondroblast (*kon-drō-blahst*). The embryonic cell forming cartilage.

chondroma (*kon-drō'-ma*). A benign tumour of cartilage cells.

chordae tendineae (*kor-dē tendi-ni-ē*). Thin musculo-tendinous bands extending between the walls of the ventricles of the heart and the tricuspid and mitral valves.

chordee (*kor-dē'*). Painful erection of penis, common in gonorrhoea.

chorditis (*kor-dī'-tis*). Inflammation of the vocal cords.

chordotomy (*kor-do-to-mē*). Division of an antero-lateral column of the spinal cord.

chorea (*ko-rē'-a*). St. Vitus' dance; involuntary twitchings of the muscles, and incoordination of movement; most common in children and rheumatic in origin.

chorion (*ko'-ri-on*). Layer enclosing embryonic structures and enveloping the foetus. *See* ALLANTOIS.

chorion epithelioma (*ko'-ri-on epi-thē-li-ō'-ma*). A malignant growth of the uterus after abortion or delivery. Especially to be dreaded after hydatidiform mole. *See* MOLE.

chorionic villi (*kor-i-ō'-nik*). Vascular processes developing on the external surface of the chorion.

choroid (*ko'-royd*). The posterior five-sixths of the middle coat of the eye, containing blood-vessels and pigment. It lies between the retina and the sclerotic.

choroid plexus (*ko-royd plek-sus*). Specialized vascular epithelium which produces the cerebrospinal fluid. One choroid plexus is situated in each of the four ventricles of the brain.

choroiditis (*kor'-oyd-ī'-tis*). Inflammation of the choroid.

choroidocyclitis (*kor-oyd-ō-sī-klī-tis*). Inflammation of the choroid and ciliary body.

Christmas disease (*kris'-mas*). Rare defect of blood coagulation.

chromatography (*krō-ma-to-gra-fi*). A method of separating different substances in solution and used in chemical analysis.

chromatosis (*krō-ma-tō-sis*). Pigmentation of the skin, *e.g.* as in Addison's disease.

chromic acid (*krō'-mik as-id*). Red crystals used as a caustic.

chromocyte (*krō'-mo-sīt*). Any coloured cell.

chromophil adenoma (*krō-mo-fil a-de-nō-ma*). Tumour of the pituitary gland found in acromegaly, *q.v.*

chromophobe adenoma (*krō-mō-fōb a-de-nō-ma*). Pituitary tumour causing hypopituitarism.

chromosomes (*krōm-o-sōmz'*). When a cell divides, the genetic material present in the nucleus becomes segregated into thread-shaped bodies which are visible under the microscope. These are known as chromosomes and consist of connected strands of D.N.A. molecules known as genes. In man there are 46 chromosomes per cell: 22 pairs of *autosomes* and two pairs of *sex chromosomes*; females have two X chromosomes, males one X and one

Y. The Y chromosome is shorter than the X chromosome.

chronic (*kron'-ik*). A lengthy disease, reverse of acute.

chrysarobin (*kris-ar'-ō-bin*). Goa powder. By oxidation is converted into chrysophanic acid. Is used, in the form of an ointment, for psoriasis. It stains linen, and the stains must be removed before the linen is sent to the wash.

Chvostek's sign (*shfos-teks*). A spasm of the facial muscles produced by tapping the facial nerve. This sign is present in tetany.

chyle (*kīl*). The milk-like fluid which is lymph draining from the villi of the small intestine.

chyluria (*kī-lū'-ri-a*). Passing of chyle in the urine.

chyme (*chīm*). Food which has been digested in the stomach.

cicatricial (*sik'-a-trish-al*). Pertaining to a scar, or cicatrix.

cicatrix (*sik'-a-triks*). The scar of a healed wound or ulcer.

cilia (*sil'-i-a*). (1) Eyelashes. (2) Hairlike processes of certain cells. *See* CILIATED EPITHELIUM.

ciliary body (*sil'-i-a-ri*). Consists of the ciliary muscle and processes, forming part of the middle coat of the eye.

ciliated epithelium (*sil'-i-ā-ted*). Epithelium with hairlike processes on the surface which waft in one direction only. It lines the respiratory tract and the Fallopian tubes.

cimex lectularius (*sē-meks lek-tū-lā-rē-us*). The common bed-bug.

cinchocaine hydrochloride (*sin-ko-kān hī-drō-klor-īd*). Local anaesthetic used for both suface analgesia and spinal analgesia.

cinchona (*sin-kō'-na*). Peruvian bark, which yields quinine. A tonic, and a valuable medicine in malaria.

cinchonism (*sin'-ko-nizm*). Intolerance to quinine, indicated by buzzing in the ears, nausea, vomiting.

cinchophen (*sin'-ko-fen*). A drug given to patients with gout. It increases the uric acid excretion in the urine, consequently lowering the amount in the blood. Caution is required in use as the drug may be toxic.

cinnamon (*sin'-na-mun*). Useful medicinally as an aromatic stimulant. Sometimes given as an astringent.

circa (*ser'-ka*). About.

circinate (*ser-kin-āt*). Ringshaped.

Circle of Willis (*wi'-lis*). Circular intercommunication of arteries supplying the brain.

circulation (*ser-kū-lā'-shon*). *See* HEART. *Systemic or General Circulation.* Arterial blood received into the left atrium passes through the mitral valve to the left ventricle. It then passes into the aorta and through its smaller branches to the capillaries—into smaller veins, then larger, until on reaching the superior and inferior venae cavae it passes into the right atrium. *Pulmonary Circulation.* The venous blood which is received into the right atrium passes through the tricuspid valve into the right ventricle. From there into the pulmonary artery, which divides into two branches, one going to each lung. The artery divides in the lung into capillaries, and here, by means of the haemoglobin in the red corpuscles, takes up oxygen from the inspired air. Oxygenated blood returns to the heart by the four pulmonary veins, two from each lung entering the left atrium. *Portal Circulation.* Veins from the pancreas, spleen, stomach, intestines, unite behind the pancreas and form the portal tube or vein. This takes blood, rich in the products of digestion, to the liver where it divides into smaller vessels and capillaries. Blood leaves the liver by the hepatic veins which enter the inferior vena cava.

circumcision (*ser-kum-si'-zhon*). Surgical removal of the foreskin.

circumduction (*duk'-shon*). Circular movement of a limb.

circumflex nerve. This arises from the brachial plexus to supply the deltoid and teres minor muscles.

circumoral (*sir-kum-or'-al*). Around the mouth. *Circumoral Pallor*, especially seen in scarlet fever, when the white area around the mouth is in great contrast to the colour of the rest of the face.

circumvallate (*ser-kum-val-lāt*). Surrounded by a wall.

cirrhosis (*sir-rō'-sis*). Chronic diffuse damage to an organ, usually applied to the liver or the lung.

cirsoid (*sir'-soyd*). Resembling a varix.

cisterna magna (*sis-ter'-na mag'-na*). A subarachnoid space at the back of the brain between cerebellum and medulla oblongata.

cisternal puncture (*sis-ter'-nal*). A puncture made with a hollow needle at the nape of the neck into a space called the cisterna magna which contains cerebrospinal fluid. Used when the fluid cannot be obtained by lumbar puncture.

citrate (*sit'-rāt*). Compound of citric acid and a base. Sodium citrate renders milk more digestible. A citrate solution added to shed blood delays clotting.

citric acid (*sit'-rik as-id*). Acid prepared from lemon juice. Antiscorbutic. Makes an astringent mouthwash.

Cl. Symbol for Chlorine.

clamps (*klamps*). Instruments used to compress vessels or to secure a grip on a structure.

claudication (*klaw-dik-ā'-shon*). Limping. *Intermittent C.* Limping with severe pain on walking which disappears with rest; due to insufficient blood supply.

claustrophobia (*klaw-'strŏ-fŏ'-bi-a*). Fear of a confined space, such as a room. Opposite of agoraphobia.

clavicle (*klav'-e-kl*). The collar-bone, going from each shoulder to the breastbone across the front of the chest.

DIAGRAM SHOWING
POSITION OF CLAVICLE

clavus (*klā-vus*). A corn.

claw foot (*klor*). The foot is shaped like a claw and has a very pronounced arch.

claw hand. Claw-shaped hand due to flexor spasm followed by contracture of the muscles flexing the fingers. Often caused by ulnar nerve damage.

cleft palate (*pal'-et*). Failure of fusion of the lip and palate during development; the line of cleavage is shown in the diagram. The cleft is variable in extent; the deformity can be remedied by plastic surgery.

cleidocranial dysostosis (*klī-dō-krā-ni-al di-so-stŏ'-sis*). Rare hereditary condition in which there is a failure of develop-

ment of membranous bone; consequently there may be partial or total absence of the clavicles and imperfect ossification of the skull in the region of the fontanelle. The striking feature is the ability to approximate the shoulders in front of the chest.

CLEFT PALATE

cleidotomy (*klī-dot'-o-mē*). Cutting the collar-bone.

climacteric (*klī-mak'-ter-ik*). Termination of reproductive period. The menopause (*q.v.*).

climatology (*klī-ma-tol'-o-ji*). The study of climates as affecting the treatment of disease.

clinic (*klin'-ik*). An institution to treat patients.

clinical (*klin'-ik-al*). Relating to the observation and treatment of a patient.

clinical thermometer (*thermom'-et-er*). *See* THERMOMETER.

Clinitest (*kli-ni-test*). Proprietary tablets containing reagent for testing urine for sugar.

clitoris (*kli'-tor-is*). A small organ of erectile tissue, found in the female in front of the urethra. The seat of sexual excitement.

cloaca (*klo-ā-ka*). Aperture through which both urine and faeces are discharged.

clonic (*klon'-ik*). Spasmodic contractions, short and irregular. They occur in the second stage of an epileptic convulsion and in certain other fits.

clonus (*klō-nus*). Reflex irregular contractions of muscles.

Clostridium (*klos-tri-di-um*). Large spore-bearing anaerobic bacilli. The genus includes *Cl. botulinum*, *Cl. tetani* and the gas gangrene group.

clotting time (*klo'-ting tīm*). Time taken for blood to clot when bleeding has occurred. Normal time is 4 to 13 minutes at 37° C.

clove hitch (*klōv hit'-ch*). Useful knot for a temporary sling.

cloxacillin (*klok-su-si-lin*). A semi-synthetic penicillin, used esp. in staphylococcal infections resistant to benzyl-penicillin.

clubbing (*klu-bing*). The appearance of fingers and sometimes toes when the normal angle at the base of the nail is lost. It results from hyperplasia of connective tissue. Clubbing is associated with longstanding respiratory or cardiovascular disease.

first position

second position

third position

CLOVE HITCH

clubfoot (*klub-foot*). *See* TALIPES.

clumping. Packing together of cells, usually red blood cells, due to loss of membrane charge resulting from reaction with antibody. *See* AGGLUTININS.

Clutton's joints (*klut'-tons joyntz*). Swelling of the knee joints found in congenital syphilis.

C.M.B. Abbreviation for Central Midwives Board (*q.v.*).

C.N.S. *See* CENTRAL NERVOUS SYSTEM.

coagulase test (*kō-a-gū-lās test*). Test used for identification of pathogenic staphylococci which depends on the demonstration of the enzyme coagulase which breaks down fibrinogen and clots plasma.

coagulation (*kō-ag-ū-lā'-shon*). Thickening of a fluid into curds or clots. Almost always applied to blood. *See* BLOOD and BLOOD TRANSFUSION.

coal-tar (*kōl-tah*). A viscid liquid, from dry distillation of bituminous coal.

coalesce (*kō-a-les*). To converge or come together as may occur with spots in a skin rash.

coarctation (*kō-ark-tā'-shon*). The compression of the walls of a vessel. When this occurs in the aorta it is narrowed where it is joined by the ductus arteriosus.

cobalt (*kō'-bawlt*). Trace element. Its absence from the diet of young animals may lead to anaemia. *C. Bomb*. Source of irradiation in deep X-ray therapy using Co^{60}.

cocaine (*ko-kān'*). A powerful local anaesthetic, much used in ophthalmology. It enlarges the pupil of the eye. Included in the Misuse of Drugs Act.

cocainism (*ko-kān'-izm*). Chronic poisoning from indulgence in the drug.

coccus (*kok'-us*). Any spheroidal-shaped micro-organism. *See* BACTERIA.

coccydynia (*kok-si-din'-i-a*) Pain in the coccyx.

coccyx (*kok'-siks*). The tail-like termination of the spine.

THE COCCYX

cochlea (*kok'-le-a*). The spiral cavity of the internal ear, containing the nerve endings of the eighth cranial or auditory nerve. *See illustration of* EAR, *p. 127.*

cock-up splints (*kok'-up*) for hand and wrist. Usually made of metal.

COCK-UP SPLINT

codeine (*kō-dēn*). One of the alkaloids of opium. It allays cough, and is used in diarrhoea for its constipating effect.

cod-liver oil (*kod-li-ver oyl'*). *Oleum Morrhuae*; contains Vitamin D. Used in the prevention and treatment of rickets. Also applied to chronic ulcers, bed-sores, burns.

coeliac (*sēl'-i-ak*). Related to the abdominal cavity.

coeliac disease (*sēl'-i-ak di-zēz*). A condition commencing in early childhood, associated with deficient absorption of fat from the intestines, resulting in the passage of loose, bulky, pale, offensive stools, abdominal enlargement, wasting and retarded development.

coelioscopy (*sē-lē-os'-ko-pē*). Also known as peritoneoscopy. Examination of the abdominal contents as follows: a small incision is made through the abdominal wall under a local anaesthetic. Air is passed into the peritoneal cavity and the contents viewed by means of a cystoscope. This method may be used when an exploratory laparotomy is unjustifiable.

coffee ground vomit. Appearance of vomit when it contains partly digested blood.

cognition. Awareness. Part of a mental process. There is cognition when there is perception or memory of a material thing or idea.

coitus (*kō-it'-us*). Sexual intercourse.

colchicum (*kol-chi-kum*). Drug used in the treatment of gout.

colectomy (*ko-lek'-to-mē*). The operation of removing the colon.

colic (*kol'-ik*). Severe abdominal pain due to muscular spasm of a hollow viscus frequently caused by obstruction. *Biliary Colic.* Intense pain due to lodging of a gallstone in the cystic or common bile duct. Sudden relief when it passes into duodenum. *Intestinal Colic.* Severe pain in the abdomen due to irritation of the gut as in food poisoning. *Renal Colic.* Same when due to a stone in the pelvis of kidney blocking up upper end of ureter. *Uterine Colic.* Spasmodic contractions of the uterus as it endeavours to expel its contents.

colicystitis (*ko-li-sist-ī'-tis*). Cystitis from the colon bacillus.

coliform (*ko'-li-form*). Resembling *bacillus coli communis*.

colitis (*ko-lī'-tis*). Inflammation of the colon. *Acute, ulcerative C.,* due to an infection, e.g. Dysentery. *Chronic ulcerative C.,* cause unknown. *Mucous C.,* thought to be of nervous origin and associated with constipation.

collagen (*kol'-a-jen*). A protein constituent of fibrous tissue.

collagen diseases. A group of diseases in which there is inflammation of the small blood-vessels, e.g.. disseminated lupus erythematosus, polyarteritis nodosa.

collapse (*kol-laps'*). Severe sudden prostration. *Symptoms: see* SHOCK. *C. massive* of one or more lobes of the lung may result from a chest wound. *C. of the lungs.* Lack of air in previously expanded air tissue.

collar-bone (*ko'-la*). Clavicle.

collateral. Accompanying or accessory.

Colles' fracture (*kol'-es*). Transverse fracture of the radius just above the wrist with displacement of the hand backwards and outwards.

Colles' law (*kol'-es*). A woman may breast-feed her baby, and this child being syphilitic may affect others and yet apparently not the mother. The explanation is—the mother is already affected, not yet showing any signs of the disease, but her Wassermann will be positive, and later in life she will show some signs of late tertiary syphilis, *e.g.* gummata, G.P.I. or tabes.

collodion (*kol-lō'-di-on*). Pyroxylin dissolved in alcohol and ether; used in surgery to form a false skin for clean wounds. Highly inflammable.

colloid (*kol'-oyd*). A substance which will not pass through an animal membrane, *e.g.* starch. Various metals can be reduced into a peculiar semi-gelatinous or colloidal state in which they are said to be very active therapeutically: *e.g.* gold, silver, copper, manganese, antimony, etc.

collutorium (*kol-ū-to'-ri-um*). A mouthwash; a gargle.

collyrium (*kol-lir'-i-um*). An eyewash.

coloboma (*kol-ob-ō'-ma*). A fissure or gap in the eyeball or in one of its component parts, *e.g.* coloboma iridis.

colocynth (*kol'-ō-sinth*). A very powerful purge, dose 120 to 300 mg.

colon (*kō'-lon*). The part of the large intestine between the caecum and the rectum. See BOWEL.

Colon Bacillus (*bas'-il-us*). *Bacillus coli communis:* a microbe present in vast numbers in the intestine, and the cause of serious diseases if it gets a foothold anywhere else in the body. See BACILLURIA.

colony (*ko'-lo-ni*). A collection of bacteria growing in culture medium.

colorimeter (*kol-or-im'-et-er*). An instrument for estimating the depth of colour of a fluid.

colostomy (*ko-lost'-o-mi*). Operation to make an artificial opening so that the colon opens out into the anterior abdominal wall.

colostrum (*ko-los'-trum*). A milky fluid flowing from the breasts the first two or three days after confinement, before the true milk comes.

colotomy (*kol-ot'-o-mi*). An incision into the colon.

colour blindness (*ku'-ler blind-nes*). Inability to distinguish certain colours, known sometimes as Daltonism.

colour index (*in'-deks*). Is a measure of the amount of haemoglobin contained in each red cell, compared to the normal amount. It is calculated thus:

$$\frac{\text{Haemoglobin percentage}}{\text{Red cell percentage}}$$

Normal $\frac{100}{100} = 1$

colpitis (*kol-pī'-tis*). Inflammation of the vagina.

colpocele (*kol'-po-sēl*). A tumour or hernia in the vagina.

colpocystopexy (*kol'pō-sis-tō-pek'-si*). Operation for stress incontinence of urine involving the suture of the bladder neck and vaginal wall to the periosteum of the pubic symphysis.

colpohysterectomy (*kol-pō-his-ter-ek'-to-mi*). Removal of the uterus through the vagina.

colpoperineorrhaphy (*kol'-po-per-i-nē-ōr'-af-i*). Operation for repairing a torn vagina and perineum.

colporrhaphy (*kol-por'-af-i*). Operation for repairing a torn vagina or for preventing prolapse of the vaginal walls. *Anterior Colporrhaphy*. Repairing the anterior vaginal wall and preventing recurrence of a cystocele. *Posterior Colporrhaphy*. Repairing the posterior vaginal wall and preventing the recurrence of a rectocele.

colpotomy (*kol-pot'-o-mi*). Incision of the vagina.

coma (*kō-ma*). Insensibility, stupor, sleep.

comatose (*kō'-ma-tōs*). In a state of coma.

comedones (*ko-me-dōns*). Accumulations of sebaceous secretions in the hair follicles, commonly called blackheads.

comma bacillus (*ko'-ma*). The bacillus which produces cholera.

commensal (*ko-men-sal*). Refers to members of different species living in close association but without influencing each other, *cf.* symbiosis.

comminuted fracture (*kom'-me-nūt-ed frak'-tūr*). See FRACTURE.

commissure (*kom-mis-sūr*). A connecting structure. Bundle of nerve fibres connecting the right and left side of the brain and spinal cord. In gynaecology the anterior and posterior commissures of the vulva are used to denote its two ends. The anterior commissure passes immediately above the clitoris, the posterior constitutes the anterior edge of the perineum.

communicable disease (*ko-mū-ni-kabl di-sēz*). A disease caused by micro-organisms transmitted indirectly or directly from one person or animal to another. How the disease spreads and its clinical and social aspects all provide fields for study.

commutator (*ko-mū-tā-ter*). A mechanical device for reversing the direction of an electric current.

compact tissue (*kom'-pakt ti-sū*). The hard, external portion of a bone. See BONE.

compatibility (*kom-pa'-ti-bil-iti*). Able to be mixed together without ill result: thus *compatible blood* is used for transfusion since it can be mixed with that of the recipient. *Compatible drugs* are those which can be mixed without producing undesirable chemical interactions. *See* BLOOD GROUPING and BLOOD TRANSFUSION.

compensation (*kom-pen-sā'-shon*). Psychiatric term for tendency to exaggerate features of behaviour opposite to those which seem to the patient to be unsatisfactory. In *Cardiac C.* the heart muscle hypertrophies to compensate for valvular defects.

Complan (*kom-plan*). A powdered food of which each 100 g contains 31 g protein, 16 g fat and 44 g carbohydrate, vitamins and essential minerals. Used in tube feeding and as a complete or supplementary food.

complement (*kom'-ple-ment*). A protein present in the blood which forms an essential component of certain antibody-antigen reactions.

complement fixation test. The disappearance of complement from the serum is used to detect antigen-antibody reactions. This complement 'fixation' forms the basis of certain serological tests such as the Wassermann reaction.

complemental air (*kom-ple-ment'-al*). The additional air drawn into the lungs on deep inspiration.

complex (*kom'-pleks*). A group of ideas with an emotional background. Partially or entirely repressed in the unconscious mind, it may be the underlying cause of mental abnormality.

complicated fracture (*kom'-plē-kā-ted frak'-tūr*). *See* FRACTURE.

complication of disease (*kom-pli-kā'-shon*). A disease occurring in the course of some other disease and more or less dependent upon it.

compos mentis (*kom-pos men'-tis*). Of sound mind.

compound (*kom-pownd*). Chemical substance made up of more than one element and having special properties.

compound fracture. *See* FRACTURE.

comprehension (*kom-prē-hen-shon*). The understanding of ideas and the relationship between them.

compress (*kom'-press*). (1) A tightly folded pad of lint, gauze, or other material used to secure local pressure. (2) A sterile dressing applied over an area which has been prepared for a surgical operation.

compression (*kom-presh'-on*). The state of being compressed. *Cerebral C.*, increased intracranial pressure from a tumour, etc.

compulsive (*kom-pul-siv*). Applied to some action which a person feels he must perform, however irrational. It may be done to work out some anxiety.

concave (kon-kāv). With outline curved like interior of a circle.

concavity (kon-kav'-i-ti). A depression.

concentration (kon-sen-trā-shon). The amount of dissolved substance in a solution and therefore its strength.

concentric (kon-sen-trik). With a common centre.

conception (kon-sep'-shon). (1) The impregnation of the ovum. (2) An idea.

concha auris (kong'-ka aw'-ris). Deepest hollow of pinna of the outer ear.

concretion (kon-krē'-shon). A calculus. An abnormal deposit in the body such as stone in the gall bladder.

concussion (kon-kush'-on). Interruption of function of the brain as the result of compression wave set up by a blow to the head. The wave of compression transmitted through the cerebrospinal fluid and the brain substance obliterates momentarily the blood capillaries supplying the brain. Recovery may take many hours.

condensation (kon-den-sā-shon). The transformation of a gas to a liquid, or a liquid to a solid.

condenser (kon-den'-ser). (1) Apparatus to cool and

thus cause condensation of gas. (2) Apparatus used to store charges of electricity. It consists of metal plates separated by non-conducting material. (3) Means of focusing light in optical apparatus.

conditioned reflex (kon-dish-ond rē-fleks). Reflex action produced by association of ideas.

condom (kon-dom). Rubber sheath for the penis preventing conception.

conduction (kon-duk'-shon). Passage of a physical disturbance through matter. Biologically, the passage of a nerve impulse.

conductor (kon-dukt'-or). An instrument used to direct surgical knives, called also a director. In electricity, a substance which allows the passage of electric currents.

condyle (kon'-dīl). A round projection at the ends of some bones. See HUMERUS.

condyloma (kon-dē-lō'-ma). Wartlike growth about the anus or pudendum.

cones, retinal (kōns). Together with rods form the vision receptor layer of the retina.

confabulation (kon-fab-ū-lā'-shon). The narration of fictitious occurrences.

confection (kon-fek'-shon). Medication with sweet covering.

confinement (kon-fīn'-ment). Childbirth.

conflict (kon-flikt'). In psychology a mental disturbance denoting antagonism between contradictory desires.

confluent smallpox (*kon-flū-ent'*). A severe form of small-pox in which the individual papules coalesce.

confusion (*kon-fū-zhon*). Inability to think clearly.

congenital (*kon-jen'-i-tal*). Existing at birth.

congenital heart disease. Heart disease present from birth. Due to developmental abnormalities of the cardiovascular system.

congestion (*kon-jest'-chon*). Hyperaemia. Accumulation of blood in a part of the body, as in the lungs or brain. *Congestion of the lungs*, pneumonia.

Congo red (*kon'-gō*). A red dye turned blue by acid substances.

conisation (*ko-nī-zā-shon*). Part of the cervix is removed, by excision or diathermy.

conjugate (*kon'-jū-gāt*). An important diameter of the pelvis, measured from the most prominent part of the upper half of the sacrum to the nearest point on the back of the symphysis pubis. This is the *true* conjugate, which should measure not less than 10·8 cm and is sometimes as large as 11·4 cm or 12·0 cm. If less than 10·8 cm, the pelvis is a deformed one. The *diagonal* conjugate is measured from the lower edge of the symphysis to the sacrum, and can be determined clinically, whereas the true conjugate cannot. The diagonal conjugate is about 1·3 cm to 1·9 cm longer than the true conjugate. The *external* conjugate is measured from the spine of the last lumbar vertebra to the front of the symphysis pubis (this can only be done with calipers), and is normally about 20 cm.

conjunctiva (*kon-junk-tī'-va*). The mucous membrane which covers the sclerotic and lines the eyelids.

conjunctivitis (*kon-junk-ti-vī'-tis*). Inflammation of the conjunctiva.

connective tissue (*kon-nek'-tiv tish'-ū*). Supporting or packing material consisting of a fibrous gel made up of collagen and elastin fibres.

Conn's syndrome (*kons sin-drōm*). Too much aldosterone.

consanguinity (*kon-san-gwin'-i-ti*). Blood relationship.

conservative (*kon-ser'-va-tiv*). Aiming at preservation or repair, *e.g.* conservative treatment of a tooth.

consolidation (*kon-sol-i-dā-shon*). Becoming solid, as with a lung in pneumonia.

constipation (*kon-sti-pā'-shon*). Undue delay in the passage of the residue of a meal.

constitutional (*kon-sti-tū'-shon-al*). Affecting the whole body, not local.

constrict (*kon-strikt*). Contract or draw together.

consumption (*kon-sum-shon*). Using up. Popular term for tuberculosis.

contact (*kon'-takt*). One who has been exposed to an infectious disease. *C. lens*, plastic lens worn directly on the cornea.

contagious (*kon-tā'-jus*). Communicable disease which is transmitted by contact, *i.e.* not communicable through atmosphere.

contraception (*kon-tra-sep'-shon*). Preventing conception.

contraceptives, oral. Drugs, usually progestogens, which inhibit ovulation. They prevent blastocyst implantation and make cervical mucus unfavourable to sperm migration.

contracted pelvis (*kon-trak'-ted pel'-vis*). A pelvis is contracted if any of its diameters is shorter than normal (*see* CONJUGATE and DIAMETERS). The commonest form of contraction is the *simple flat* pelvis, in which the true conjugate is the only diameter materially shortened. Other common forms are the *generally contracted* or *small round* pelvis; and the *generally contracted flat* pelvis. The obliquely distorted, the triradiate, the osteomalacic, the spondylolisthetic and others are rare. A contracted pelvis may lead to difficulty during delivery.

contraction (*kon-trak'-shon*). Shortening. A drawing together.

contraction ring. *See* RETRACTION RING.

contracture (*kon-trak-tūr*). Permanent contraction of structure due to the formation of fibrous tissue which is inelastic. *Dupuytren's C.* Localized thickening of palmar fascia which involves the overlying skin of the palm. There is a strong tendency for this to contract, drawing the affected fingers into rigid flexion.

contra-indication (*kon-tra-in-di-kā'-shon*). Sign that a particular treatment is unsuitable.

contralateral (*kon-tra-la'-te-ral*). On the opposite side.

contre-coup (*kon-tr-koo*). Injury through transmission of force of the blow, remote from original point of contact.

Controlled Drugs. *See* MISUSE OF DRUGS ACT.

contusion (*kon-tū'-zhon*). A bruise.

convalescence (*kon-val-es-enz*). Period of regaining full health after an illness.

convection (*kon-vek'-shon*). The heat of liquids and gases transmitted by a circulation of heated particles.

conversion (*kon-ver'-shon*). In psychology when an emotion becomes transformed into a physical manifestation.

convex (*kon-veks*). With outline curved like exterior of circle.

convolutions (*kon-vo-lū'-shons*). The folds and twists of the brain or the intestines. *See* BOWEL and BRAIN.

convulsions (*kon-vul'-shons*). Violent spasms of alternate muscular contraction and relaxation, due to disturbance of cerebral function. A fit.

convulsive therapy (*kon-vul-sif the-ru-pē*). Electroplexy. Shock treatment given by electrical apparatus to psychiatric patients. *See* ELECTROCONVULSIVE THERAPY.

Coombs' test (*kooms*). Coombs' reagent detects the presence of any antibody coating the red cell, i.e. in a newborn baby with haemolytic disease and following a mis-matched blood transfusion.

copper sulphate (*sul'-fāt*). Blue stone, blue vitriol. It is emetic and astringent.

copulation (*kop-ū-lā-shon*). Sexual intercourse.

cor pulmonale (*kor-pul-mon-ah-lē*). Heart disease resulting from affection of the lung.

coracoid (*kor'-a-koyd*). A process of bone on the scapula which resembles a crow's beak. *See* SCAPULA.

Coramine (*kor-a'-mēn*). *See* NIKETHAMIDE.

cord (*kawd*). Any string-like body such as the spinal cord or umbilical cord.

cordotomy. *See* CHORDOTOMY.

corium or dermis (*ko'-re-um*). Internal layer of the skin. The true skin.

corn (*kawn*). A local thickening of the skin due to pressure such as found on the feet.

cornea (*kor'-ne-a*). Transparent epidermis and connective tissue which forms the front surface of the eye.

corneal graft (*kor-nē-al grah-ft*). Healthy cornea is given by grafting to replace a diseased cornea.

cornu (*kaw-nū*). Horn-like.

corona dentis. Crown of a tooth.

coronal suture (*ko-rō'-nal sū'-tūr*). The suture which joins the parietal and frontal bones of the skull.

coronary (*ko-ron'-a-ri*). Encircling as a vessel. *C. Arteries* supply the heart muscle; narrowing and spasm of these produce angina pectoris. There are also coronary arteries in the stomach. *C. Sinus*, a passage for the venous blood into the right atrium.

coronoid (*ko-ro-noyd*). Like a crow's beak as with certain bony processes.

corpora quadrigemina (*kor'-por-ah kwod-ri-jem'-in-ah*). Four rounded bodies consisting chiefly of grey matter in the midbrain.

corpulency (*kaw'-pū-len-si*). Undue fatness. Obesity.

corpus callosum (*kal-ō-sum*). The band of nervous tissue which connects the two hemispheres of the cerebrum.

corpus luteum (*loo-tē-um*). A temporary organ secreting the hormone progesterone which favours the establishment and continuity of a pregnancy. It is formed under the influence of luteinizing hormone of the pituitary, by growth of the wall of a Graafian follicle after ovulation. If ovulation does not result in fertilization, the corpus luteum degenerates, but if fertilization occurs, the corpus luteum persists.

corpus striatum (*strē-ā-tum*). Basal ganglion in the midbrain.

corpuscle (*kor'-pusl*). A minute protoplasmic body—for instance, the red and white corpuscles of the blood. *See* BLOOD.

corrective (*kor-rek'-tiv*). A drug which modifies the action of another drug, *e.g.* hyoscyamus, mixed with colocynth, prevents the griping action of the latter in pil. colocynth et hyoscyamus—a purgative.

Corrigan's pulse (*ko'-rig-anz puls*). Known also as water-hammer pulse, occurs in aortic regurgitation. The artery distends forcibly and then appears to empty suddenly and completely.

corrosive (*kor-rō'-siv*). Eating into, consuming.

corrosive sublimate (*sub'-li-māt*). Perchloride of mercury. Powerful, very poisonous antiseptic. For douches is used in strengths of 1 in 1,000 to 1 in 10,000. Itself colourless, it is generally coloured blue to distinguish it.

cortex (*kaw'-teks*). The outer layer of an organ.

Corti's organ (*kaw-tēz aw'-gan*). The collection of nerve endings of the auditory nerve in the cochlea.

corticosteroids (*kor-ti-kō-ste-royds*). Steroidal hormones from the adrenal cortex.

corticotrophin (*kor-ti-kō-trō'-fin*). ACTH. Hormone from the anterior pituitary gland stimulating the adrenal cortex.

cortisone (*kaw'-ti-zōn*). One of the hormones of the adrenal cortex. Used in the treatment of rheumatoid arthritis, Addison's disease, etc.

Corynebacterium Diphtheriae (*ko-rin-e-bak-tār-ium dif-thā'-ri-ā*). The bacillus causing diphtheria.

coryza (*ko-rī'-za*). Cold in the head, nasal catarrh.

cosmetic (*kos-me-tik*). Improving the appearance. *C. operation.* Operation designed to improve the appearance of disfigured or unsightly part.

costal (*ko'-stal*). Relating to the ribs.

costive (*ko'-stiv*). Constipated.

cotyledon (*kot-i-lē'-don*). One of the constituent portions of the placenta.

counter-extension (*kown'-ter eks-ten'-shon*). Extension by means of holding back the upper part of a limb while the lower is pulled down.

counter-irritation (*kown'-ter-i-ri-tā-shon*). The application of an irritant stimulus to the skin in order to divert attention from sensory information coming from another site, *e.g.* application of hot water bottle to relieve abdominal pain.

coupling (*ku'-pling*). Abnormal heart beat which occurs in overdose of digitalis. The normal heart beat is followed by an extra ventricular contraction (ventricular extrasystole). The latter may be too weak to transmit a pulse.

Cowper's glands (*koo'-perz*). Two small glands near the bulb of the urethra in the male.

cowpox. See VACCINIA.

coxa (*kok'-sa*). The hip joint.

coxalgia (*koks-al-ji-a*). Pain in the hip joint.

coxa valga (*koks'-a val'-ga*). Deformity of the hip joint in which the angle made by the neck and shaft of the femur is greater than normal. *C. Vara.* In this case the angle is less than normal. (*See illustration of* FEMUR.)

Coxsackie virus (*kok-sa-ki vī-rus*). Group of viruses which may cause epidemic myalgia (Bornholm disease) and benign lymphocytic meningitis, and possibly other relatively mild diseases.

crab louse (*krab' lows*). The phthirus pubis which infests the pubic region.

cracked nipple (*krakt*). Fissure in mother's nipple due to overfull breasts and aggressive sucking by infant. If untreated leads to mastitis.

cramp (*kramp*). Sudden painful tonic contraction of the muscles.

craniometry (*krā-nē-o'-me-tri*). Measurement of skulls.

craniotabes (*krā-ni-ō-tā'-bēz*). Thinning of the bones of the vault of the skull; occurs in rickets.

craniotomy (*krā-ni-ot'-o-mi*). Operation in which the skull is opened.

cranium (*krā'-nē-um*). The skull.

creatine (*krē'-at-in*). A nitrogenous constituent of muscle. *Blood C.* is raised in hyperthyroidism.

creatinine (*krē-at'-in-in*). A substance formed from creatine and excreted in the urine. *Blood C.* may rise in kidney disease.

Crede's method (*kred'-āz meth-od*). Expelling the placenta by means of compression of the fundus of uterus.

crepitation, crepitus (*krep-i-tā'-shon*). 1. The grating of ends of a fractured bone. 2. Type of 'clicking' sound heard on auscultation of the chest when the alveoli contain fluid.

cresol (*krē'-sol*). An antiseptic, similar to phenol, and obtained from coal-tar.

cretinism (*kret'-in-izm*). Congenital deficient thyroid secretion, causing impaired mentality, small stature, coarseness of skin and hair and deposition of fat on the body. Treated early with thyroid extract, great improvement may result.

cribriform (*kri'-bri-form*). Perforated like a sieve.

cricoid cartilage (*kri'-koyd kar'-ti-lāj*). A ring-shaped cartilage below the thyroid.

crisis (*krī'-sis*). The deciding point of a disease, from which the patient either begins to recover or sinks rapidly; often marked by a long sleep, profuse perspiration, or other phenomena.

Crohn's disease (*krōns*). Chronic form of enteritis affecting the terminal part of the ileum. Syn. regional ileitis.

crossed laterality (*krost la-te-ral'-iti*). Combination of either right-handedness with left eyedness or of left-handedness with right eyedness.

cross-infection. Hazard in hospitals where, owing to proximity of patients to each other, infection is easily transferred. Particularly dangerous in surgical and obstetric wards where wound infection is a problem despite stringent efforts to minimize the spread of bacteria.

cross-resistance. Micro-organisms which are resistant to one antibiotic, tend to have resistance to other antibiotics of the same type.

croup (*kroop*). Dyspnoea and stridor due to obstruction of the larynx. It may be due to

inflammation, or spasm of the muscles.

crucial (*kroo'-shul*). Critical or decisive.

cruciate (*kroo-shē-āt*). Cross-shaped.

crural (*krū'-ral*). Relating to the thigh.

crus (*kroos*). Latin for leg. A limb-like structure.

crush syndrome (*krush sin-drōm*). As the result of extensive crushing of muscles, toxic substances pass into the circulation which cause the medullary circulation of the kidney to be opened up so that blood is diverted from the glomeruli in the renal cortex. This results in oliguria.

crutch paralysis (*kru'-tch pa-ral'-is-sis*). Caused by pressure on the axillary nerves and vessels by a crutch.

cryosurgery (*krī-ō-ser-je-ri*). Surgery which entails the use of freezing as for replacement of detached retina, removal of lens in cataract operation.

cryptomenorrhoea (*krip-to-men'-o-re-a*). Apparent amenorrhea due to obstruction to the flow of menstrual blood.

cryptorchid (*krip-tor'-kid*). A male in whom one or both testicles have failed to reach the scrotum.

crypts of Lieberkühn (*kripts of lē-ber-koon*). Glands found in the mucous membrane of the small intestine. They secrete a mixture of digestive enzymes collectively termed intestinal juice.

crystalline lens (*kris-ta-lin*). Lens of the eye, *q.v.*

crystalloids (*kris'-tal-loyds*). Substances which will pass through an animal membrane. They easily crystallize and are readily soluble, *e.g.* salt, sugar.

crystalluria (*kris-ta-lū-ri-a*). Crystals which are found in the urine esp. when patient's intake of water is too small when sulpha drugs are prescribed.

cubit (*kū'-bit*), **cubitus.** (1) The forearm. (2) The elbow.

cuirass respirator (*kyor-as*). Respirator, fitting over patient's chest and abdomen like a breastplate, used in poliomyelitis.

culdoscope (*kul-dos-kŏp*). Instrument passed through the posterior vaginal wall to view the pelvic cavity.

culture (*kul'-cher*). The artificial cultivation of tissues, cells or viruses.

culture media (*mē'-dia*). Substances used for cultivating bacteria, *e.g.* gelatin, broth.

cumulative action (*kū'-mu-la-tiv*). A term applied to the prolonged use of certain drugs which are excreted slowly. After several doses have been given, symptoms of poisoning may arise, *e.g.* mercury, digitalis.

cuneiform (*kū-nē-form*). Wedge-shaped. Three of the tarsal bones.

curare (*kū'-rah'-rē*). A poison derived from a South American plant. It paralyses motor nerves. Used by anaesthetists to produce muscular relaxation, thus reducing the amount of anaesthetic required.

curettage (*kū-re-tahj*). The operation of scraping with a curette; most commonly the uterus is the seat of operation.

curette (*kū-ret'*). A spoon-shaped instrument. *C., suction.* Hollow tube of metal, glass or plastic, connected to a vacuum pump and used to terminate pregnancy in the early stages.

UTERINE CURETTE

ADENOID CURETTE

curie (*kū'-rē*). Unit of radioactivity.

Cushing's disease (*ku'-shings di-zēz*). Adenoma of the pituitary with hypersecretion of ACTH resulting in adrenal cortical overactivity.

Cushing's syndrome (*ku'-shings sin'-drŏm*). Syndrome due to oversecretion of adreno-cortical hormones and characterized by moon-face, redistribution of body fat, polycythaemia, hirsutism, acne, amenorrhoea, osteoporosis, glycosuria, hypertension, purpura, muscular weakness and occasionally mental derangement.

cusp (*kusp*). Projection, esp. on crown of tooth; also applied to part of heart valve.

cutaneous (*kū-tā'-ne-us*). Pertaining to the skin.

cuticle (*kū'-ti-kl*). The external, or scurf skin.

cutis (*kū'-tis*). True skin or derma.

cyanide poisoning. *See* APPENDIX, p. 388.

cyanocobalamin (*sī-an-ō-kō-bal-a-min*). Vitamin B$_{12}$, the antipernicious anaemia principle of liver extract.

cyanosis (*sī-an-ō'-sis*). Blue appearance; due to deficient oxygenation of the blood. It occurs in heart failure, diseases of the respiratory tract, and congenital heart disease. *See* BLUE BABY.

cycle (*sī-kl*). Repeated series of events, *e.g.* cardiac cycle, menstrual cycle.

cyclical vomiting (*sik'-li-kal*). Recurrent attacks of vomiting occurring in childhood, usually with headache, and signs of acidosis.

cyclitis (*sīk-lī'-tis*). Inflammation of ciliary body of the eye.

cyclobarbitone (*sī-klō-bah'-bi-tōn*). A short-acting barbiturate.

cyclodialysis (*sī-klō-dī-a-li-sis*). Ophthalmic operation to drain the anterior chamber of the eye.

cycloplegia (*sī-klō-plē'-ji-a*). Paralysis of the ciliary muscle of the eye.

cyclopropane (*sī-klō'-prō-pān*). A gas that is used to produce general anaesthesia. It must be used in a closed circuit. Used for operations on the chest as it causes the minimum respiratory movement.

cyclothymia (*sī-klō-thī'-mia*). A mental state in which depression alternates with exuberance.

cyclotomy (*sī-klot-o-mē*). Incision through the ciliary body of the eye.

cyesis (*sī-ē-sis*). Pregnancy.

cyst (*sist*). A tumour containing fluid in a membranous sac. *Daughter C.* One developed from the walls of a large one.

cystadenoma (*sis-tad-e-nō'-ma*). Benign growth containing cysts.

cystectomy (*sis-tek'-to-mi*). Removal of the urinary bladder.

cystic disease of the lung. Congenital disease in which the pancreas is first affected and then the lung. There is bronchiectasis.

cystic duct (*sis'-tik*). The duct leading from the gall bladder to the common bile duct.

cysticercosis (*sis-ti-ser-kō'-sis*). Normally the cysticercus stage of the tapeworm occurs in the pig. Occasionally it develops in the muscle or nervous system of man producing serious symptoms, *e.g.* epilepsy.

cystine (*sis'-tin*). A sulphur-containing amino-acid, *q.v.*

cystitis (*sis-ti'-tis*). Inflammation of the urinary bladder.

cystitome (*sis-ti-tōm*). Knife used by ophthalmic surgeon in operation for cataract.

cystobubonocele (*sis-to-bū-bo'-nō-sēl*). Hernia involving the bladder.

cystocele (*sis'-tō-sēl*). Hernia of the bladder into the vagina.

cystogram (*sis-tō-gram*). X-ray of urinary bladder.

cystolithiasis (*sis-to-li-thi'-a-sis*). Stone in the bladder.

cystometry (*sis-to-me-tri*). Measurement of tone of the bladder.

cystoscope (*sis'-to-skōp*). An instrument for examining the bladder.

CYSTOSCOPE IN THE BLADDER

cystostomy (*sis-tos'-to-mi*). Operation of producing an opening from the bladder to the exterior.

cystotomy (*sis-tot'-o-mi*). Incision of the bladder or division of the anterior capsule of the lens of the eye.

Cytamen (*si-ta-men.*) Cyanocobalamin, *q.v.*

cytology (*si-tol'-o-ji*). The study of cells. *Exfoliative C.* The study of shed cells used in the diagnosis of premalignant disease.

cytolysis (*si-tol'-is-is*). Cell disintegration.

cytometer (*si-tom'-et-er*). An instrument for counting cells.

cytoplasm (*si-to-pla-sm*). Protoplasm.

cytotoxic (*si-tō-tōk-sik*). Substance which damages cells. *C. drugs.* Used in malignant disease to destroy cancer cells.

cytotoxin (*si-tō-tok-sin*). Antibody inhibiting a cell's normal activity.

D

Dacron (*dak-ron*). Man-made fibre used in vascular surgery.

dacryadenitis (*dak-ri-ad-en-i'-tis*). Inflammation of the lacrimal gland.

dacryocystitis (*dak'-ri-ō-sis-ti'-tis*). Inflammation of the tear sac.

dacryocystorhinostomy (*dak-ri-ō-sis-tō-ri-nos'-to-mi*). Operation to establish a communication between the tear (lacrimal) sac and the nose.

dacryolith (*dak'-ri-ō-lith*). Stone in the lacrimal duct.

dacryoma (*dak-ri-ō'-mah*). Benign tumour arising from lacrimal epithelium.

dactyl (*dak-til'*). A digit of the hand or foot.

dactylion (*dak-til-i'-on*). Webbed fingers or toes.

dactylitis (*dak-ti-lī'-tis*). Inflammation of the fingers or toes. Generally used of the bones only.

dactylology (*dak-ti-lol'-o-jē*). Talking by the fingers; deaf and dumb language.

Dakin's solution (*dā'-kinz*). An antiseptic solution containing sodium hypochlorite and boric acid used to irrigate wounds.

Daltonism (*dal'-tōn-izm*). Colour blindness.

dandruff (*dan'-druf*). Scurf at the hair roots.

dandy fever. *See* DENGUE.

dapsone (*dap-zōn*). Sulphone drug used in the treatment of leprosy and other skin diseases.

Daptazole (*dap-ta-zōl*). *See* AMIPHENAZOLE.

day hospital. Hospital for patients, esp. the elderly and psychiatric patients, who go home at night.

Darwinism (*dar'-win-izm*). The theory of descent by evolution as taught by Charles Darwin in the nineteenth century.

D.D.A. Dangerous Drugs Act, regulated sale and prescribing of the following poisons: morphia, heroin, cocaine, Indian hemp, pethidine, amidone (proprietary name Physeptone), phenadoxone (proprietary name Heptalgin). Now replaced by the Misuse of Drugs Act 1971.

D.D.T. A synthetic insecticide.

deaf mute (*def mūt*). An individual who is both deaf and dumb.

deafness (*def-nes*). Lack of hearing. *Word D*. Agnosia.

deamination (*dē-am-in-ā-shon*). The breaking down of aminoacids in the liver.

debility (*de-bil'-i-ti*). Weakness, loss of power.

debridement (*dā-brēd'-mo*). Thorough cleansing of a wound and excision of the edges.

decalcification (*dē-kal-sif-i-kā'-shon*). Loss or removal of calcium salts from bone.

decapitation (*dē'-kap-e-tā'-shon*). The operation of severing the fetal head from the body, very occasionally necessary in cases of obstructed labour.

decapsulation (*dē-kap-sū-lā'-shon*). Removal of the capsule of an organ, *e.g.* of the kidney.

Decicain. Amethocaine hydrochloride (*q.v.*).

decidua (*de-sid'-ū-a*). The thickened lining of the uterus formed to receive the fertilized ovum. As the ovum grows larger, the decidua covering it is called the *deci-*

dua reflexa; the part where it is attached to the uterine wall and which later becomes the placenta, the *decidua basalis*; while that lining the rest of the uterine cavity is the *decidua vera*.

deciduoma malignum (*de-sid-ū-ō-ma ma-lig'-num*). *See* CHORION EPITHELIOMA.

decompensation (*dē-kom-pen-sā'-shon*). Failure of compensation, as of the heart.

decomposition (*dē-kom-pō-zish'-on*). (1) Putrefaction. (2) Breakdown of substances by hydrolytic enzymes.

decompression (*dē-kom-presh'-on*). An operation performed to relieve internal pressure, *e.g.* trephining of the skull. *D. sickness.* Caisson disease, *q.v.*

decortication (*dē-kor-ti-kā'-shon*). Removal of the cortex or external covering from an organ, *e.g.* of the cerebrum or of the kidney. *D., Pulmonary*, pleurectomy: removal of one or more ribs and the visceral layer of the pleura.

decubitus (*de-kū'-bit-us*). The recumbent or horizontal position.

decussation (*dē-kus-ā'-shon*). (1) An interlacing or crossing of fellow parts. (2) The point at which the crossing occurs. *D. of the Pyramids.* The crossing of the motor fibres from one side of the medulla to the other.

deep X-ray therapy. *See* X-RAYS.

defaecation (*dē-fē-kā'-shon*). The act of evacuating the bowels.

defibrillator (*dē-fi-bri-lā-tor*). Apparatus which applies electrical impulses to the heart. Designed to stop fibrillation, *q.v.*, and restore the normal cardiac cycle.

deficiency diseases (*de-fish'-en-sē*). Due to an inadequate supply of vitamins in the diet, *e.g.* rickets, scurvy, beriberi.

deformed pelvis (*dē-fawm'd*). *See* CONTRACTED PELVIS.

degeneration (*dē-je-ner-ā'-shon*). Deterioration in structure or function of tissue. When the structural changes are marked, descriptive terms are sometimes used, *e.g.* colloid, fatty, hyaline, etc.

deglutition (*deg-lū-tish'-on*). Act of swallowing.

dehydration (*dē-hī-drā'-shon*). Loss of water.

déjà vu phenomenon (*dā-ja vū fe-no-me-non*). Illusion of familiarity when experiencing something new.

Delhi boil (*del'-ē*). A form of boil prevailing in the East. Cutaneous leishmaniasis.

delinquent (*de-lin-kwent*). One who acts against the accepted moral code.

deliquescent (*de-li-kwe-sent*). Able to absorb moisture and become fluid.

delirium (*de-lir'-i-um*). Extravagant talking, raving, generally due to high fever.

delirium tremens (*de-lir'-i-um tre'-menz*). An acute psychosis usually associated with chronic alcoholism. The patient is disorientated, has hallucinations and is excited. There is a coarse tremor of the fingers, tongue and facial muscles.

delivery (*de-li'-ver-i*). Parturition. Childbirth.

deltoid (*del'-toyd*). The muscle which covers the prominence of the shoulder.

THE DELTOID MUSCLE

delusion (*de-lū'-zhon*). A false idea, entirely without foundation in the facts of the environment.

demarcation (*de-mar-kā'-shon*). The marking of a boundary. *Line of D.*, red line which forms between dead and living tissue in gangrene.

dementia (*de-men'-she-a*). Feebleness of the mental faculties, inconsequent ideas.

A form of insanity. An acquired condition. *D. Praecox*, schizophrenia, *q.v.*

demographic (*de-mō-gra-fik*). Relating to vital statistics and social science.

demulcents (*de-mul'-sents*). Agents which protect sensitive surfaces from irritation.

dendron, dendrite (*den'drīt*). A protoplasmic process of a nerve cell.

denervated (*de-ner-vā-ted*). Deprived of nerve supply.

dengue (*deng'-ge*). A virus disease of the tropics, transmitted by mosquitoes and characterised by fever, headache, pains in the limbs, and a rash.

Denis Browne splints. A number of splints designed to correct congenital deformity, as that of the hip, bear this surgeon's name. His padded metal splints to correct congenital talipes equinovarus are widely used.

dens. A tooth.

density (*den'-si-ti*). Compactness. The amount of matter contained in a given space.

dental (*den'-tal*). Pertaining to the teeth.

dentine (*den'-tēn*). The substance which forms the body of a tooth. *See* TEETH.

dentition (*den-tish'-on*). Teething. *See* TEETH.

denture (*den'-tūr*). A set of artificial teeth.

deodorant, deodorizer (*dē-ō'-dor-ī-zer*). Destroyer of

smells; the chief deodorants are chloride of lime, sulphurous acid, nitrous acid, chlorophyll, iodoform, scents, and fumigating pastilles. They are all more or less disinfectants.

deoxidation (*dē-ok-si-dā'-shon*). The removal of oxygen from a substance.

deoxycorticosterone (*dē-ok-si-kaw-ti-kos'-te-rōn*). A constituent of suprarenal cortex extract, prescribed in Addison's disease.

deoxyribonucleic acid (*dē-ok-si-ri-bo-nū-klā-ik a-sid*). D.N.A. A complex chemical found in the cell nucleus and containing the genetic information.

depersonalization (*dē-per-son-al-i-zā-shon*). A neurotic state when the person feels that he has no reality in existence but is only an onlooker at his own behaviour and actions.

depilatory (*dē-pil'-a-to-ri*). An agent for removing superfluous hairs from the body.

depletion (*dē-plē'-shon*). Act of emptying; bleeding; purging.

deposit (*de-poz'-it*). A sediment.

depressant (*de-pres'-ant*). An agent reducing functional activity.

depression (*dē-pre'-shon*). A feeling of gloom due to disappointment, loss or failure. In *reactive depression*, due to stress, the patient does not lose touch with reality.

Severe depression is a psychotic state and there is usually a predisposition to it in the person's make-up. He then loses all touch with reality and needs expert help. *Involutional depression* occasionally occurs at the menopause.

depressor (*de-pres'-or*). (1) Down-drawing muscle. (2) An instrument for depressing a part.

Derbyshire neck (*dah-bi-shu nek*). Term used to describe a swollen neck due to goitre. Once common in Derby.

derealization (*dē-rē-al-i-zā-shon*). A feeling that the world is unreal and strange.

derma, dermis (*der'-ma*). The cutis or true skin.

dermalgia (*der-mal'-jia*). Pain of the skin.

dermatitis (*der-ma-ti'-tis*). Inflammation of the skin. The numerous causes may be of external or internal origin. Some common external irritants are dyes, metals, disinfectants, flowers.

dermatology (*der-ma-tol'-oji*). The science of the skin and its diseases.

dermatome (*der-ma-tōm*). Instrument for cutting a skin graft.

dermatomycosis (*der-mat-o-mī-kō'-sis*). A skin disease caused by a fungus.

dermatophyte (*der-ma-tō-fīt*). Group of fungi on skin and mucous membranes.

dermatosis (*der-ma-tō'-sis*). Any skin disease.

dermis (*der'-mis*). The true skin which lies below the epidermis.

dermographism (*der-mo'-graf'-izm*). The production of wheals on the skin, resembling urticaria, on gently stroking the skin.

dermoid cyst (*der-moyd sist'*). A cyst containing epithelial substances, especially hair, teeth, and sebaceous material.

DERMOID CYST OF OVARY

Descemet's membrane *des-e-mā*). Lining membrane behind the cornea of the eye.

desensitization (*de-sen-si-ti-zā'-shon*). To remove sensitivity to a substance. A method of treatment used for the allergic state, *q.v.*

desiccation (*des-ik-ā'-shon*). The act of drying.

desmoid (*des'-moyd*). Like a bundle. Fibrous tissue.

desquamation (*des-kwa-mā'-shon*). Peeling off of the skin, *e.g.* after scarlet fever.

detergent (*de-ter'-jent*). Substance which effectively lowers the surface tension of a fluid. Used for cleansing purposes.

deterioration (*dē-tār-i-or-ā'-shon*). A worsening condition.

detoxicated (*dē-toks-i-kā'-ted*). With toxic properties removed.

detritus (*de-trē'-tus*). Debris. Accumulation of disintegrated material.

detrusor (*dē-trū-sor*). An expelling muscle.

Dettol (*de'-tol*). Official name: Liq. Chloroxylenol. An antiseptic lotion.

dexamphetamine (*deks-am-fet-a-mēn*). Similar to amphetamine, *q.v.*

dexter (*dek'-ster*). Right. Upon the right side.

dextran (*deks'-tran*). A blood-plasma substitute. Used as 6% solution.

dextrin (*deks'-trin*). An intermediate product in the conversion of starch into sugar.

dextrocardia (*dek-stro-kar'-dia*). Congenital transposition of the heart from the left to the right side of chest.

dextrose (*deks-'trōs*). Grape sugar. Glucose. For rectal or intravenous injection, 5 per cent. solution, *i.e.* 1 oz. to 1 pint, of water is the usual strength.

dhobie itch (*dō'-bē*). Ringworm, mainly in the inguino-crural region. Also called tinea cruris.

diabetes insipidus (*dī-a-bē'-tēz*). Syndrome cause by deficient secretion of anti-diuretic hormone (A.D.H.) by the pituitary gland and characterized by the passage of enormous quantities of pale urine of low specific gravity, containing no sugar.

diabetes mellitus. A disease marked by an excessive flow of urine containing sugar, and thirst. It is due to failure of the pancreas to manufacture insulin; this being necessary for the metabolism of carbohydrates. The nurse will have to measure and test urine. The specific gravity may be as high as 1030 to 1045. The treatment is dietetic with the administration of the prescribed amount of insulin. *See* URINE TESTING in Appendix, p. 383.

diabetic diets. *See* Appendix, pp. 420–424.

diacetic acid (*dī-as-ē'-tik*). Aceto-acetic acid. This is a substance occasionally present in the urine: especially in serious cases of diabetes. *See* ACETONE, TEST FOR. *See* Appendix, p. 383.

diagnosis (*dī-ag-no'-sis*). The decision as to the nature of an illness, arrived at by studying the case.

dialysis (*dī-al'-is-is*). The separation of certain substances from a mixture by passing the latter through a membrane. Usually applied to dialysis of blood to remove toxic waste in cases of renal insufficiency (kidney machine). *See* HAEMODIALYSIS.

diameters of pelvis (*dī-am'-et-erz*). Besides the three conjugate diameters (described under CONJUGATE), the most important pelvic measurements are as follows: *The right and left oblique*, from the right and left sacro-iliac joints to the left and right pectineal eminences respectively; these should measure 12–13 cm. The *transverse*, which at the brim measure 12 cm and at the outlet about 10 cm. *The distance between the anterior superior spines* of the ilia should be not less than 25 cm, and *between the iliac crests* at least 2·5 cm more than this.

diameters of skull. The important diameters of the fetal skull at term are as follows: Sub-occipito-bregmatic, 9 cm; cervico-bregmatic, 9 cm; fronto-mental, 8 cm; occipito-mental, 13 cm; supra-occipito-mental, 14 cm; occipito-frontal, 11 cm; sub-occipito-frontal, 10 cm, biparietal, 9 cm; bitemporal, 8 cm (Jellett).

diamorphine (*dī-ah-mor'-fin*). An alkaloid obtained by the action of acetic anhydride on morphine. It allays cough, induces sleep and does not leave the depressing after-effects of morphia, but its narcotic action is less. (Synonym, Heroin.) Addiction is a constant risk.

Diamox (*dī-a-moks*). *See* ACETAZOLAMIDE.

diapedesis (*dī-a-ped-ē'-sis*). The passage of leucocytes through the walls of blood-vessels. It occurs in inflammation.

diaphoresis (*dī-a-fo-rē'-sis*). Perspiration.

diaphoretics (*dī-a-for-et'-iks*). Agents which increase perspiration, *e.g.* pilocarpine.

diaphragm (*dī'-a-fram*). The muscular septum separating the chest from the abdomen. *See* illustration.

Xiphoid process of Sternum

Vena caval opening

Oesophegeal opening

Aortic opening

Central tendon

Lumbar vertebrae

THE ABDOMINAL SURFACE OF THE DIAPHRAGM

diaphragmatic hernia (*dī-a-frag-ma-tik her-ni-a*). Herniation of abdominal viscera through the diaphragm into the chest. Usually due to a congenital defect of the diaphragm.

diaphysis (*dī-af'-fe-sis*). The middle part of long bones; the shaft, *cf.* epiphysis.

diarrhoea (*dī-ar-rē'-a*). Frequent loose stools.

diarthrosis (*dī-ar-thrō'-sis*). A freely movable joint permitting movement in any direction.

diastase (*dī'-as-tās*). An enzyme which converts starch into sugar with intermediate dextrins.

diastasis (*dī-as'-tā-sis*). Forcible separation of bones without fracture; dislocation.

diastole (*dī-as'-tō-lē*). That part of cardiac cycle when the ventricles fill with blood, *cf.* systole.

diastolic (*dī-as-tol'-ik*). Connected with diastole. Thus a *diastolic murmur* is one produced during the relaxation or diastole, of the heart.

diathermy (*dī-ath-er'-mi*). The passage of high frequency electric current through a tissue. Because of the electrical resistance of the tissue, heat is generated. This is diffuse when large electrodes are used, as in physiotherapy. Tissues may be cauterized by using a small electrode. Diathermy is used so that tissues are destroyed, *e.g.* as in removal of superficial new growths. It is also used as a cautery to arrest bleeding.

diathesis (*dī-ath'-e-sis*). Constitutional disposition to a particular disease.

dichotomy (*dī-kot'-o-mi*). Division into two parts.

dicrotic pulse (*dī-krot'-ik*). Having two beats. Usually applies to secondary pulse wave due to the closure of semilunar valves since, when this is marked as in conditions associated with vasodilatation, *e.g.* high fever, it gives the impression of a double pulse.

didactyle (*dī-dak'-tīl*). Having only two fingers, or two toes.

didymitis (*did-i-mī'-tis*). Inflammation of the testicle.

dielectric (*dī-e-lek'-trik*). The non-conducting material separating the conducting surface in an electrical condenser.

diet (*dī'-et*). System of food.

dietetics (*dī-e-tet'-iks*). The study of food values.

Dietl's crises (*dē'-tl*). Severe attacks of renal pain accompanied by scanty, bloodstained urine. Occurs in some cases of movable kidney probably due to kinking of the ureter.

differential blood count (*di-feren'-shal*). The determination of the proportion of each type of white cell in the blood, carried out by microscopical examination. Useful in diagnosis.

differential diagnosis. Discrimination between diseases with similar symptoms.

diffusion (*di-fū'-zhon*). The process by which gases and liquids of different densities mix when brought into contact with one another.

digestion (*dī-jest'-chon*). Process of converting food into

simple substances capable of absorption into the blood.

digit (*di-jit*). A finger or two.

digitalis (*dij-i-tā'-lis*). The foxglove; a cardiac tonic, used chiefly in auricular fibrillation. It slows, strengthens, regulates the heart beat and increases the output of blood per beat. It is indirectly a diuretic. Action, cumulative; poison. Decrease or marked intermittence of pulse, vomiting, or cardiac pain to be immediately reported.

digitoxin (*dij-i-tok'-sin*). Chief active principle of the digitalis leaves.

digoxin (*dij-ok-sin*). Chief active constituent of Austrian foxglove. May be given orally or by intravenous injection.

diguanides (*dī-gwa-nīds*). Type of oral hypoglycaemic drug, *e.g.* metformin and phenformin, antidiabetic agents.

dilatation (*dil-a-ta'-shon*). In-increase in size, enlargement. The operation of stretching.

dilator (*dī-lā'-tor*). An instrument for dilating any narrow passage, as the rectum, uterus, urethra.

dill. Dried ripe fruit of Anethum graveolens. Its distilled water sometimes given to infants for flatulence.

dilution (*dī-lū-shon*). A liquid whose strength has been lowered by the addition of water.

dimenhydrinate (*dī-men-hī-drināt*). Antihistamine drug used as an anti-emetic. Proprietary name Dramamine.

dimercaprol (*dī-mer-ka-prol*). See B.A.L.

diodone (*dī-ō-dōn*). Intravenous contrast agent; similar to iodoxyl, q.v. but less irritant.

dioptre (*dī-op'-ter*). The unit of refractive power of lens. A lens of one dioptre has a focal length of 1 metre.

dioxide (*dī-ok'-sīd*). A compound containing two atoms of oxygen, e.g. carbon dioxide (CO_2).

diphtheria (*dif-the'-ri-a*). A serious infectious disease, caused by corynebacterium diphtheriae. Any mucous membrane may be attacked but usually that of the throat or nose. A false grey membrane develops. There is severe general malaise. An antitoxin is given and the patient kept at rest to avoid heart complications. *D. immunization*, a toxoid is injected prophylactically and all children from a year old should thus be protected against the disease.

diplegia (*dī-plē-ji-ah*). Paralysis of both sides of the body.

diplococci (*dip-lō-ko-kī*). Micrococci which are arranged in pairs. See BACTERIA.

diploe (*dip'-lō-ē*). A cellular osseous tissue separating the two cranial tables.

diplopia (*dī-plō'-pi-a*). Double vision.

dipsomania (*dip-so-mā'-ni-a*). Pathological craving for alcohol.

director (*dī-rek'-tur*). A grooved surgical instrument used to guide another instrument (*see below*).

DIRECTOR

Disablement Resettlement Officer. D.R.O. Officer appointed by Department of Employment and Productivity to provide disabled persons with suitable jobs.

disaccharide (*dī-sak'-ar-īd*). Any carbohydrate formed by the condensation of two monosaccharides, e.g. cane sugar.

disarticulation (*dis-ar-tik-ū-lā'-shon*). Amputation at a joint.

disc (*di'-sk*). A circular plate or surface. (1) That part of the optic nerve which is seen with the ophthalmoscope as it enters the eyeball. (2) *Intervertebral D.*, the fibro-cartilaginous layer between the vertebrae.

discharge (*dis-charj*). Emission of material, e.g. fluid, pus, light, etc.

discission (*dis-sish'-on*). Also called needling. Surgical rupture of the lens capsule of the eye.

discrete (*dis-krēt'*). Separate, distinct; opposed to confluent.

disease (*di-sēz*). A process which disturbs the structure or functions of the body.

disinfectants (*dis-in-fek'-tants*). Agents which destroy micro-organisms; such as sunlight, heat, carbolic acid, sulphur dioxide, chlorine.

disinfection (*dis-in-fek'-shon*). See FUMIGATION.

disinfestation (*di-sin-fes-tā-shon*). Riddance of animal parasites, *e.g.* lice.

dislocation (*dis-lō-kā'-shon*). Displacement of the articular surface of a bone. Treatment, reduction under anaesthesia and immobilization. *Congenital dislocation of the hip joint.* The acetabulum is shallow and does not accommodate the head of the femur. The child has a waddling gait. Treatment must be early and is generally the Lorenz method by which after manipulation the hip is immobilized in plaster for many months. The thigh is abducted at a right angle to the trunk.

(see diagram of elbow-joint for normal position of humerus)

DISLOCATION OF THE ELBOW JOINT

disorientation (*dis-or-ien-tā'-shon*). Loss of the ability to locate one's position in the environment, or the mental confusion seen in psychic disorders.

dispensing (*dis-pen'-sing*). The mixing and preparing of medicines.

disproportion (*dis-pro-por'-shon*). General term to indicate that the ratio between the size of the foetal head and the size of the maternal pelvis is abnormally large.

dissection (*dīs-sek'-shon*). A separation by cutting of parts of the body.

disseminated (*dis-em'-in-ā-ted*) Scattered throughout an organ or throughout the body. *D. Sclerosis,* a chronic, degenerative disease of the nervous system. Also known as mutiple sclerosis and insular sclerosis.

dissociation (*di-sōs-si-ā'-shon*). Abnormal mental state in which the patient fails to recognize certain, frequently unpalatable, facts relating to himself.

dissolution (*dis-so-lū'-shon*). Decomposition.

distal (*dis'-tal*). Situated away from the centre.

distichiasis (*dis-ti-kī'-a-sis*). A double row of eyelashes, causing irritation and inflammation.

distillation (*dis-til-ā'-shon*). The process of vaporizing a substance and condensing the vapour. *Fractional D.*

Successive distillations are carried out.

dithranol (*di-thra-nol*). Used as an ointment to treat psoriasis, ringworm etc. Benzene will remove dithranol stains from clothes.

diuresis (*dī-ū-rē'-sis*). An increased secretion of urine.

diuretics (*dī-ū-ret'-iks*). Drugs which increase the volume of urine secreted, *e.g.* caffeine.

diurnal (*dī-er-nal*). Daily.

divaricator (*dī-va-ri-kā-tor*). Hinged splint used to treat congenital dislocation of hip.

diverticulitis (*dī-ver-tik-ū-lī'-tis*). Inflammation of a diverticulum. Specially applied to inflammation of diverticula, often very many in number, of the pelvic colon.

diverticulosis (*dī-ver-tik-ū-lō'-sis*). Presence of numerous diverticula of the intestine.

diverticulum (*dī-ver-tik'-ū-lum*). A pouch-like process from a hollow organ, *e.g.* oesophagus, intestine, urinary bladder.

D.N.A. *See* DEOXYRIBO-NUCLEIC ACID.

DOCA. Deoxycorticosterone (*q.v.*).

Döderlein's bacillus (*der-der-līns*). Non-pathogenic bacillus present in secretions of the vagina.

dolor (*dol'-or*). Pain.

domette (*do'-met*). A soft cotton and woollen fabric used for bandages.

dominance (*do'-mi-nanz*). A factor present in the left cerebral hemisphere of humans, which makes people right- or left-handed. This lateral dominance is established early in childhood.

donor (*dō-nor*). Individual from whom tissue is removed for transfer to another, *e.g.* blood transfusion, grafting.

dorsal (*daw'-sal*). Relating to the back or the posterior part of an organ.

dorsiflexion (*dor-si-flek-shon*). Bending backwards or in a dorsal direction.

dorsum (*daw'-sum*). The back.

dosis (*dō-sis*). A dose.

douche (*doosh*). A shower of water usually used to irrigate a cavity of the body. Hot douche 112° F (44° C); cold douche 60° F (16° C).

Douglas's pouch (*dug'-las*). The peritoneal pouch between the back of the uterus and the front of the rectum.

Dover's powder (*dō'-verz*). A sedative medicine of which the chief ingredients are ipecacuanha and opium. It increases perspiration. Dose, 300 to 600 mg.

Down's syndrome. *See* MONGOLISM.

Doyen's gag (*dwah'-yan*). A mouth gag much used by anaesthetists.

Doyen's speculum. A self-retaining speculum for keeping the incision widely open during abdominal operations.

DOYEN'S GAG

drachm (*dram*). Weight of 60 gr. = 3·888 g, or in fluid measure 60 min. (about one teaspoonful).

dracontiasis (*dra-kon-tī-a-sis*). Infestation by the guinea-worm, common parasite in tropical countries.

drainage tubes (*drān'-āj*). Tubes made of various materials which are inserted into operation wounds to allow material such as blood to drain from the wound.

drastic (*dras'-tik*). Strong, severe.

draught (*drah-ft*). A quantity of fluid to be taken at one time.

drawsheet (*draw'-shēt*). A sheet so arranged that it can be removed easily from under a patient lying upon it.

Drinker's apparatus (*drin'-kerz*). A mechanical respirator, used to carry out artificial respiration when the respiratory muscles are paralysed, popularly known as the iron lung. The patient lies in a receptacle with his head only outside. A negative pressure is created in the receptacle by means of a suction pump;

this draws air through the respiratory passages into the lungs. A similar type is the Both.

drip, intravenous (*intra-vēn-us*). The administration into a vein of saline, plasma or blood.

drive (*drīv*). In psychology, an urge to satisfy a basic need, such as hunger.

droplet infection. Droplets sprayed from a person's mouth, especially when talking, which infect other people.

dropsy (*drop'-si*). An unnatural effusion of watery fluid into the tissues or cavities of the body. Common causes are heart failure, renal failure.

drug. Substance used as a medicine. *D. addiction.* A dependence on drugs which is beyond the subject's control. *D. eruption.* Rash due to sensitivity to a drug. *D. reaction.* General reaction to a drug. This may include fever, malaise, joint pains, rashes, jaundice, etc. *D. resistance.* Strains of micro-organisms resistant to the action of antibiotics.

Duchenne's disease (*dū-shen'*). Progressive muscular atrophy, a disease of the spinal cord.

Ducrey's bacillus (*doo-krā'*). The cause of soft sore or chancroid; a venereal disease. Small oval streptobacillus.

duct. Passage lined by epithelium.

ductless glands. *See* ENDO-CRINE.

ductus (*duk'-tus*). A duct; a little canal of the body. *D. arteriosus*, connects the pulmonary artery and the aorta in fetal life. Occasionally this remains patent.

Dulcolax. A proprietary laxative which does not cause griping.

dum-dum fever. Same as Kala-azar (*q.v.*).

dumping syndrome. Palpitations and gastric discomfort sometimes felt by the patient after gastrectomy.

duodenal (*dū-ō-dē'-nal*). Belonging to the duodenum.

duodenostomy (*dū-ō-dē-nos'-to-mi*). Surgical establishment of a communication between the duodenum and another structure.

duodenum (*dū-ō-dē'-num*). The first 10 in. of the small intestine, beginning at the pyloric orifice of the stomach.

Gall bladder
Bile duct
Stomach
Pyloric sphincter
Duodeno-jejunal flexure
Duodenum
Pancreatic duct

DUODENUM

Dupuytren's contracture (*dū-pwē'-trenz*). A contracture

affecting especially the ring and little fingers, which bends them down into the palm so that they cannot be extended.

dura mater (*dūra mā'-ter*). The outer membrane lining the interior of the cranium and spinal column.

dwarf (*dworf*). Individual of stunted growth.

dys (*dis*). A prefix meaning difficult, painful, abnormal.

dysaesthesia (*dis-es-thē-zi-a*). Partial loss of feeling.

dysarthria (*dis-ar'-thri-a*). Impairment of speech.

dyschezia (*dis-che-si-a*). Painful defaecation.

dyschondroplasia (*dis-kon-drō plā-si-a*). Multiple enchondromas. Cartilage is deposited in the shaft of some bone(s). Those affected, which are often in the hands and feet, are short and deformed.

dyscoria (*dis-ko-ri-a*). Abnormality in the shape of the pupil.

dyschromatopsia (*dis-krō-mat-op'-si-a*). Loss of vision for colour.

dysdiadokinesis (*dis-dī-a-dō-kī-nē'-sis*). Inability to carry out rapid alternating movements, such as rotating the hands. A sign of cerebellar disease.

dysentery (*dis'-en-ter-i*). Inflammation of the large intestine. There are two kinds of dysentery, bacillary and amoebic; the former due to a bacillus, the latter to a *entamoeba histolytica*.

dysfunction (*dis'-funk-shon*). Abnormal or impaired function.

dyskinesia (*dis-kĭn-ē'-zi-a*). Impairment of voluntary movement.

dyslalia (*dis-la'-li-a*). Mechanical speech defect, *cf.* dysphasia.

dyslexia (*dis-lek-si-a*). Difficulty in reading.

dysmenorrhoea (*dis-men-o-re'-a*). Painful or difficult menstruation.

dysorexia (*dis-o-rek-si-a*). A depraved or unnatural appetite.

dyspareunia (*dis-par-ū'-ni-a*). Painful coitus.

dyspepsia (*dis-pep'-si-a*). Indigestion.

dysphagia (*dis-fā'-ji-a*). Difficulty in swallowing.

dysphasia (*dis-fā-si-a*). Difficulty in speaking.

dysplasia, polyosteotic fibrous (*displā-si-a po-li-os-tē-o-tik fĭ-brus*). Metabolic defect in the calcification of bone.

dyspnoea (*disp-ne'-a*). Difficult breathing.

dystaxia (*dis-tak-si-a*). Difficulty in controlling voluntary movements. *See also* ATAXIA.

dystocia (*dis-tō'-ki-a* or *dis-tō'-se-a*). A difficult labour (obstetric).

dystrophia adiposo-genitalis (*dis-trō-fi-a a-di-pō-sō-je-ni-tā-lis*). *See* FRÖHLICH'S SYNDROME.

dystrophy (*dis'-tro-fē*). Defective structure due to shortage of essential factors.

dysuria (*dis-ū'-ri-a*). Painful micturition.

E

E.3. Lachesine chloride. Atropine substitute for eye drops in case of atropine irritation.

ear (*ē-r*). The organ of hearing. It consists of external, middle and internal ear.

The *external ear* comprises the auricle and external auditory canal, and is separated from the middle ear by the tympanic membrane.

The *middle ear* is an irregular cavity in the temporal bone. In front it communi-

SECTION OF EAR

cates with the eustachian tube which forms an open channel between the middle ear and the cavity of the nasopharynx. Behind, the middle ear opens into the mastoid antrum, and this in turn communicates with the mastoid cells. There are two openings into the inner ear, both of which are covered with membrane. A string of tiny bones, joined together, extends from the tympanum to the *foramen ovale* of the internal ear. These bones are, from the tympanum— (1) malleus, (2) incus, (3) stapes.

The *internal ear* comprises (1) the organ of hearing or cochlea in which are the endings of the auditory nerve, and (2) the organ of equilibrium or balance consisting of the three semicircular canals, arranged mutually at right angles.

ear drum. The tympanum.

ear wax. *See* CERUMEN.

eau (*ō*) water; *eau-de-vie* is brandy (*ō-de-vē*).

Eberth's bacillus (*eb-erts bas-il-us*). The typhoid bacillus.

ecbolic (*ek-bol'-ik*). An agent used to stimulate the uterus and thus accelerate the expulsion of the foetus, *e.g.* pituitary extract.

ecchondroma (*ek-on-drō'-ma*). A tumour composed of cartilage.

ecchymosis (*ek-i-mō'-sis*). A bruise; an effusion of blood under the skin.

E.C.G. *See* ELECTROCARDIO-GRAM.

Echinococcus (*e-kī-nō-kok'-us*). One of the species of tape worm. In its adult stage it infests dogs. In its larval stage it produces hydatid cysts in man.

ECHO virus (*e-kō vī-rus*). Enteropathic, cytopathic human orphan virus. *See* ADENOVIRUS. May cause benign lymphocytic meningitis and Bornholm disease.

echolalia (*ek-ko-lal'-i-a*). Repetition of everything said.

eclampsia (*ek-lamp'-si-a*). Convulsions arising from severe toxaemia of pregnancy.

ecmnesia (*ek-nē'-zi-a*). A lapse in memory, the memory before and after the lapse being normal.

ECMO virus (*ek-mō vī-rus*). Enteropathic, cytopathic monkey orphan virus. *See* ADENOVIRUS.

ecraseur (*ek-rah-ser*). Instrument with wire loop used to remove a polypus.

E.C.T. Abbreviation for electroconvulsive therapy (*q.v.*).

ectasis (*ek-ta-sis*). Distension, as in bronchiectasis when the bronchial tubes are dilated.

ecthyma (*ek-thī'-ma*). A pustular skin disease, a form of impetigo.

ectoderm (*ek'-tō-derm*). The outer layer of the primitive embryo. From it are developed the skin and its appendages, and the nervous system.

ectogenous (*ek-toj'-en-us*). Originating outside the body.

ectomy (*ek'-tom-i*). A suffix denoting removal.

ectoparasite (*ek-tō-pa-ra-sīt*). Parasite living on the surface of its host.

ectopia (*ek-tō'-pi-a*). Not in the usual place.

ectopic gestation (*ek-top'-ik jes-tā-shon*). Pregnancy in which the fertilized ovum is not situated in the uterus. The ovum may lie in one of the Fallopian tubes or in the

right Fallopian tube
containing embryo

left Fallopian
tube

uterus

right
ovary

FERTILIZED OVUM IN
THE FALLOPIAN TUBE

abdominal cavity. In course of time the gestation sac is apt to rupture, causing profuse haemorrhage into the abdominal cavity and necessitating immediate operation.

ectrodactylia (*ek-trō-dak-til'-i-a*). Absence from birth of one or more toes or fingers.

ectropion (*ek-tro'-pi-on*). Eversion of the eyelid.

eczema (*ek'-ze-ma*). Inflammation of the skin, acute or chronic. There is redness and

vesicles may appear which weep and form crusts.

E.D.T.A. Ethylenediamine tetra-acetic acid. A chelating agent, *q.v.* used especially in the treatment of lead poisoning.

E.E.G. *See* ELECTROENCE-PHALOGRAPHY.

effector (*ef-fek-tor*). Nerve endings found in muscles, glands, etc., and which effect the functioning of the organ.

efferent (*ef'-fer-ent*). Conveying from the centre, *e.g.* the motor nerves which convey impulses from the brain and spinal cord to muscles and glands, *cf.* afferent.

effervescent (*ef-fer-ves'-ent*). Bubbling. Giving off small bubbles of gas.

effleurage (*ef-fler'-arj*). Movement performed in physiotherapy. The tips of the fingers or the whole surface of the hand are moved along the course of the blood vessels and lymphatics stimulating the circulation and lymphatic drainage.

effluent (*ef-loo-ent*). Liquid end-product of any process, *e.g.* sewage.

effort syndrome (*ef-fort sin-drōm*). Also called da Costa's syndrome, disordered action of the heart, soldier's heart. A form of anxiety neurosis characterized by symptoms referable to the heart.

effusion (*ef-fū'-zhon*). An escape of fluid from one part to another.

egocentric (*ē-gō-sen'-trik*). With every idea centred on oneself.

Ehrlich's theory (*ār'-lik*). A theory explaining the process of immunity against disease. The cells of the body are supposed to contain certain molecules, consisting of a stable central group, to which are attached less stable 'lateral chains' of molecules or *receptors*. These side chains have the power of combining with and thus neutralizing the poisons produced by invading micro-organisms, but in the process the receptors themselves are destroyed. However, as this destruction of receptors proceeds, the central group is stimulated to produce fresh side chains or receptors.

There are two kinds of receptors, namely, *uniceptors* or *antitoxins*, such as antigens, and *amboceptors* or *cytolysins*. The uniceptors or antitoxins act in the way mentioned above by combining with and thus neutralizing the toxins. The amboceptors or cytolysins have two affinities, one for the invading bacteria and one for a body called the *complement*, which exists in the fluids of the body. The complement when united with the bacteria by means of the amboceptor or cytolysin is capable of causing solution and destruction of the bacteria.

ejaculation (*ē-jak-ū-lā'-shon*). Forcible, sudden expulsion, especially of semen.

elastin (*e-las-tin*). Fibrous protein laid down by fibroblasts in connective tissue ground substance. It is structurally similar to collagen and is found particularly in structures which require to withstand mechanical stresses, *e.g.* walls of large arteries.

Elastoplast bandage (*e-las-tō'-plast*). An adhesive bandage containing zinc oxide, which has astringent and slightly germicidal properties.

elation (*e-lā-shon*). A happy and exalted state of mind.

elbow (*el'-bō*). The joint between the arm and forearm. The bones forming the joint are the humerus above, and the radius and ulna below.

Humerus

Radius

Olecranon

Ulna

ELBOW JOINT

Electra complex (*e-lek-tra kom-pleks*). Excessive love for a father by a daughter who hates her mother. Named after Electra in Greek mythology.

electric shock (*e-lek'-trik shok*). *See* Appendix VI, p. 441.

electrocardiogram (*e-lek-trō-kar-di-ō-gram*). E.C.G. Recording of electrical events occurring in the heart muscle. The recording is made by attaching electrodes to the skin and amplifying the electrical signal. The oscillations may be recorded by a pen writer.

electrocardiophonography (*e-lek-trō-kar-di-ō-fō-no'-gra-fi*). Recording of heart sounds electrically by a phonocardiograph.

electroconvulsive therapy (*e-lek-trō-kon-vul-siv the-ra-pi*). E.C.T. Therapy used especially in depressive mental illness, consisting of passing a low amperage electric current between electrodes placed on the side of the head. The reaction is modified by general anaesthesia and muscle relaxant drugs given before the shock treatment.

electrode (*e-lek'-trōd*). The point where an electric current enters or leaves the battery or the body of the patient.

electro-encephalography (*en-ke-fa-log'-ra-fi*). Recording of electric currents characteristic of cerebral activity.

electrolysis (*e-lek-trol'-i-sis*). 1. Separation of ions by placing them in an electric field. 2. Destruction of hair follicles by the passage of an electric current.

electrolytes (*el-ek-trō-līts*). Substances, such as sodium chloride or potassium carbonate, which, dissolved in water, dissociate into ions, *q.v.* The water becomes a conductor of electricity. *E. balance*. Balance of relative amounts of electrolytes, *e.g.* sodium, potassium, chloride, in body fluids, usually blood.

electro-magnetic spectrum (*e-lek-trō-mag-ne-tik spek'-trum*). Wide range of radiations which are transmitted by photons distributed in a frequency pattern known as electro-magnetic waves, including radio waves, light, X-rays and gamma rays.

electromotive force (E.M.F.) (*mō'-tiv*). The measure of the tendency of an electric current to flow from one point to another. The unit of E.M.F. is the volt.

electromyography (*e-lek-trō-mī-o-gra-fi*). E.M.G. The recording of electrical events occurring in muscle.

electron (*e-lek-tron*). A negatively charged atomic particle of mass 0.00055 units. *E. microscopy*. The use of electrons instead of light to visualize microscopic objects. The apparatus is complex but allows very much greater resolution to be obtained and therefore more details to be seen.

electroplexy (*el-ek-trō-ple'-ksi*). *See* ELECTROCONVULSIVE THERAPY.

electroretinogram (*e-lek-trō-re-ti-no'-gram*). Recording of electrical variations in the retina on exposure to light.

element (*el'-e-ment*). A primary part. A substance which cannot be decomposed further by ordinary chemical means, apart from radio-activity or bombardment of atoms.

elephantiasis (*el-e-fan-tī'-a-sis*) or **filariasis**. A parasitic disease of the lymphatic vessels, causing great enlargement of the limb or limbs affected. It is chronic, and the skin thickens until it somewhat resembles an elephant's hide. The parasite is the *Filaria*.

ELEPHANTIASIS

elevator (*el'-e-vā-ter*). (1) A muscle which raises a limb. (2) An instrument used for raising depressed bone, etc.

elimination (*el-im-in-ā'-shon*). The expulsion of poisons or waste products from the body.

elixir (*e-lik'-ser*). A term sometimes applied to certain preparations having a sweet taste.

emaciation (*e-mā-sē-ā'-shon*). The act of wasting or becoming thin.

emanation (*em-an-ā'-shon*). The act of flowing out. Applied especially to the rays given out by radioactive substances.

emasculation (*e-mas-kū-lā'-shon*). Castration of the male.

embolectomy (*em-bol-ek'-to-mi*). Removal of an embolus.

embolism (*em'-bo-lizm*). Obstruction of blood vessel, usually an artery by a body, *e.g.* thrombus, fat cells, air, transported in the bloodstream. If the clot, or embolus, is large enough to block completely any of the valvular orifices of the right side of the heart, sudden death is the result: if small enough to pass through the right side of the heart, the embolus may be arrested somewhere in the pulmonary artery or in one of its subdivisions, giving rise to an infarct of the lung, with symptoms of intense sudden pain in the chest, coughing of blood, and great distress. In certain cases of valvular disease of the heart, pieces of clot formed upon the affected valve break off and are carried away in the bloodstream. When such an embolus reaches an artery too small for it, an embolism results, with symptoms according to the organ affected. Embolism of an artery of the brain may result in immediate death or in paralysis.

embolus (*em'-bō-lus*). A blood clot or other foreign body in the bloodstream.

embrocation (*em-bro-kā'-shon*). A lotion for rubbing on the skin.

embryo (*em'-bri-ō*). Animal in process of development from the fertilized ovum.

embryology *(em-brē-o'-lo-ji)*. Science of the development of the embryo.

embryoma *(em-brē-ō'-ma)*. Teratoma. An ovarian tumour, often a dermoid cyst, *q.v.*

embryotome *(em'-bri-o-tōm)*. An instrument for destroying any part of the child during birth for the purpose of facilitating delivery.

embryotomy *(em'-brē-ot'-o-mi)*. Destruction of the foetus.

emesis *(em'-e-sis)*. Vomiting.

emetic *(e-met'-ik)*. Any means used to produce vomiting. Tickling the throat with a feather; large draughts of tepid water, salt water, mustard and water; ipecacuanha, or zinc sulphate. Apomorphine, given hypodermically, is the quickest and surest method.

emetine *(em-et-in')*. An alkaloid contained in ipecacuanha. It is a powerful irritant and nauseant. Specific for amoebic dysentery.

emission *(ē-mish'-on)*. Discharge, especially of semen.

emmenagogue *(em-en'-a-gog)*. A medicine which promotes the flow of the menses, *e.g.* ergot, rue and all ecbolics.

emmetropia *(em-e-tro'-pi-a)*. Normal sight.

emollients *(e-mol'-li-ents)*. Softening and soothing applications or liniments.

emotion *(e-mō-shon)*. A response of mind and body to stimuli; such as anger or fear.

empathy *(em-pa-thi)*. A form of fantasy when one imagines oneself 'in someone else's shoes' and feels intensely with that person.

emphysema *(em-fi-sē'-ma)*. *Pulmonary e.* The overdistension of the lungs by air. Three types occur: obstructive, compensatory and chronic vesicular emphysema. *Surgical e.* Air bubbles in the subcutaneous tissues following trauma.

empirical *(em-pi'-ri-kal)*. Term applied to treatment founded on experience only not on reasoning.

emplastrum *(em-plas'-trum)*. A plaster.

empyema *(em-pī-ē'-ma)*. A collection of pus in a cavity, most commonly referring to the pleural cavity. The term is also used for collections of pus in the maxillary antrum, frontal sinus, and other cavities.

emulsion *(e-mul'-shon)*. Fine suspension in a fluid of particles of an immiscible fluid, *e.g.* milk is an emulsion of fat in water.

enamel *(en-am'-el)*. The hard outer coating of the tooth. See TEETH.

enarthrosis *(en-ar-thrō'-sis)*. A ball-and-socket joint.

encephalitis *(en-kef-al-ī'-tis)*. Inflammation of the brain. *See* MENINGITIS. *E. lethargica.* Encephalitis associated with profound disturbance of sleep rhythm.

encephalocele (*en-kef'-a-lō-sēl*). Protrusion of the brain through the skull.

encephalography (*en-ke-fal-o'-gra-fi*). Also called ventriculography. The X-ray examination of the brain after air, which is radiolucent, has been introduced into the cerebral ventricles.

encephaloid (*en-kef'-a-loyd*). Brainlike.

encephaloma (*en-ke-fa-lō'-ma*). A brain tumour.

encephalomalacia (*en-kef'-al-ō-mal-ās'-e-ah*). Softening of the brain.

encephalomyelitis (*en-kef'-al-ō-mī-el-i'-tis*). Inflammation of the brain and spinal cord.

encephalon (*en-kef'-a-lon*). The brain.

encephalopathy (*en-ke-fa-lo'-pa-thi*). Disease of the brain.

encephalotomy (*en-ke-fa-lo-to-mi*). Dissection of the brain.

enchondroma (*en-kon-drō'-ma*). A tumour of cartilage.

encopresis (*en-kō-prē-sis*). Incontinence of faeces.

encysted (*en-sis'-ted*). Enclosed in a sac or cyst.

endarteritis (*en-dar-te-rī-tis*). Inflammation of the lining membrane of the arteries.

endemic (*en-dem'-ik*). Occurring frequently in a particular locality.

endocarditis (*en-dō-kar-dī'-tis*). Inflammation of the lining membrane of the heart. The valves are affected in conse-quence. Often a complication of acute rheumatism, chorea or other fevers. In bacterial or malignant endocarditis, fungating growths develop on the valves.

endocardium (*en-dō-kar'-di-um*). The lining membrane of the heart.

endocervicitis (*en-dō-ser-vi-sī'-tis*). Inflammation of the mucous membrane lining the canal of the cervix uteri.

endocolpitis (*en-dō-kol-pī'-tis*). Inflammation of inner coat of the vagina.

endocrine (*en'-dō-krēn*). The term used in describing the ductless glands giving rise to an internal secretion. Some of the internal secretion organs have both an internal and an external secretion, and so may have ducts. The endocrines are—suprarenals, thymus, thyroid, parathyroids, pituitary, pancreas, ovaries, and testicles.

endocrinology (*en-dō-krin-ol-o-ji*). Science of the endocrine glands.

endoderm (*en-dō-derm*). Germ layer of embryo composed, as is mesoderm, of cells which have migrated from the surface to the interior of the embryo during gastrulation, *q.v.*, and from which the alimentary tract is largely derived.

endogenous (*en-do-jen-us*). Produced within the body, *e.g.* endogenous infection.

endolymph (*en-dō-limf*). Fluid of the membranous labyrinth of the ear.

endometrioma (*en-dō-mē-tri-ō'-ma*). Tumour, from tissue like that of the endometrium, but found outside it in myometrium, ovary, uterine ligaments, rectovaginal septum, peritoneum, caecum, pelvic colon, umbilicus and laparotomy scars.

endometriosis (*en-dō-mē-tri-ō'-sis*). The presence of endometriomata (plural of endometrioma).

endometritis (*en-dō-mē-trī'-tis*). Inflammation of the endometrium.

endometrium. The lining membrane of the uterus.

endoneurium (*en-dō-nū-ri-um*). Fine connective tissue found round each nerve fibre.

end-organ (*end-aw-gan*). Collection of cells connected to the peripheral nervous system which act as a transducer, transforming a stimulus into a nerve discharge (receptor), or a nerve discharge into a stimulus, *e.g.* end-plate, *q.v.*

endoscope (*en'-dos-kōp*). An instrument for the inspection of the interior of a hollow organ.

endosteoma (*en-dos-tē-ō'-ma*). Tumour within a bone cavity.

endosteum (*en-dos'-te-um*). The medullary membrane of bone. *See* BONE.

endothelioma (*en-dō-thē-li-ō-ma*). A malignant growth originating in endothelium.

endothelium (*en-dō-thē'-lē-um*). The lining membrane of serous cavities, blood-vessels and lymphatics.

endotoxin (*en-dō-toks'-in*). An intracellular toxin, *i.e.* retained within the bacteria. When the bacteria are disintegrated the toxin is liberated.

endotracheal (*en-dō-tra-kē'-al*). Within the trachea.

end-plate (*end plāt*). Accumulation of muscle cytoplasm and nuclei in association with the terminal branches of a motor nerve through which the nerve discharge stimulates contraction of muscle.

enema (*en'-em-a*). An injection into the bowel. It can be given with a rectal tube and funnel but glycerin suppositories and disposable enemas are replacing those given by tube and funnel. Some forms of enemata are: *Enema Saponis.*—Dissolve an ounce of yellow soap in 20 oz. of water, temp. 99° F. *Castor-oil Enema.*—Add 1 oz. of castor oil to a soap-and-water enema; or it can be mixed with 16 oz. of thin starch. *Enema terebinthinae.*—Mix 1 oz. of turpentine with 12 oz. of thin starch or add to an enema saponis.

enervating (*en-er-vā-ting*). Weakening.

engagement of head (*en-gāj-ment*). Descent of fetal head into the cavity of the pelvis. Normally occurs two to four weeks before term in the primigravida but in multi-gravida may not occur until labour.

engorgement (*en-gawj'-ment*). Vascular congestion.

enophthalmos (*en-of-thal-mos*). Recession of the eyeball into the orbit.

enostosis (*en-os-tō'-sis*). A tumour in a bone.

ensiform cartilage (*kar'-til-āj*). The sword-shaped process at the lower end of the sternum.

Entamoeba histolytica (*ent-am-ē'-ba his-to-lit-ika*). The parasite which causes amoebic dysentery.

enteral (*en'-ter-al*). Intestinal.

enterectomy (*en-ter-ek'-to-mi*). Excision of part of the intestine.

enteric fevers (*en-te'-rik*). A term now used to include three separate but closely allied diseases: typhoid, paratyphoid A, paratyphoid B fevers.

enteritis (*en-te-rī'-tis*). Inflammation of the small intestine.

Enterobius vermicularis (*en-te-rō-bi-us ver-mi-kū-lā-ris*). Threadworm.

enterocele (*en'-ter-ō-sēl*). Hernia containing a piece of bowel.

enterococcus (*en'-ter-ō-kok-us*). Streptococcus found in intestinal tract.

enterocolitis (*en-te-rō-ko-lī'-tis*). Acute inflammation of the ileum, caecum and ascending colon giving rise to symptoms similar to appendicitis.

enterokinase (*en-ter-ō-kin'-ās*). An activating enzyme of the succus entericus which converts trypsinogen into trypsin.

enterolith (*en'-te-rō-lith*). Stone in the intestines.

enteron (*en-ter-on*). The intestine.

enteropexy (*en-ter-ō-peks'-i*). Suturing of the intestines to the abdominal wall.

enteroptosis (*en-ter-op-tō'-sis*). Prolapse of the intestines due to stretching of the mesenteric attachment.

enterorrhaphy (*en-te-ro'-raf-i*). The suturing of a rent in the intestine.

enterospasm (*en'-ter-ō-spasm*). Spasm of the intestine. Colic.

enterostenosis (*en-te-rō-ste-nō'-sis*). Stricture of the intestines.

enterostomy (*en-te-ros'-to-mi*). Surgically established opening between the small intestine and another surface, *e.g.* gastro-enterostomy, a connection between the stomach and the small intestine.

enterotomy (*en-ter-ot'-o-mi*). Incision into the small intestine.

enteroviruses (*en-te-rō-vī-ru-sez*). Viruses belonging to the pico RNA virus group. *Es.* enter the body by the alimentary tract and comprise the three polio viruses, the Coxsackie virus causing Bornholm disease and the ECHO viruses causing aseptic meningitis.

entropion (*en-tro'-pi-on*). Inversion of the margin of the eyelid.

enucleation (*e-nū-klē-ā-shon*). (1) Removal of the nucleus. (2) Removal of a central structure, *e.g.* tumour without its surrounding structures.

enuresis (*en-ū-rē'-sis*). Incontinence of urine. *Nocturnal E.* Bedwetting at night.

envelope (*en'-vel-ōp*). Bunyan-Stannard. Treatment for burns. A resin-coated silk bag envelops the burn and a 1–200 sol. of 1% electrolytic sodium hypochlorite is run over the wound at intervals.

environment. The external influences which surround a person or thing.

enzyme (*en'-zīm*). Protein which acts as a catalyst, *q.v.* There are many different kinds of enzyme which increase the reactivity of certain substances.

eosin (*ē'-o-sin*). An acid dye used extensively for staining histological sections.

eosinophilia (*ē-ō-si-nō-fi-li-a*). (1) Property of being stained by acid dyes such as eosin which combine with basic groups in the tissue. (2) Term used to denote an increase above the normal 2 to 5 per cent in the numbers of polymorpho-nuclear leucocytes in the blood which stain deeply with eosin.

Epanutin (*ep-an'-ū-tin*). Phenytoin sodium, *q.v.*

ependyma (*e-pen'-di-ma*). The lining membrane of the cerebral cavities and spinal canal.

ependymoma (*e-pen-dē-mō'-ma*). A tumour arising from ependymal cells.

ephedrine (*ef'-e-drēn*). An alkaloid from the plant ephedra vulgaris. It is closely related to adrenaline, and acts similarly. It is administered orally.

ephelis (*e-fe-lis*). A freckle.

epiblepharon (*e-pi-ble-fa-ron*). See EPICANTHUS.

epicanthus (*ep-i-kan-thus*). Projection of the nasal fold to the eyelid.

epicardium (*ep-i-kar'-di-um*). Visceral layer of the pericardium.

epicondyle (*e-pi-kon'-dīl*). Bony eminence as upon the femoral condyles.

epicranium (*ep-i-krā'-nē-um*). The integuments which lie over the cranium.

epidemic (*ep-i-dem'-ik*). An infectious or contagious disease attacking a number of people in the same neighbourhood at one time.

epidemiology (*e-pi-dē-mē-ol'-oji*). The study of epidemics.

epidermis (*ep-i-der'-mis*). The outermost layer of the skin. See SKIN.

epidermophytosis (*ep-i-der-mō-fī-tō'-sis*). An infection of the skin by fungi, the hands and feet being principally affected. Often termed 'Athlete's Foot' as it is frequently contracted in public gymnasia or swimming baths.

epididymis (*ep-i-di′-di-mis*). A long convoluted tube through which sperm pass between the testis and the vas deferens. It forms a mass at the upper pole of the testis.

epididymitis (*ep′-i-did-i-mī′-tis*). Inflammation of the epididymis.

epididymo-orchitis (*e-pi-did-ē-mō-or-kī′-tis*). Inflammation of the epididymis and testes.

epidural analgesia. *See* CAUDAL ANALGESIA.

epigastrium (*ep-i-gas′-tri-um*). Surface marking on anterior abdominal wall over the region occupied by the stomach. *See* ABDOMEN.

epiglottis (*ep-i-glot′-tis*). The flap of cartilage which guards the entrance to the glottis or windpipe. *See* LARYNX.

epilation (*e-pi-lā-shon*). Removal of hair with destruction of the hair follicle.

epilepsy (*ep′-il-ep-si*). A disorder of the brain marked by the occurrence of convulsive fits. *Idiopathic E.*, typical epilepsy. In many cases the fit is preceded by a warning or aura. This is usually a sensory disturbance. The two main types are (1) petit mal, momentary loss of consciousness with no convulsion. (2) Grand mal, loss of consciousness, tonic and clonic convulsions. *Jacksonian E.* Local spasm, *e.g.* of one limb or one side of the body, due to irritation of the cerebral cor-

tex. It is important to observe in which group of muscles the movements first commence in order that the cerebral lesion may be located.

epileptiform (*e-pi-lep′-ti-form*). Like the convulsions of epilepsy.

epiloia (*e-pi-loy′-a*). Tuberous sclerosis. Inherited defect characterized by sebaceous adenoma of the face, multiple gliomas in the brain and tumours of the heart, kidneys and retina. Fits are the earliest signs of the disease and mental deficiency usually follows.

epimenorrhoea (*e-pē-me-nor-rē′-a*). Menstrual periods of frequent recurrence.

epinephrectomy (*e-pē-nef-rek′-to-mi*). Excision of suprarenal gland.

epinephrine (*ep-i-nef′-rin*). Adrenaline (*q.v.*). A hormone from the medulla of the suprarenal glands; a powerful vaso-constrictor. It is injected hypodermically. *See* SUPRARENAL.

epineurium (*ep-in-ūr′-i-um*). The sheath of a nerve.

epiphora (*e-pif′-o-ra*). An excessive flow of tears.

epiphysis (*e-pif′-i-sis*). The separately ossified end of growing bone separated from the shaft, diaphysis, *q.v.*, by a cartilaginous plate (epiphyseal plate). When growth is completed the epiphysis and diaphysis fuse.

epiphysitis (*ep-if-is-ī′-tis*). Inflammation of an epiphysis.

epiplocele (*ep-ip'-lo-sēl*). A hernia containing omentum.

epiploon (*e-pi-plo-on*). The omentum.

episcleritis (*ep-is-kler-ī'-tis*). Inflammation of the outer layers of the sclera. *See* EYE.

episiotomy (*ep-i-si-ot'-om-i*). Incision of the perineum just at the end of the second stage of labour, sometimes performed to avoid extensive laceration of the perineum.

epispadias (*ep-is-pa'-di-as*). A congenital malformation in which the urethra opens on the dorsum of the penis.

epispastics (*ep-i-spas'-tiks*). Agents applied to the skin to produce discharge, such as blisters or vesicatories. *See* CANTHARIDES.

epistaxis (*ep-is-taks'-is*). Bleeding from the nose.

epithelial casts (*ep-ith-ēl'-ial kar-sts*). Filaments of renal epithelium found in the urine in certain diseases, when examined under the microscope. They are chiefly cylindrical, are finely granular, and the cells have large nuclei. If in considerable quantity, they signify nephritis, or some other disease of the kidneys.

epithelioma (*ep-ith-ēl-i'-ō-ma*). Tumour of epithelium.

epithelium (*e-pi-thē-li-um*). Sheet of coherent cells forming the lining of tubes, cavities and surfaces, except if derived embryologically from mesoderm when it is termed endothelium or mesothelium. Epithelia are classified according to thickness of the sheet and the shape or function of the cells composing them. Epithelium may be mucous, keratinizing, simple (one cell thick), stratified (many cells thick), squamous (flat cells), cubical and columnar (tall cells).

epitrochlea (*ep-i-trok'-lea*). The inner round projection at the lower end of the humerus.

eponym (*e-po-nim*). Name of disease or organ which is called after a person or place, *e.g.* Bornholm disease.

Epsom salts (*ep'-sum*). Sulphate of magnesium.

epulis (*e-pū'-lis*). Tumour on the gums.

erasion (*e-rā'-zhon*). Scraping.

Erb's paralysis. The muscles of the upper arm are paralysed due to a lesion of the fifth and sixth cervical nerve roots. May result from excessive traction on the arm during labour. It hangs limply, rotated internally from the shoulder, elbow extended, forearm pronated and palm of hand turned outwards.

erectile tissue (*e-rek'tīl tis-sū*). Specialized vascular tissue which becomes rigid when filled with blood, *e.g.* penis.

erector (*e-rek-tor*). A muscle which raises a part.

erepsin (*er-ep'-sin*). A ferment of the succus entericus (secretion of the small intestines). It completes the digestion of the proteins.

ergograph (*er'-gō-grarf*). An instrument for recording the amount of work done by muscular action.

ergosterol (*er-go-ster'-ōl*). A sterol found in fats and present in the skin which is converted into vitamin D by irradiation with ultra-violet light.

ergot (*er'-got*). A drug got from a fungus which grows on rye; it is used especially after labour cases to contract the uterus and arrest haemorrhage. Active principles are ergometrine, ergotoxine and ergotamine.

ergotism (*er'-go-tism*). Poisoning by alkaloids present in the fungus *Claviceps purpurea* which is found in cereals. One of the alkaloids, ergometrine, is used in obstetrics to control postpartum haemorrhage; another, ergotamine is used in the treatment of migraine.

erosion (*e-rō'-zhon*). Ulceration. *Cervical e.* Vaginal epithelium is replaced by columnar epithelium growing down from the cervical canal. As the secretion of the vagina is acid, this epithelium tends to ulcerate and bleed.

erotic (*e-ro-tik*). Pertaining to sexual love.

eructation (*e-ruk-tā'-shon*). Flatulency, with passage of gas from stomach through mouth.

eruption (*e-rup'-shon*). A breaking out on the skin.

erysipelas (*er-i-sip'-e-las*). Acute streptococcal infection of the skin.

erythema (*e-ri-thē'-ma*). Red skin, due to vasodilatation in the dermis. *E. multiforme.* Lesions consisting of raised red lesions of varying size and shape which may blister. The cause is unknown but it may represent an abnormal immune response. *E. nodosum.* Red tender skin nodules on the legs which may occur in conjunction with certain conditions such as tuberculosis and sarcoidosis.

erythrasmia (*er-ith-raz'-mi-a*). An infection of the skin due to a fungus.

erythroblast (*e-ri-thrō-blast*). Nucleated red blood cell normally found in the bone marrow and which gives rise to a red blood corpuscle.

erythroblastosis foetalis (*e-rith-rō-blas-tō-sis fē-tā'-lis*). *See* HAEMOLYTIC DISEASE OF THE NEWBORN.

erythrocytes (*er'-ith-rō-sīts*). Red blood corpuscles.

erythrocythaemia (*e-rith-rō-sī-tē'-mi-a*). Increased number of red blood cells.

erythrocytopaenia (*e-rith-rō-sī-tō-pē-ni-a*). Diminished number of red blood cells.

erythrocytosis (*e-rith-rō'-sī-tō'-sis*). *See* POLYCYTHAEMIA.

erythromycin (*eri-thro-mī-sin*). An antibiotic. A useful alternative when infection is resistant to penicillin.

erythropoiesis (*e-ri-thrŏ-pō-ē-sis*). The manufacture of red-blood cells.

Esbach's albuminometer (*es'-baks al-bū-min-om'-et-er*). A graduated tube used to estimate the quantity of albumin in urine. *See* URINE TESTING in Appendix, p. 382.

eschar (*es'-kar*). A dry healing scab on a wound; generally the result of the use of caustic. Also the mortified part in dry gangrene.

Eschatin (*es-kāt-in*). An extract made from the cortex of the suprarenal gland. Used by injection in the treatment of Addison's disease.

eserine, or **physostigmine**. A drug extracted from Calabar bean. It contracts the pupils and stimulates peristalsis. Used in the treatment of myasthenia gravis.

Esmarch's method (*es'-marches*). A bloodless method for operations. An india-rubber bandage is tightly applied to the limb, beginning at the extremity, and when it has reached above the point of operation a stout tube is wound round the limb and fastened.

esoteric (*ē-sō-te'-rik*). For the initiate only.

esotropia (*ē-so-trō-pi-a*). Converging squint.

E.S.R. Erythrocyte sedimentation rate. The rate at which red blood cells stick together and sediment to the bottom of a graduated tube. An increased rate is found in infection.

essentiae (*es-en'-shi-ē*). Essences; strong solutions of one part volatile oil in five of rectified spirits. Usually given in a few drops on sugar.

essential oil (*es-en'-shal*). A volatile oil distilled from an odoriferous vegetable substance, *e.g.* oil of cloves.

ethanolamine oleate (*e-tha-no-la-mēn ō-lē-āt*). Drug used for injection in treatment of varicose veins.

ether (*ē'-ther*). A volatile liquid much used as an anaesthetic. It must never be used near an uncovered flame, as it is highly inflammable.

ethics (*e-thiks*). Moral principles governing our life.

ethinyloestradiol (*e-thi-nil-ēs-trā-dē-ol*). Potent oestrogenic substance given orally.

ethisterone. A compound similar to progesterone, but active orally.

ethmoid (*eth'-moyd*). A bone of the nose through which the olfactory nerves pass.

ethnology (*eth-nol-o-ji*). The science of the races of mankind.

ethopropazine (*e-thō-pro-pa-zēn*). Drug used to relieve spasm in Parkinson's disease.

ethyl biscoumacetate (*e-thil bis-koo-ma'-se-tāt*). Anticoagulant effective orally and with more rapid action than dicoumarol.

ethyl carbamate (*e-thil kar-ba-māt*). Urethane. Has a cytotoxic action but is less potent than nitrogen mustard.

ethyl chloride (*e-thil klaw-rīd*). Anaesthetic, used in dental and other minor operations. Also used locally to freeze the tissues and so render them insensitive.

ethylene (*e-thi-lēn*). A hydrocarbon gas, sometimes used as an anaesthetic.

etiology (*ēt-i-ol'-o-ji*). The science of the causation of disease. Syn. aetiology.

eucaine (*ū-kān*). A local anaesthetic.

eucalyptus (*ū-ka-lip'-tus*). An antiseptic inhaled in catarrhal affections. It is a colourless, oily liquid, with a pungent, resinous smell. It is made into an ointment with paraffin and used for healing ulcers.

Eucortone (*ū-kor-tōn'*). A solution of active principles of adrenal cortex, given by injection.

eugenics (*ū-jen'-iks*). The study and cultivation of conditions that will improve the human race.

eugenol (*ū-jen-ol*). The principal constituent of oil of cloves.

Eumydrin (*ū'-mi-drin*). Official name, atropine methonitrate. Prescribed for babies with pyloric stenosis. It relaxes the pyloric sphincter. The preparation used is a 0·6 per cent solution in rectified spirit. The dose is 1 minim 15 minutes before feeds.

eunuch (*ū-nuk*). A castrated human male.

euonymus (*ū-on'-i-mus*). A drug used as a mild purgative.

euphoria (*ū-for'-i-a*). Exaggerated sense of well-being.

eusol (*ū-sol*). An antiseptic containing hypochlorous acid. Used for septic wounds.

Eustachian tube (*ū-stā'-shi-an*). The canal from the throat to the ear. *See* EAR.

euthanasia (*ū-tha-nā'-si-a*). A painless death procured by the use of drugs.

eutocia (*ū-tō'-sē-a*). Easy labour (obstetric).

evacuation (*ē-vak-ū-ā'-shon*). Discharge of excrement from the body. *See* MOTIONS.

evaporating lotions (*ē-vap-o-rā'-ting lō-shon*). Used to procure local coldness. Lead lotion, or eau-de-Cologne and water, are most common.

Eve's method. A method of artificial respiration. By placing the patient in a special rocking apparatus, the diaphragm is forced up and down.

eventration (*ē-ven-trā'-shon*). Protrusion of the intestines.

eversion (*e-ver'-shon*). Folding outwards.

Evipan (*e'-vi-pan*). Official name, hexobarbitone. A short-acting barbiturate with rapid action. Sleep is induced within 10 to 20 minutes and may last from 3 to 6 hours.

evisceration (*e'-vis-ser-ā'-shon*). Removal of the abdominal contents.

evolution (*ē-vol-ū'-shon*). Spontaneous evolution means the delivery without obstetric assistance of a foetus in the transverse lie; it is as a rule only possible in the case of a premature or dead foetus.

evulsion (*ē-vul'-shon*). A tearing apart.

Ewing's tumour (*ū-wings tū-mer*). Malignant tumour of bone occurring in young adults.

exacerbation (*eg-zas-er-bā'-shon*). An increase in the severity of symptoms; a paroxysm of disease.

exanthemata (*ek-san-thē-ma'-ta*). Diseases accompanied by specific rashes.

exchange transfusion (*eks-chanj tran-sfu-zhon*). Transfusion of the newborn when the whole circulatory volume of the infant's blood is removed and replaced by donor blood. This is necessary in severe haemolysis of the baby's blood in Rhesus group incompatibility. *See* BLOOD GROUPING.

exarteritis (*eks-ar-te-rī'-tis*). Inflammation of the external coat of an artery.

excipient (*ek-sip'-i-ent*). The substance used as a medium for giving a medicament.

excision (*ek-siz'-zhon*). A cutting out.

excitability (*ek-sī-ta-bi-li-ti*). (1) Reaction to a stimulus. (2) A state of being unduly excited.

excitement (*ek-sīt'-ment*). Increased activity of an organ or organism.

excoriation (*eks-ko-rē-ā'-shon*). Abrasions of the skin.

excrement (*eks-kre-ment*). Faecal matter.

excrescence (*eks-kres'-sens*). An unnatural protruding growth.

excreta (*ek-skrē'-ta*). The natural discharges from the body, urine, faeces, sweat.

exenteration (*eks-en-ter-ā'-shon*). Removal of all contents. *E. of orbit.* Removal of all contents of the bony orbit. *E. of pelvis.* Removal of pelvic contents and transplantations of ureters onto the sigmoid colon.

exfoliation (*eks-fō-lē-ā-shon*). Loss of flakes of material from a surface.

exhibitionism (*eks-hi-bi'-shon-izm*). Behaving in a way to attract attention and term used in psychiatry for sex perversion such as indecent exposure.

exhumation (*ek-sū-mā'-shon*). Disinterment of the body.

exogenous (*eks-o'-jen-us*). Due to an external cause.

exomphalos (*eks-om'-fal-os*). Umbilical hernia of congenital origin.

exophthalmos, exophthalmia (*eks-of-thal'-mos*). Protrusion of the eyeball. *See also* GOITRE.

exostosis (*eks-os-tō'-sis*). A bony tumour growing from bone.

exotoxin (*ek-sō-tok'-sin*). Toxin released from exterior of an organism, *cf.* endotoxin.

expectorant (*ek-spek'-to-rant*). A drug which increases expectoration, *e.g.* ipecacuanha.

expectoration (*eks-pek-to-rā'-shon*). The coughing up of sputum.

exploration (*eks-plo-rā'-shon*). Operative surgical investigation.

expression (*eks-pre-shon*). (1) The act of expulsion. (2) Facial appearance.

exsanguinate (*ek-san'-gwin-āt*). To make bloodless.

extension (*ek-sten'-shon*). (1) A certain pull or weight applied to a fractured, dislocated, or contracted limb to keep it straight. There are two methods, (a) Skin traction applied as follows: A long piece of strapping, about 2 in. wide, with a stirrup, consisting of a square piece of wood the same width as that of the foot at the ankle, and with a hole in the middle, is required; also some short narrower pieces of strapping. To apply it, the stirrup should be about 4 in. below the foot, and the strapping attached to it should be carried up the inside and outside of the leg well above the knee: the short pieces of strapping are put round the leg from the ankle to below the knee. A knotted piece of cord is passed through the hole in the wood over a pulley at the foot of the bed. Weights are attached to the cord, the number varying according to the age of the patient and condition for which it is applied. For a fractured femur $\frac{1}{7}$ of the body weight is usually satisfactory. The

EXTENSION APPARATUS

foot of the bed should be slightly raised. (b) Skeletal traction, a Steinmann's pin or Kirschner wire is passed through the lower fragment of the bone or an ice-tong caliper may be inserted. (*See* p. 456, PLATE B, and CALIPER.) (2) The straightening of a flexed limb or part.

extensor (*eks-ten'-sor*). A muscle which extends a part.

external conjugate (*kon'-jū-gāt*). *See* CONJUGATE.

external os. *See* OS EXTERNAL.

external version (*ver-shon*). A method of changing the lie or presentation of the foetus by manipulation of the uterus through the abdominal wall.

extirpate (*ek-ster-pāt*). To remove completely.

extra. Latin for outside.

extracapsular (*eks-tra-kap'-sū-la*). Outside a capsule.

extracellular fluid (*eks-tra-sel-ū-la*). That part of the body fluid not contained in cells nor the blood.

extract (*ek'-strakt*). Concentrated preparation of a drug: it may be in a liquid or solid form, *e.g.* extract of cascara.

extrapyramidal (*eks-tra-pi-ra'-mi-dal*). Motor nerve tracts and associated centres which do not directly communicate with the main motor pathway (pyramidal tract). It is a very complex system with many functions, one of which is to regulate muscle tone.

extrasystoles (*ek-stra-sis-to-lēs*). Systolic contraction of the heart the impulse for which originates in a focus other than the sino-atrial node, and is therefore outside the normal chain of events in the cardiac cycle.

extra-uterine gestation (*ek-stra-ū'-te-rīn jes-tā'-shon*). Pregnancy outside the uterus. *See* ECTOPIC GESTATION.

extravasation (*eks-trav-a-sā'-shon*). Escape of fluid from its proper channel into surrounding tissue.

extravert (*eks-tra-vert*). *See* EXTROVERT.

extremity (*eks-tre-mi-ti*). The end part of any organ. A limb.

extrinsic (*ek-strin'-sik*). External. From without. *E. factor*. *See* PERNICIOUS ANAEMIA.

extrovert (*eks-strō-vert*). Thinking of things other than one-

HORIZONTAL SECTION OF THE RIGHT EYE

self. The opposite kind of temperament to introvert.

exudation (*eks-ū-dā'-shon*). Oozing; slow escape of liquid.

eye (*i*). The organ of vision. *See* illustration, p. 145.

eye-strain (*i-strān*). Headache due to effort required to focus on near objects when the refractive properties of the lens are defective.

eye-teeth (*i'-tēth*). The canines.

F

F. Abbreviation for Fahrenheit, *q.v.*

face presentation (*fās pres-en-tā-shon*). The advance of the foetus face first into the pelvis during labour. It is usually due to some degree of pelvic contraction. The majority of such cases are delivered naturally.

facet (*fas'-et*). A small, smooth, flattened surface of bone.

facial (*fā-shi-al*). Relating to the face. *F. nerve.* Seventh cranial nerve supplying the salivary glands and superficial muscles of the face. *F. paralysis.* Paralysis of the muscles of the face caused by injury or disease involving the facial nerves.

facies (*fa'-si-ēs*). Facial expression, *e.g.* adenoid facies, mouth partly open, vacant, unintelligent look in the eyes.

facultative (*fa-kul-ta-tiv*). Able to live under varying conditions.

faecal (*fē'-kal*). Relating to the faeces.

faecalith (*fē-ka-lith*). Stone-like body composed of compacted faeces.

faeces (*fē'-sēs*). The discharge from the bowels. Common abnormalities to be noted are *Colour*—Black may indicate the presence of altered blood or the patient may be taking iron. Green stools occur in enteritis. Clay-coloured stools in jaundice. *Consistency*—Loose watery stools occur in diarrhoea, hard dry stools in constipation. Foreign bodies such as worms may be present. Unaltered blood may be due to haemorrhoids. Mucus and blood may be due to colitis or intussusception.

Fahrenheit (*fa'-ren-hit*). Temperature scale used in the graduation of many clinical thermometers in the United Kingdom. *See* p. 19.

faint (*fā-nt*). Syncope.

falciform (*fa'-si-form*). Sickle-shaped. Applied to certain ligaments and other structures.

fall out (*fawl owt*). Particulate matter containing radioactive material which falls from clouds containing the debris of atomic explosion.

Fallopian tubes (*fal-lo'-pi-an tubes*). Two trumpet-like canals, about 7.5 cm long, passing from the ovaries to the uterus. *See* UTERUS and SALPINGITIS.

Fallot's tetralogy (*fa'-loz*). A group of congenital heart defects consisting of dextra-position of the aorta, right ventricle hypertrophy, intra-ventricular septal defect and stenosis of the pulmonary artery.

falx cerebri (*falks se-re-brē*). The fold of dura between the two cerebral hemispheres.

familial (*fam-il'-ial*). Affecting several members of one family.

fanaticism (*fa-na-ti-sizm*). Zeal for some belief or cause carried to excess.

fantasy (*fan'-ta-si*). A world of imagination controlled by the whim of the individual.

Fantus test. Test for the presence of chloride in the urine.

farad (*fa'-rad*). A unit of electrical capacity.

faradism *far'-a-dizm*). The interrupted, as opposed to the constant, electric current.

farinaceous (*far-i-nā'-shi-us*). Containing flour or grain. Farinaceous diet consists of milk puddings, gruel, bread, and other starchy foods.

fascia (*fa-shi-a*). A fibrous structure separating one compartment of the body from another, or one muscle from another.

fascicle (*fas'-i-kl*). A little bundle of fibres.

fastigium (*fa-sti-ji-um*). The summit or height, e.g. of a fever.

fat. Oily substance necessary in human diet. *See* p. 417. Mother's milk contains about

4 per cent. of fat in finely divided globules. Cow's milk contains about 3·6 per cent of fat. Cream contains up to 20 per cent.

fatigue (*fa-tēg*). Tiredness.

fatty degeneration (*dē-jen-e-rā'-shon*). Term applied to the appearance of certain cells which as a result of damage take on an appearance of having droplets of fat in their cytoplasm.

fauces (*faw'-sēs*). The short passage between the back of the mouth and the pharynx.

favus (*fā-vus*). A type of ring-worm infection.

Fe. Chemical symbol for iron.

febrile (*fe'-bril*). Relating to fever.

fecundation (*fe-kun-dā'-shon*). Impregnation. Fertilization.

fecundity (*fe-kun'-di-ti*). Power of producing young.

feeble-minded. Subnormal mentality. No longer an official classification.

Fehling's solution. Sulphate of copper and potassium hydrate are the chief ingredients; the solution was used as a test for sugar in the urine. For other tests, *see* p. 383.

fel. Bile.

felon (*fe-lon*). A whitlow.

Felty's syndrome (*fel-tis sin-drŏm*). chronic arthritis and leucopenia and splenomegaly.

female (*fē-māl*). Applied to the sex that bears young.

femoral artery (*fem'-o-ral ar'-te-ri*). The artery of the thigh, from the groin to the knee.

femoral canal (*ka-nal'*). The small canal internal to the femoral vein. The site of a femoral hernia.

femoral vein, thrombosis of. *See* PHLEGMASIA ALBA DOLENS.

femur (*fē'-mer*). The thigh bone.

pit for ligament — head
neck
greater trochanter
lesser trochanter
linea aspera on back of shaft
intercondylar notch
medial condyle — lateral condyle

FEMUR
(Posterior View)

fenestra (*fen-es'-tra*). A window, applied to certain apertures.

fenestration (*fe-nes-trā'-shon*). Making a window artificially such as that made in the inner ear to help to relieve deafness in otosclerosis.

Fergusson's speculum. *See under* SPECULUM.

ferment (*fer'-ment*). *See* ENZYME.

fermentation (*fer-men-tā'-shon*). Decomposition of organic material by enzymes present in certain organisms, *e.g.* yeasts and bacteria.

ferric (*fe-rik*). Applied to compounds of iron with a valency of more than two.

ferrous. Applied to compounds containing bivalent iron.

ferrum (*fe'-rum*). Iron, *q.v.*

fertility (*fer-ti-li-ti*). Ability to produce young.

fertilization (*fer-ti-lī-zā'-shon*). Union of male and female germ cells whereby reproduction takes place.

fester (*fes'-ter*). Inflammation, with collection of pus.

festination (*fe-sti-nā-shon*). Propulsive gait as in Parkinsonism.

fetishism. The worship of an inanimate object which symbolizes a loved person.

fetus (*fē-tus*). The unborn child. Formerly frequently spelt foetus.

fever (*fē-ver*). A rise in body temperature above normal. There is quick pulse, lassitude, often delirium, and inhibition of the secretory glands. The nursing treatment is rest, freedom from chills, and light nourishing diet with abundant fluids.

fibre (*fī'-ber*). Threadlike structure.

fibrillation (*fī-bri-lā-shon*). Unco-ordinated contraction of heart muscle. May affect the atria only (atrial fibrillation) or the ventricles (ventricular fibrillation).

fibrin (*fī'-brin*). Protein which forms a fibrous gel matrix as a basis for a blood clot. It is formed from the soluble plasma protein fibrinogen by the action of thrombin.

fibrinogen (*fī-bri-nō-jen*). Blood protein which is converted into fibrin, *q.v.*

fibrinolysin (*fī-bri-nō-lī'-sin*). Enzyme which dissolves fibrin.

fibro-adenoma (*fī-brō-ad-en-ō-ma*). A tumour composed of mixed fibrous and glandular elements.

fibroblast (*fī-brō-blast*). A cell that forms new fibrous tissue.

fibrocartilage (*fī-brō-kar-ti-lāj*). Cartilage with fibrous tissue.

fibrochondritis (*fī-brō-kon-drī'-tis*). Inflamed fibrocartilage.

fibrocystic disease (*fī-bro-sis-tik di-sēz*). Mucoviscidosis. A disease due to a defect in salt retention in mucous and sweat glands. As a result the mucopolysaccharide secretions, *e.g.* in the respiratory tract and from the pancreas, become excessively viscous, resulting in the formation of retention cysts which become fibrosed.

fibroelastosis (*fī-brō-ē-las-tō'-sis*). Rare disorder affecting the heart. Excess collagen and elastin form under the endocardium.

fibroid (*fī'-broyd*). A tumour composed of fibrous tissue. *See also* FIBROMYOMA.

fibroma (*fī'-brō-ma*). Benign tumour of fibrous tissue.

fibromyoma (*fī-brō-mī-ō'-ma*). A tumour composed of mixed muscular and fibrous tissue. Especially common in the uterus, and commonly spoken of as 'fibroids'.

fibrosis (*fī-brō'-sis*). Decomposition of fibrous connective tissue and usually occurring in regions which have been damaged by some trauma.

fibrositis (*fī-brō-sī'-tis*). Inflammation of fibrous tissue. *See* LUMBAGO.

fibula (*fib'-ū-la*). The small bone on the outer side of the leg.

field of vision (*vi'-zhon*). The area which can be seen without movement of the eye.

filament (*fil'-a-ment*). Thread-like piece of fibre.

Filaria (*fil-ar-ia*). Parasitic thread-like worm which may cause lymphatic obstruction. *See* ELEPHANTIASIS.

filiform. Threadlike. *F. bougie.* A slender bougie.

filipuncture (*fil-i-punkt'-ūr*). A method of treating aneurysm by inserting a fine wire thread. This acts as a foreign body, and the blood inside the sac clots.

filix mas (*fē-liks mas*). Male fern; a worm-expelling drug specific for the tape worm. Dose 3 to 6 ml of liq. ext.

filter (*fil'-ter*). Device used for removing a certain substance whilst allowing others to pass through. Optical filters made from different types of glass allow only light in certain parts of the spectrum to pass through. Fluid filters, according to their pore-size, are used to remove viruses, bacteria or other suspended impurities.

filterable, filtrable (*fil-trabl*). Able to pass through a filter.

filtration (*fil-trā'-shon*). Passage through a filter.

filum (*fē-lum*). A structure resembling a thread. *F. Terminale.* The tapering end of the enlargement of the lumbar spinal cord.

fimbria (*fim-bria*). A fringe, especially the fringe-like end of the Fallopian tube.

finger (*fing'-ger*). One of the digits of the hand.

first intention (*ferst in-ten'-shon*). A surgical term for aseptic healing of a wound by bringing the edges directly together.

first stage (*ferst stāj'*) (of labour). The act of parturition from the first pains up to the full dilatation of the cervix.

fission (*fi-shon*). Division into two or more parts: a mode of reproduction for bacteria and protozoa. *Nuclear F.* The splitting of an atomic nucleus, thus releasing energy.

fissure (*fi-sher*). A split or cleft.

fissure in ano (*fi-sher in ā'-nō*). Anal fissure. Small ulcerated cleft in the mucous membrane of the anus.

fistula (*fis'-tū-la*). Any unnatural passage communicating with two epithelialized surfaces. *Fistula in Ano,* anal fistula: any sinus connected with the anus and therefore discharging faeces. *See* ISCHIO-RECTAL ABSCESS. *Faecal Fistula.* A communication between the bowel and the surface; this may be a complication of an abdominal operation. General peritonitis seldom occurs, as track of the discharge from bowel to surface becomes walled off by adhesions. They tend to close spontaneously, but take some weeks. *Internal Fistula* is an artificial opening between two viscera—*e.g.* (1) Biliary Fistula, between the gall bladder and intestine. (2) *A Vesico-Vaginal F.,* a communication between the bladder and the vagina; this may be a complication of an extensive operation on the female generative organs.

fit. Convulsion usually with loss of consciousness.

fixation (*fik-sā-shon*). (1) Focusing the eyes on an object so that the image falls on the retina. (2) Learning something so that it is fixed in the memory or becomes a motor habit as after learning to ride a bicycle. In psychology abnormal attachment to a thing or person such as a parent so that new interests and attachments do not develop.

flaccid (*flak'-sid*). Soft, lacking rigidity.

flagellum (*fla-je-lum*). (Plu. flagella). Fine, thread-like structure projecting from surface of certain cells, *e.g.* spermatozoa, which by a lashing movement propels the cell, *cf.* cilia.

flap. A piece of skin cut to fold over the stump in an operation for amputation.

flatfoot. Flattening or total loss of arches of the foot. It then rests completely on the ground, giving characteristic appearance and walk.

flat or flattened pelvis. *See* CONTRACTED PELVIS.

flatulence (*flat'-ū-lens*). Gas in the alimentary canal, usually refers to the stomach. It may be produced by simply swallowing air or by the fermentation of food. Carminatives give relief.

flatus (*flā-tus*). Gas in the alimentary canal, usually refers to the bowel. It may be relieved by passing a flatus tube or by giving a turpentine or ox bile enema or a hypodermic injection of Pituitrin or eserine.

flavine. (*flā'-vēn*). *See* ACRIFLAVINE.

flea (*flē*). The human flea is *Pulex irritans*. It is without wings and sucks blood, giving rise to irritation and sepsis.

flexion (*flek'-shon*). Being bent; the opposite of extension.

Flexner bacillus (*fleks'-ner*). One of the Shigella group of

bacteria causing bacillary dysentery.

flexor (*fleks'-or*). A muscle which causes flexion.

flexure (*flek'-sur*). A bend. A curvature of an organ, *e.g. Hepatic F.* Bend of the colon beneath the liver.

floating ribs (*flō'-ting ribz*). The two lower pairs of ribs.

flooding (*flud'-ing*). Excessive bleeding from the uterus.

fluctuation (*fluk-tū-ā-shon*). A wavelike motion felt on palpation of an abscess or a cyst containing fluid.

fluke (*flook*). Any of the trematode class of worm.

fluorescein (*flor-e-sēn*). A coaltar derivative which stains cornea a vivid green if there is any loss of surface epithelium—*e.g.* in an abrasion or ulcer.

fluorescence (*flo-re-sens*). Emission of light at a wavelength which is different from that of the incident light. The emitted light has a lower energy, *i.e.*, is of longer wave-length, from the incident irradiation which is absorbed.

fluorescent screen (*flo-res'-ent skrēn'*). A screen coated with materials which fluoresce when exposed to X-rays.

fluoridation (*floor-ī-dā'-shon*). The addition of fluoride, such as when added to drinking water.

fluorine (*floo-o-rēn*). A halogen element. If added in minute quantities to drinking water it may cause a lessened incidence of dental decay.

fluoroscopy (*flo-ro-sko-pi*). Use of fluorescent screen to view X-ray images.

flying squad (*flī-ing skwod*). Emergency obstetric unit which can travel rapidly to domiciliary cases of complicated labour.

focus (*fō'-kus*). Point of maximum intensity.

foetor (*fē-tur*). Strong unpleasant smell.

foetus (*fē'-tus*). See FETUS.

foetus papyraceus (*pap-ī-rā'-sē-us*). A fetus which has been retained within the uterus for months after its death, and has undergone a kind of natural mummification.

folic acid (*fō-lik a-sid*). Pteroylglutamic acid, part of the vitamin B complex found in liver, yeast, spinach, etc. Essential for blood formation.

folie à deux (*fo-lē ah-der*). Delusion shared by two persons.

follicle (*fol'-li-kl*). A minute bag containing some secretion.

follicle stimulating hormone (*fo-li-kl sti-mū-lā-ting hor-mōn*). F.S.H. Hormone secreted by the anterior lobe of the pituitary gland. In the female it stimulates the growth of ovarian follicles and the production of oestrogens. In the male it promotes the development of spermatozoa in the testis.

follicular tonsillitis (*fol-lik'-ū-lar*). Pus in the follicles of the tonsils. The tonsils are red and swollen and covered with small yellow spots.

fomentations (*fō-men-tā'-shons*). Lint or flannel wrung out in some boiling fluid and applied for the alleviation of pain. It must be wrung out thoroughly and shaken to allow escape of steam and applied as hot as can be borne; cover lint with a slightly larger piece of jaconet and then a still larger piece of wool, and bandage whole securely. For a turpentine fomentation, sprinkle half an ounce of turpentine on the flannel before pouring on the boiling water. When applied to a septic wound, some surgeons prefer to omit the jaconet.

fomites (*fō'-mīts*). Articles of clothing or bedding which have been in contact with a patient ill with a contagious disease.

fontanelle (*fon-ta-nel'*). A soft space in the skull of an infant before the skull has completely ossified. The anterior fontanelle, or bregma, is where the coronal, frontal and sagittal sutures meet. The posterior fontanelle is where the lambdoid and sagittal sutures meet. The anterior fontanelle should be closed by 2 years of age. Delay is a sign of rickets. *See* p. 153.

food poisoning. Diarrhoea and/or vomiting from eating infected food. Symptoms may

THE FONTANELLES

be caused by the preformed toxins of *Staphylococcus aureus* or *Clostridium welchii* or from infection by organisms of the *Salmonella group* or rarely by *botulinus* toxin. Infected foods are usually meat products or confectionary containing eggs, which have been allowed to remain in warm rooms. Another source of infection may be the unwashed hands of those handling food.

foot. That part of the leg below the ankle.

foot and mouth disease. Virus disease well-known in cattle. It occasionally affects man, causing blistering of the buccal mucosa and similar lesions on the hands and feet, especially round the nails.

foot drop. Inability to keep a foot bent at right angles with the leg. The toes and foot drop and walking becomes difficult. Caused by pressure of bedclothes, or inadequate support to under side of foot when leg is in a splint for a long time, or from paralysis of the muscles which produce dorsiflexion of the ankle.

foramen (*fo-rā'-men*). An opening. *F. magnum.* Opening in the back of the skull through which the spinal cord passes. *F. ovale.* Opening between the right and left atria in the foetus which allows oxygenated venous blood from the placenta to pass into the left side of the heart thus bypassing the pulmonary circulation. It normally closes at birth. *Optic f.*, where the optic nerve enters the skull.

forceps (*for'-seps*). Surgical pincers used for lifting and moving instead of using the fingers. *See* below and p. 154.

BONE-HOLDING FORCEPS

a. DISSECTING FORCEPS
b. DRESSING FORCEPS

PEDICLE FORCEPS

SPONGE-HOLDING FORCEPS

BAYONET FORCEPS

SINUS FORCEPS

SPENCER WELLS
ARTERY FORCEPS

TONGUE FORCEPS

SEQUESTRUM FORCEPS

TOOTH-EXTRACTING
FORCEPS FOR LOWER
TEETH

forebrain. Cerebrum.

forensic medicine (*fo-ren'-sik*). Medicine in so far as it has to do with the law.

foreskin (*for'-skin*). The prepuce, or skin covering the end of the male penis.

formaldehyde (*for-mal'-dē-hīd*). A powerful antiseptic. Its gas is used to disinfect unoccupied rooms.

formication (*for-mi-kā'-shon*). A sensation as of ants creeping over the body. Used almost entirely to denote tingling sensation in a nerve recovering from pressure or injury, and therefore after nerve injury is a sign of regeneration.

formula (*for'-mū-la*). A prescription. Statement of constituents which form a compound.

formulary (*for-mū-la-ri*). A collection of formulae (pl. of formula), for medical preparations such as those found in the British Pharmacopoeia.

fornix (*for'-niks*). An arch. Applied to various anatomical structures, but especially to the roof of the vagina. Pl. **fornices.**

fossa (*fo'-sa*). Little depressions of the body, such as *fossa lacrimalis*, the hollow of the frontal bone, which holds the lacrimal gland. *Iliac fossae*. Concavities of the iliac bones of the pelvis.

Fothergill's operation (*fo'-thergilz*). Repair of the anterior and posterior vaginal walls and amputation of the cervix.

fourchette (*foor-shet*). A thin fold of skin behind the vulva.

fovea (*fō'-vea*). A small fossa or cup. In the eye, shallow depression in the retina. It is the site of maximum visual stimulation and the region on which the image is focused when the eyes are fixed.

fractional distillation (*frak'-shon-al dis-til-ā'-shon*). *See* DISTILLATION.

fractional test meal (*frak-shon-al test'-mēl*). Performed to examine the gastric contents and to estimate the rate of emptying of the stomach. The patient fasts for 10 hours. A Ryle's tube is passed into the stomach and secured to the side of the cheek by strapping. A syringe is attached and a sample of the gastric juice present in the empty stomach is withdrawn. This is called the resting juice. A meal of gruel is then given, after which about 15 to 20 ml. are withdrawn by means of the syringe every fifteen minutes till the stomach is empty. The specimens are put into small numbered containers. To make the meal—take two tablespoonfuls of fine oatmeal to 2 pt. of water. Simmer down to 1 pt. and strain. A little sugar may be added but no salt. (The histamine test meal is now more usual than the fractional test meal.)

fracture (*frak-tūr*). A break in a bone. The symptoms are—pain, swelling, deformity, loss of function, unnatural mobility, shortening, crepitus. A fracture may be: (1) *Simple or closed*, not connected with an external wound. (2) *Compound or open*, communicating with the surface. (3) *Greenstick*, when the bone is fractured half through on the convex side of the bend as in a green twig. Only seen in children. (4) *Comminuted*, where bone is broken into more than two pieces. (5) *Impacted*, where one fragment is driven into the other. (6) *Complicated*, where fracture is combined with injury to another important structure, *e.g.* artery, nerve, or organ. The type of break may be: (1) *Transverse*, due to direct violence applied at point of fracture. (2)

transverse   *oblique*

spiral

comminuted   *greenstick*

FRACTURES

Oblique, due to indirect violence, when a force applied at a distance causes the bone to break at its weakest part. (3) *Spiral*, when a limb is violently rotated. (4) *Depressed Fracture*, only of skull, when bone is driven inwards: it may be *guttershaped* with sharp depressed edge, or *pond-shaped* with sloping edge; the latter is only in infants and due to birth injury. *See* COLLES' FRACTURE, POTT'S FRACTURE, SPLINTS, SPONTANEOUS FRACTURE.

fraenum (*frā'-num*). A small membranous fold attached to certain organs, and acting as a check. *F. Linguae.* That under the tongue.

fragilitas ossium (*fra-jil'-i-tas os-ium*). Abnormal brittleness of the bones.

framboesia (*fram-bē'-zia*). A contagious tropical disease called yaws. Fungus-like masses are formed on the face, hands and feet.

free association. In psycho-analysis, when the patient gives the first word which a stimulus brings to his mind, or a train of ideas.

fremitus (*fre'-mit-us*). A vibration perceived by palpation, always applied to a vibration in the chest.

Freud (*froyd*). A famous Austrian psycho-analyst (1856-1939).

Freudian (*froy-di-an*). According to Freud's teaching. He taught that psychological dis-

orders often resulted from unconscious sexual impressions during childhood. These he brought to consciousness through psycho-analysis. Dreams he said were the wish-fulfilment of repressed desires.

Friar's balsam (*fri'-arz*). Compound tincture of benzoin.

friction (*frik'-shon*). (1) A circular movement in massage performed with the tips of the fingers or thumb as deeply as possible over joints; the object being to break down adhesions. (2) The sound heard in auscultation when two dry, roughened surfaces rub together as in pleurisy.

Friedman's test (*frēd-manz*). Pregnancy test. The urine of pregnant women contains an excess of secretion from the trophoblast. chorionic gonadotrophin, or APL principle. The urine is injected into an immature virgin rabbit. The rabbit is killed in 48 hours. If the woman is pregnant, characteristic changes will be seen in the ovaries of the rabbit.

Friedreich's ataxia (*frēd-rīks a-tak-si-a*). Inherited degenerative disease of the nervous system. The onset is in childhood and is progressive. There is clumsiness, unsteady gait, weakness, dysarthria and other neurological disturbances.

frigidity (*fri-ji-di-ti*). Lack of sexual desire.

Fröhlich's syndrome (*frer-liks sin-drōm*). A disorder with obesity, sexual infantilism, disturbances of sleep and temperature regulation and diabetes insipidus due to damage of the pituitary and hypothalamus.

frontal (*frun'-tal*). Relating to the forehead.

frontal bone (*frun'-tal bōn*). One of the bones of the skull. *F. Sinus. See* SINUS.

frostbite (*frost-bīt*). Injury of the skin or a part from extreme cold. There is redness, swelling and pain and necrosis may result.

fructose (*frūk-tōz*). Fruit sugar.

frustration (*fru-strā'-shon*). Disappointment experienced by a person who is thwarted and prevented by circumstances from achieving some desired object.

F.S.H. *See* FOLLICLE STIMULATING HORMONE.

fugue (*fū'g*). A fleeing from reality as in hysteria. The patient has no recollection of his actions during this time.

full time or term. The fetus is said to be at term when it is 20 to 21 in. long, has both testicles descended (if a boy), and has finger-nails and toe-nails reaching to the ends of the digits. Such a child should weigh anything from 7 lb. upwards, and have been developing in the uterus for not less than forty weeks.

Fuller's earth (*ful-erz erth'*). Chiefly consists of silica, alumina, and oxide of iron. Very absorbent.

fulminant, fulminating (*ful'-mi-nā-ting*). Sudden, severe, rapid in course, as fulminant glaucoma.

fumigation (*fū-mi-gā'-shon*). Sterilization of rooms by disinfectant vapour.

function (*funk'-shon*). The normal special work of an organ.

functional disorder (*funk'-shon-al*). The malfunctioning of an organ or organs when no organic disease is present.

fundus (*fun'-dus*). The enlarged part of a hollow organ farthest removed from the orifice; thus the fundus oculi is the interior of the eye behind the lens and pupil, visible with an ophthalmoscope; the fundus uteri is the top of the uterus.

fungi (*fun-gī*) (Sing. fungus). A subdivision of Thallophyta including moulds, mushrooms, rusts, yeasts, etc. Fungi are used as a source of protein and vitamins, certain enzymes, used in baking and brewing and antibiotics, notably penicillin. A few fungi cause disease in man.

fungicide. Any substance used for the destruction of fungi.

funiculitis (*fū-nik-ū-lī'-tis*). Inflammation of the spermatic cord.

funnel chest. Also called pectus excavatum. A developmental deformity in which the sternum is depressed and the ribs and costal cartilages curve inwards.

furuncle (*fŭ-rung-kl*). A boil, q.v.

furunculosis (*fŭ-run-kŭ-lō'-sis*). The appearance of one or more boils.

fusiform (*fŭ-zi-form*). Spindle-shaped. *See* ANEURYSM.

fusion (*fŭ-zhon*). Joining together.

G

Gaertner bacillus (*gărt'-ner*). *See* SALMONELLA.

gag. An instrument for keeping the mouth open. *See* DOYEN'S GAG.

gait (*gāt*). Manner of walking.

galactagogue (*gal-ak'-tag-og*). An agent that causes an increased flow of milk.

galactocele (*ga-lak'-tō-sēl*). A cyst of the breast containing milk.

galactorrhoea (*ga-lak-to-re'-a*). Excessive flow of milk.

galactosaemia (*gal-ak-tō-zē-mea*). A metabolic disorder characterized by presence of galactose in the blood stream.

galactose (*ga-lak'-tōz*). A hexose sugar which, in combination with glucose, forms the disaccharide lactose which is present in breast milk.

gall (*gawl*), or **bile**. The secretion of the liver; it accumulates in the gall bladder.

gall bladder (*gawl'-bla'-der*). The membranous sac which holds the bile. *See* BILIARY DUCTS.

gallamine (*ga-la-mēn*). Drug used to relax muscles especially in abdominal surgery. Antidotes are neostigmine methylsulphate and atropine sulphate.

gallipot (*ga-li-pot*). Small pot for containing medical preparations.

gallon (*ga'-lon*). Liquid measure holding 4 qt.

gallstone (*gawl'stōn*). Calculus in the gall bladder. If the stone passes into the cystic or common bile duct there is great pain, and if in the common bile duct, jaundice. *See* COLIC.

galvanism (*gal'-van-izm*). Therapeutic use of direct electric current, either continuous, or interrupted. Interrupted galvanism is used to stimulate denervated muscle.

galvanofaradization (*gal'-van-ō-fa-rad-i-zā'-shon*). A combination of galvanic and faradic treatment.

galvanometer (*gal-van-om'-e-ter*). An instrument for measuring the flow of a galvanic current.

gamete (*gam'-ēt*). A sexual reproductive cell, *e.g.* sperm, ovum.

gamgee tissue (*gam'-jē tis-yŭ*). Absorbent wool between two layers of gauze.

gamma rays (*gam'-a rāz*). Electromagnetic waves of

extremely short wave length emitted by radio-active substances; similar to X-rays, but shorter. Employed for dry, cold sterilization of any articles which would be destroyed by moisture or heat.

gammaglobulin (*ga-ma-glo-bū-lin*). Protein fraction of plasma, rich in antibodies against infection.

Gammexane (*ga-meks-ān*). Insect powder. An insecticide used on clothing and on animals but not for cage birds, chickens or cats.

ganglion (*gang-glē-on*). (1) A collection of nerve cells forming a semi-independent nerve centre. They are found in the sympathetic nervous system and in other parts of the nervous system. (2) Surgically, a chronic synovial cyst generally connected with a tendon sheath; most common site, back of hand, near the wrist.

ganglionectomy (*gan-glē-ō-nek-to-mi*). Excision of a ganglion.

gangrene (*gang'-grēn*). Massive necrosis of tissue as the result of reduced blood supply. *Dry G.* The arterial supply is increasingly diminished, the veins remaining patent. The part becomes dry and mummified. The commonest cause is senility. *Wet G.* is caused by a sudden interference with the arterial supply and the venous return, as may occur if a tourniquet

is left on too long. The part readily becomes infected. *Gas G.*, due to infection by a group of anaerobic gas-forming organisms of which the bacillus Welchii is the best known. Wounds which have been in contact with soil are likely to be infected. The signs are a rise in the pulse-rate after recovery from the initial shock, discoloration, oedema, discharge, and gas felt in the tissues. Anti-gas gangrene serum is given as a prophylactic and curative measure. Sulphapyridine or sulphanilamide or penicillin are also prescribed.

Gantrisin (*gan'-tris-in*). A sulphonamide of value in urinary infections.

gargarisma (*gar'-gar-iz-ma*). A gargle.

gargle (*gar'-gl*). A liquid medicine for washing out the throat.

gargoylism (*gar-goy'-lism*). Hurler's syndrome. A defect of skeletal development in which the skull is grossly deformed and the digital bones are bulbous, the hands assuming a claw-like appearance. There is often associated congenital heart disease and intellectual impairment.

gas gangrene (*gas gan'-grēn*). *See* GANGRENE.

Gasserian ganglion (*gas-ē'-rian gan'-gli-on*). A ganglion of the sensory root of the fifth cranial nerve deeply situated in the skull. It is sometimes operated on for the relief of intractable trigeminal neuralgia.

gastrectomy (*gas-trek'-tom-i*). Removal of the stomach.

gastric (*gas-trik*). Relating to the stomach. *G. aspiration.* Also called *g. suction.* Performed post-operatively after operations on the alimentary tract to prevent dilatation of the stomach. A Ryle's tube is passed and the contents aspirated at frequent intervals or continuously. *G. juice.* The digestive fluid of the stomach. *G. lavage.*

Washing out the stomach: a procedure used in the treatment of poisoning.

gastric ulcer (*ul-ser*). Ulceration of the mucosa lining the stomach. Acute ulceration may be caused by ingested substances, *e.g.* aspirin. Chronic ulceration may be due to reduced capacity of the epithelium to withstand the acid gastric secretion or to a tumour of the epithelium.

gastrin (*gas-trin*). A hormone released by cells in the wall of the pyloric antrum, when

negative pressure created by bottle slowly emptying (or by suction pump)

water

suction

clip

drip chamber

glass connection

suction

negative pressure

Ryle's tube

water + gastric contents

stomach

CONTINUOUS GASTRIC SUCTION

it is distended. This stimulates the secretion of gastric juice by the secretory cells in the rest of the stomach.

gastritis (*gas-trī'-tis*). Inflammation of the epithelium lining the stomach.

gastrocele (*gas'-trō-sēl*). Hernia of the stomach.

gastrocnemius (*gas-trō-knē'-me-us*). A large muscle of the calf of the leg.

Femur

Lateral head — Medial head

Gastrocnemius

Fibula — Tibia
Achilles tendon

Talus

Calcaneum

GASTROCNEMIUS MUSCLE

gastrocolic reflex (*gas-trō-ko-lik rē-fleks*). Reflex peristaltic contractions in the colon occurring as the result of filling the stomach.

gastroduodenostomy (*gas'-trō-dū-ō-den-ost'-omi*), **gastro-enterostomy** (*en-te-ros'-to-mi*), **gastrojejunostomy** (*je-jŭn-os'-*

to-mi). The operation of making an artificial passage direct from the stomach to the duodenum or the jejunum.

gastroenteritis (*gas'-trō-en-ter-ī'-tis*). Inflammation of the stomach and intestines.

gastrogastrostomy (*gas-trō-gas-tros'-to-mi*), **gastrolysis** (*gas-trol'-i-sis*), **gastroplasty** (*gas'-trō-plas-ti*). Operations for the cure of hour-glass contractions of the stomach.

gastrointestinal tract (*gas-trō-in-tes-tī-nal trakt*). The gut including the mouth, oesophagus, stomach, small and large intestine, rectum and anus and the associated structures.

gastropexy (*gas-trō-peks-i*). Fixing a displaced stomach to the abdominal wall by surgery.

gastroptosis (*gas-trop-tō-sis*). Downward displacement of the stomach.

gastroscope (*gas'-tros-kōp*). An instrument for inspecting the cavity of the stomach. It has a light at the end and is passed per oesophagus.

gastrostaxis (*gas-trō-stak'-sis*). Haemorrhage from the stomach.

gastrostomy (*gas-tros'-to-mi*). Making an artificial opening into the stomach through which patient is fed by pouring nourishment through a tube directly into the stomach. Performed for stricture, usually malignant, of the oesophagus.

gastrulation (*gas-trū-lā-shon*). Embryological term used to describe the complex movements of cells of the embryo in which the cells which give rise to the internal organs migrate inside the embryo.

Gaucher's disease (*gow-cherz*). Enlargement of the spleen with anaemia.

gauze (*gawz*). Open mesh material used in surgical dressings.

gavage (*gav'-ahj*). Forced feeding.

Geiger-Muller counter (*gī-ger moo-ler kown-ter*). Machine which detects and registers radio-activity.

gelatin (*je'-lat-in*). A jelly-like protein obtained by boiling bones, cartilage, and muscle of animals.

gemmellus (*je-mel'-lus*). Twin, the name of two muscles in the buttock.

gene (*jēn*). Chromosomal factor transmitting hereditary characteristics.

general paralysis of the insane. Also called G.P.I. Dementia due to involvement of the brain in syphilis.

generation (*jen-er-ā'-shon*). (1) Reproduction. The begetting of children. (2) Specific group of individuals resulting from a mating.

genetic (*jen-et'-ik*). Pertaining to generation.

genetics (*je-ne-tiks*). Study of heredity and its variations.

genitalia (*jen-it-ā'-li-a*). The generative organs.

genotype (*je-nō'-tīp*). The genetic make-up of an individual, *i.e.*, the set of alleles inherited by the individual.

gentian (*jen'-shan*). A useful drug, bitter, acts as a stomachic tonic.

gentian violet (*jen-shan vī-ō-let*). An antiseptic dye, used as a paint or lotion, strength 1–100 to 1–1000.

genu (*jen-ū'*). The knee.

genu-pectoral position (*jen-ū-pek'-tor-al po-si-shon*). The knee-chest position—the patient resting upon the knees and chest.

GENU-PECTORAL POSITION

genu valgum (*jen-ū val'-gum*). Knock-knee, knees are bent inwards. *G. Varum.* bow-legged. *See illustration*, p. 163.

geriatrics (*je-rē-a-triks*). The study of disease among the elderly.

germ (*jerm*). A microbe, bacillus.

German measles (*jer'-man mēz-lz*). *See* RUBELLA.

germicide (*jer'-mi-sīd*). An agent that destroys micro-organisms, *e.g.* lysol.

gerontology (*je-ron-to-lo-ji*). The study of ageing.

GENU VALGUM

Gesell's development charts (*je-sels*). Charts showing the expected motor activity, manipulation, adaptive behaviour, language, social and play reactions in children at certain ages.

gestation (*jes-tā'-shon*). Pregnancy.

gestation sac. The fetus with its enveloping membranes, decidua, etc. The contents of a pregnant uterus.

Ghon's focus (*gŏns fō-kus*). Small focus of infection found in primary infection by tubercle bacillus.

giardiasis (*gi-a-dī-a-sis*). *See* LAMBLIASIS.

gigantism (*jī-gan'-tizm*). Abnormal overgrowth of the body or of a limb, due to overactivity of the anterior lobe of the pituitary in young people. *See* ACROMEGALY.

Gigli's saw (*jēl-yēs*). An instrument for sawing through bone. *See* below.

gill (*jil*). A measure, ¼ pint.

ginger (*jin'-jer*). Carminative and stimulant.

gingival (*jin-jī'-val*). Relating to the gums.

gingivitis (*jin-ji-vī'-tis*). Inflammation of the gums.

ginglymus (*jin'-gli-mus*). A hinge joint such as elbow or knee.

girdle (*ger-dl*). Band encircling the body.

glabella (*gla-bel'-la*). Triangular space between the eyebrows.

glairy (*glār-i*). Slimy, albuminous.

gland. A secreting organ. Some have ducts to carry away their secretion, *e.g.* the salivary glands. Others are ductless, *e.g.* the thyroid (*see* ENDOCRINE). Lymphatic glands manufacture leucocytes, filter the lymph and prevent the spread of infection.

glanders (*glan'-ders*). A febrile disease with inflammation of the nasal cavities, communicable to man from the horse, ass and mule. Often fatal.

GIGLI'S SAW

glandular fever (*glan-dū-la fḗ-ver*). Fever with enlargement and tenderness of the lymphatic glands. The cause is uncertain.

glans. Bulbous extremity of the penis and clitoris.

Glauber's salt (*glaw'-berz*). Sulphate of soda, a purge.

glaucoma (*glaw'-kō-ma*). A disease of the eye with hardening of the globe, due to an increase in the intraocular pressure; acute forms of this disease may lead to complete loss of sight in a few days. *Treatment*. Eserine drops and trephine. *See* TREPHINE.

Glenard's disease (*glā'-narz*). A general slackening of the supporting ligaments in the abdomen, leading to slipping down of the viscera: *e.g.* stomach, kidney, and intestines.

glenoid (*gle'-noyd*). A cavity, a term applied to the socket of the shoulder joint.

glioma (*glī-ō-ma*). A tumour composed of neuroglia, nerve connective tissue. It may develop in the brain or spinal cord.

gliomyoma (*glī-ō-mī-ō'-ma*). A tumour composed of nerve and muscle tissue.

Glisson's capsule (*glis-onz kap'-sūl*). The connective tissue capsule of the liver, enveloping the portal vein, hepatic artery, hepatic ducts.

globulin (*glob'-ū-lin*). Group of proteins widely distributed in the body with numerous specialized functions. One group, the gamma-globulins, are antibodies.

globus hystericus (*glō'-bus his-te'-ri-kus*). Hysterical choking feeling as if of a ball in the throat.

glomerulonephritis (*glo-me-roo-lō-nef-rī-tis*). Acute inflammation of the kidney affecting all the glomeruli.

glomerulus (*glo-me-roo-lus*). The filtration unit of a nephron. It consists of a coil of fine capillaries apposed to an expansion of urinary epithelium.

glossal (*glos'-sal*). Relating to the tongue.

glossectomy (*glo-sek-to-mi*). Surgical removal of the tongue.

glossitis (*glos-sī'-tis*). Inflammation of the tongue.

glossodynia (*glos-sō-di-ni-a*). Pain in the tongue sometimes associated with trigeminal neuralgia but often of unknown origin.

glossopharyngeal (*glo-sō-fa-rin-je-al*). Relating to tongue and pharynx. *G. nerve* is the ninth cranial nerve.

glossoplegia (*glos-sō-plē'-ji-a*). Paralysis of the tongue.

glottis (*glot'-tis*). The aperture between the vocal cords in the larynx.

glucose (*glū'-kōz*). Dextrose. A hexose sugar, *i.e.* containing six carbon atoms, which is widely distributed in nature in disaccharides like sucrose and lactose and poly-saccharides such as starch. Glucose is the currency of energy production in metabolism.

gluteal (*glū'-tē-al*). Pertaining to the buttock.

THE GLUTEAL MUSCLES

gluteal bandage (*glū'-tē-al bandāj*). Triangular bandage of the hip.

gluten (*glū'-ten*). A protein constituent of certain cereals which acts as an antigen in coeliac disease.

gluteus (*glū-te'-us*). G. maximus, G. medius, G. minimus— the three large muscles of the buttock.

glycerin (*glis'-er-in*). A sweet, colourless liquid, obtained from oils and fats and by-product in the manufacture of soap. Used as an emollient in skin preparations.

glyceryl trinitrate (*gli-ser-il trī-nī-trāt*). Drug used in treatment of angina pectoris.

glycine (*glī-sin*). An amino acid.

glycogen (*glī'-kō-jen*). A special form of starch in which glucose is stored in the liver.

glycoside (*glī-kō-sīd*). Organic substance yielding sugar and a glucone on hydrolysis.

glycosuria (*glī-kō-sū'-ri-a*). Grape sugar or glucose in the urine, a symptom in diabetes. Sometimes a transitory state only.

glycyrrhiza (*glis-ir-ī'-zah*). Liquorice. Used to hide the taste of nasty medicines. Compound liquorice powder contains also senna and sulphur and so is a purgative.

gnathic (*nath'-ik*). Relating to the jaw or cheek.

G.N.C. Abbreviation for General Nursing Council.

goblet cells (*go'-blet selz*). Pear-shaped cells in certain epithelia which secrete mucin.

goitre (*goy'-ter*). Enlargement of the thyroid gland. *Exophthalmic Goitre.* Activity of the gland is increased, there is protrusion of the eyes,

GOITRE

basal metabolic rate is high, increased pulse rate, tremor, sweating, nervousness, diarrhoea. *Parenchymatous Goitre*, uniform enlargement of the thyroid, very common in young people. *Cystic Goitre* may be (1) enlargement of a single vesicle, or (2) liquefaction of an adenoma. *Adenomatous Goitre*, encephaloid masses in gland substance which may be solid or cystic. *Malignant Goitre*, a malignant growth of the thyroid.

gold therapy (*gō-ld the-ra-pi*). Gold salts were believed to penetrate the lipoid covering of the tubercle bacillus and kill it; the present view is that any beneficial effect is due to the reaction in the patient's tissues set up by the introduction of the metal. Gold may be used in the treatment of rheumatoid arthritis.

golden ointment (*oynt'-ment*). The popular name of ung. hyd. ox. flav., or yellow oxide of mercury ointment. Used as an eye-salve.

Golgi's cells (*gol-jēs selz*). Nerve cells with short processes found in the brain and spinal cord.

gomphiasis (*gom-fī-a-sis*). Looseness of teeth.

gomphosis (*gom-fō-sis*). Joint when bony eminence fits into a socket.

gonadotrophic (*gon-ad-ō-tro'-fik*). Promoting the activity of the gonads.

gonadotrophins (*gō-na-dō-trō-fins*). Hormones which stimu-

late the gonads, *e.g.* F.S.H., L.H.

gonads (*gō-nads*). Reproductive glands: ovary of the female, testis of the male.

gonococcus (*gon-o-kok'-us*). The microbe of gonorrhoea. It is a Gram negative intracellular diplococcus. *See* BACTERIA.

gonorrhoea (*gon-or-rē'a*). An acute inflammation, starting nearly always in the cervix or urethra, and due to the gonococcus. This disease is highly contagious. It may cause ophthalmia neonatorum, *q.v.* It may also cause ophthalmia in adults. By an ascending infection, in the female it may pass to the Fallopian tubes and then cause peritonitis. The chief secondary complication of gonorrhoea is gonococcal arthritis, affecting mainly the large joints. The chief symptoms of gonorrhoea are profuse discharge and pain on passing water. Penicillin is administered.

Goodpasture's syndrome (*good-pas-tūrs sin-drōm*). Haemorrhagic lung disorder and glomerulonephritis.

Gordh needle (*gawd*). Needle through which repeated intravenous injections may be given.

G.O.T. Glutamic oxalo-acetic transaminase. Increase of transaminase occurs in liver damage and heart muscle damage.

gouge (*gowj*). A grooved instrument of steel used to scoop out dead bone.

gout (*gowt*). Inherited defect of purine metabolism in which uric acid is in excess in the tissues. During acute attacks it is characterized by painful swelling of a joint, classically the big toe.

G.P.I. *See* GENERAL PARALYSIS.

G.P.T. Glutamic pyruvic transaminase. The transaminases are increased in acute liver disease.

Graafian follicles (*grah'-fian*). Small bodies lying on the surface of the ovary, containing fluid and the egg cell. When the egg cell matures the follicle ruptures, setting it free to make its way to the fimbriated end of the Fallopian tube along which it travels.

Graefe's knife (*gräfs*). Small knife used in operations for cataract.

GRAEFE'S KNIFE

graft (*grahft*). Transplanted living tissue, *e.g.* skin, bone. *Skin G.* may be: (1) *Thiersch.* Large pieces of epidermis with some dermis used chiefly for large areas. (2) *Wolfe.* The whole thickness of the skin is taken, used chiefly for small wounds. (3) *Pedicle*, used to reconstruct after burns or other severe injuries. The skin and underlying tissue is transplanted in stages. The graft retains its blood supply throughout. *Bone graft*, piece of bone removed, usually from the tibia, and secured to replace bone lost elsewhere.

grain (*grān*). In troy weight the twenty-fourth part of a penny-weight. In apothecaries' weight the twentieth part of a scruple or 0·065 of a gram.

gram (*gram'*). Metric unit of weight, equivalent to 15·43 gr. apothecaries. 30 grams are approximately equivalent to 1 oz. avoirdupois.

Gram's solution. Iodine 1 g, potassium iodide 2 g in 300 ml water.

Gram's stain. Bacteria which resist decolorization by alcohol after staining with methyl violet and Gram's solution are termed Gram positive, *e.g.* staphylococci, pneumococci. Those which are decolorized by alcohol are termed Gram negative, *e.g.* B. coli, gonococci.

gramicidin (*gra-mi-sī-din*). Drug extracted from tyrothricin. Used for local application to ulcers, wounds, burns, etc. It has no action against Gram negative bacteria.

grand mal (*gro-mal*). *See* EPILEPSY.

granular (*gra'-nū-la*). Composed of grains or granulations.

granular layer (*gra-nū-la lār*). Region in keratinizing epithelia where the cytoplasm of the cells appears granular.

granulation (*gran-ū-lā'-shon*). The process by which tiny granules of flesh form on the face of a wound during its healing. Called healing by second intention.

granule (*gran'-ūl*). Small particle or grain.

granuloma (*gran-ū-lō'-ma*). A tumour composed of granulation tissue.

grape sugar. Glucose.

graph (*grahf*). A diagrammatic record of given information.

gravel (*gra'-vel*). A popular term for small concretions formed in the kidney or bladder.

Graves' disease. Exophthalmic goitre. *See* GOITRE.

gravid (*grav'-id*). Pregnant.

gravitational ulcer. Ulcer of lower leg, often a complication of varicose veins.

gravity. Weight. *See* SPECIFIC GRAVITY.

Grawitz tumour (*grah-wits*). A malignant epithelial tumour of the kidney.

greenstick fracture. *See* FRACTURE.

grey matter. Tissue of the C.N.S. in which are situated numerous cell bodies of nerves, dendritic processes, glial cells, etc.

grey powder. Mercury and chalk: an aperient and intestinal disinfectant. Not now given to children as it may cause pink disease.

grid radiotherapy. Irradiation through a sieve-like screen, *e.g.* lead, to improve tissue tolerance in palliative radiotherapy.

grip, grippe. Influenza.

griseofulvin (*grē-sē-ō-fool'-vin*). Oral drug used in the treatment of ringworm infection, particularly of scalp and nails.

grocer's itch. Eczema of the hands, caused by frequent contact with flour and sugar.

groin (*groyn*). Juncture of the thigh and abdomen.

gruel (*groo-el*). Hot drink for invalids.

guaiacum (*gwī-ak-um*). Used to detect presence of blood in the urine. *See* URINE TESTING in the Appendix, p. 382.

guillotine (*gil'-lō-tēn*). An instrument for excising the tonsils.

guinea worm (*gi-nee werm*). Nematode worm which may infest man. The female migrates into the subcutaneous tissues.

gullet (*gul'-let*). The oesophagus.

gum acacia (*a-kā'-she-ah*). A gummy exudation from the stem and branches of acacia. Formerly a solution in normal saline was given intravenously to counteract shock. Largely superseded by plasma.

gumma (*gum'-ma*). A soft tumour occurring in the tertiary stage of syphilis. This may ulcerate. The characteristics of a gummatous ulcer are: it has a vertical, punched out edge, the surrounding tissues are healthy, the base is formed by a 'wash-leather' slough; it is painless and very slow to heal. *See* SYPHILIS.

gum resins. Used as antiseptics.

gustatory (*gus'-tā-tor-i*). Pertaining to taste.

gut. The intestine.

gutta. A drop.

guttatim. Drop by drop. Abbreviation, *gtt.*

gutter splints. For limbs, made of wood, tin or some malleable metal, and grooved to fit the limb, and often lined with felt.

gynaecology (*gī-nē-kol'-o-ji*). The study and practice of the management and treatment of disorders affecting female organs, *e.g.*, ovaries, uterus, vagina.

gypsum (*jip-sum*). Calcium sulphate (plaster of Paris).

gyrus (*jī'-rus*). A convolution, such as the convolutions of the brain.

H

H. Symbol for hydrogen.

habit. Constant and often involuntary action established by frequent repetition.

habitat. The natural abode of an animal or plant.

hacking (*hak'-ing*). Short and chopping stroke used in physiotherapy.

haem, haema, haemo, haemato. Prefixes pertaining to blood.

haemangioma (*hē-man-jē-ō'-ma*). Abnormal growth of blood vessels.

haemarthrosis (*hē-mar-thrō'-sis*). Effusion of blood into a joint cavity.

haematemesis (*hē-ma-tem'-ē-sis*). Vomiting blood from the stomach. The blood is dark, non-frothy, generally acid, and is mixed with traces of food. Common causes are ulcers or growths of the stomach.

haematin (*hē'-ma-tin*). The iron containing pigment of haemoglobin.

haematinic (*hē-ma-tin'-ik*). A substance which increases the amount of haemoglobin in the blood, *e.g.* iron.

haematocele (*hē-ma-tō-sēl*). A tumour containing extravasated blood. *Pelvic Haematocele*, a collection of blood in the pouch of Douglas, walled off by adhesions, usually caused by the leaking from a Fallopian tube, the seat of an ectopic gestation.

haematocolpos (*hē-ma-tō-kol'-pos*). Collection of menses in the vagina due to the presence of a septum.

haematocrit (*hē-ma-tō-krit*). Packed cell volume (P.V.C.). A measurement of the circulating blood occupied by red blood corpuscles.

haematology (*hē-mat-ol'-o-ji*). The science of the blood.

haematoma (*hē-ma-tō'-ma*). A swelling composed of blood. A bruise.

haematometra (*hē-ma-to-mē'-tra*). Accumulation of blood in the uterus.

haematomyelia (*hē-ma-tō-mī-ē'-le-ah*). Haemorrhage into the spinal cord.

haematoporphyrin (*hē-mat-o-por'-fir-in*). A pigment sometimes present in urine, derived from haemoglobin.

haematorrachis (*hē-ma-tō-ra-kis*). Haemorrhage into the extramedullary region of the spinal cord.

haematosalpinx. Distension of the Fallopian tube with blood.

haematoxylin (*hē-ma-tok-si-lin*). Basic dye prepared from logwood. It stains acid groups in tissue, particularly nucleic acids, and is much used in histology.

haematozoa (*hē-ma-to-zō'-a*). Protozoan parasites in the blood stream.

haematuria (*hē-ma-tū'-ri-a*). Blood in the urine, which may be due to lesions of the kidney, or urinary tract. During menstruation some blood may escape into the urine and thus cause suspicion of true haematuria. In appearance the urine may be bright or dark red if much blood be present, smoky if rather less. Albumin will be present. For test, *see* URINE TESTING in Appendix, p. 382.

haemochromatosis (*hē-mō'-krō-ma-tō-sis*). Called also pigmentary cirrhosis or bronzed diabetes. The skin is pigmented and there is sclerosis of tissue, loss of axillary hair and diabetes.

haemoconcentration. Concentration of the blood.

haemocytometer (*hē-mō-sīt'-om-et-er*). An instrument to measure average diameter of red blood cells.

haemodialysis (*hē-mō-dī-a'-li-sis*). The removal of waste products such as urea and salts from the blood by circulating it through a dialyser for patients with renal failure.

haemoglobin (*hē-mo-glō'-bin*). The colouring matter of red blood corpuscles, and the agent whereby oxygen is taken up from the air in the lungs and carried to the tissues. The amount of haemoglobin present in the blood can be estimated by a colour test, normal amount (14·6 grams per 100 ml) being called 100 per cent haemoglobin.

haemoglobinometer (*hē-mo-glō-bin-om'-e-ter*). An instrument for estimating the haemoglobin in the blood.

haemolysin (*hē-mol'-i-sin*). Agent causing the breakdown of the red cell membrane.

haemolytic (*hē-mo-lit'-ik*). Having the power to destroy red blood cells. *H. Anaemia*, resulting from destruction of red cells as in forms of poisoning, or by the action of antibodies. *H. Disease of the Newborn*, jaundice in a Rhesus positive infant caused by red cell destruction by anti-Rhesus antibodies generated in the Rhesus-negative mother's circulation during pregnancy. *See* BLOOD GROUPING.

haemopericardium (*hē-mō-peri-kar'-di-um*). An effusion of blood into the pericardial sac, which may be due to injury or disease.

haemophilia (*hē-mo-fi'-li-a*). A congenital tendency to haemorrhage, the clotting power of the blood being deficient. It occurs only in males, but is transmitted through the females of the family.

haemophiliac. A person suffering from haemophilia.

Haemophilus (*hē-mo-fi-lus*). Bacillus causing respiratory disorders such as the *H. influenzae*. H. pertussis is the cause of whooping cough.

haemophthalmia (*hē-mof-thal-mi-a*). Haemorrhage into the eye.

haemopoiesis (*hē-mō-poy-ē-sis*). The process of formation of the blood cells, particularly the red blood corpuscles. In the fetus, haemopoiesis occurs in the spleen and liver; in the adult, in the bone marrow.

haemopoietin (*hē-mo-poy-ē'-tin*). A hormone produced by the action of the intrinsic factor in the gastric juice on the extrinsic factor, present in food. It is stored in the liver and activates the red bone marrow to manufacture red blood cells.

haemoptysis (*hē-mop'-ti-sis*). Coughing up of blood.

haemorrhage (*hem'-or-āj*). A flow of blood. It may be (1) *arterial*, occurring in spurts, and bright red in colour; (2) *venous*, occurring in a steady stream and dark in colour; (3) *capillary*, oozing from a large wound surface. Haemorrhage may be (1) *primary*, at time of injury; (2) *reactionary*, within twenty-four hours of injury due to a rise in the blood pressure; (3) *secondary*, usually within seven to ten days of injury, due to sepsis. Haemorrhage may be (1) *visible* or (2) *concealed*, into one of the cavities of the body and not appearing at the surface. The symptoms of concealed haemorrhage are pallor of skin and mucous membranes, quick, sighing respiration, rapid, small, weak pulse. Restlessness, subnormal temperature, coldness, sweating and collapse. *See illustration* for pressure points for the arrest of haemorrhage, p. 172.

haemorrhagic disease of newborn (*he-mo-ra-jik*). Congenital abnormality of vitamin K metabolism which results in deficiency of prothrombin

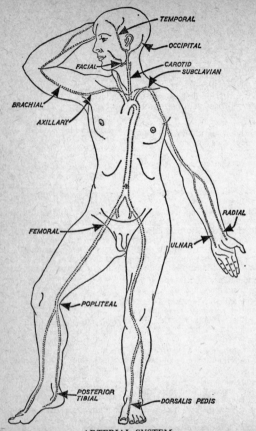

ARTERIAL SYSTEM
The arrows indicate points at which pressure may be applied to check haemorrhage.

in the blood. As a result haemorrhages occur in the body following even slight trauma.

haemorrhoidectomy (*he-mo-roy-dek'-to-mi*). Surgical removal of haemorrhoids.

haemorrhoids (*hem-o-roydz*). Varicose rectal veins (piles).

haemostasis (*hē-mos'-tā-sis*). The prevention of haemorrhage or the measures taken for its arrest.

haemostatic (*hē-mō-sta'-tik*). An agent to arrest a flow of blood.

haemothorax (*hē-mō-tho'-raks*). Escape of blood into the cavity of the chest.

hair follicle (*hār fol'-le-kl*). Little pit in the skin in which the root of the hair is fixed. *See* SKIN.

half-life. The time in which the total radiation emitted by a radio-active substance is reduced by decay to half its original value. It is a constant for each isotope and is independent of the quantity.

halibut liver oil. Oil from the liver of halibut; rich in vitamins A and D.

halitosis (*ha-li-tō'-sis*). Foul breath.

hallucinations (*hal-lū-si-nā'-shons*). The patient perceives something for which there is no sensory stimulus, *i.e.* the sights and sounds are entirely imaginary, *cf.* delusion.

hallucinogens (*ha-lū-si-nō-jens*). Term applied to drugs such as LSD which cause hallucinations.

hallux. The great toe.

hallux valgus. Displacement of the great toe outwards towards the other toes.

HALLUX VALGUS

halogens (*hal-ō'-jens*). Non-metallic elements of the series fluorine, chlorine, bromine, iodine. They are anionic in solution and combine with metals to form salts.

hamamelis (*hā-ma'-me-lis*). Witch-hazel, a haemostatic prescribed for piles, and as a bladder lavage to arrest haemorrhage.

hamate bone. One of the wrist bones.

hammer toe. A deformity of a toe in which there is permanent dorsal flexion of the first phalanx and plantar flexion of the second and third phalanges.

hamstrings. The tendons traversing the popliteal region.

hand. End of the arm. Its bones are the carpal, metacarpal and phalanges.

handicapped (*han-di-kapt*). Mentally or physically disabled.

Hanot's disease (*u-nōz*). A rare type of cirrhosis of the liver of unknown origin.

haploid (*hap-loyd*). Having a set of unpaired chromosomes in the nucleus, characteristic of gametes, *q.v.*

hard chancre (*shan'-ker*). True primary syphilitic sore.

hare lip. A congenital slit in the upper lip, frequently associated with 'cleft palate', *q.v.*

Harrison's sulcus. A groove extending from the level of the ensiform cartilage toward the axillae. It is produced in rickets.

Hartmann's solution. A saline solution containing sodium lactate. Used in acidosis.

Hashimoto's disease (*ha-shē-mō-to*). A chronic thyroiditis due to autoimmunity to thyroglobulin. It causes myxoedema.

hashish (*hash'-ēsh*). An extract of Indian hemp, a drug included in the Misuse of Drugs Act. *See* CANNABIS INDICA.

haustrations (*haw-strā-shons*). Sacculations of the colon as seen on X-ray.

Haversian canals. The minute canals which permeate bone. *See* BONE, illustration, p. 73.

hay fever. Allergic rhinitis caused by exposure of sensitized respiratory epithelium to certain dusts and pollens.

head (*hed*). That part of the body in which is the brain.

headache (*hed-āk*). Pain in the head.

healing (*hē-ling*). Any procedure which cures. The repair of broken tissue.

health (*helth*). A state of well-being with mind and body functioning at their optimum.

heart. The muscular organ which pumps the blood through the system. The heart is situated behind the sternum, rather to the left, the apex of the heart being under the left breast. If the ear or a stethoscope be placed over a healthy heart, a dull thudding sound is heard, immediately followed by a short, sharper, crisper sound; a short pause follows, and then the two sounds occur again. Each pair of sounds

DIAGRAM OF FLOW OF BLOOD THROUGH THE HEART

corresponds to one beat of the heart. *See* DIASTOLE and SYSTOLE. The heart consists of four chambers, the right and left atria and the right and left ventricles. The chambers are lined with the endocardium. Folds of endocardium form the valves of the heart. The heart is enclosed in a membranous sac, the pericardium. *See* CIRCULATION.

heart block. State of partial or complete prevention of the passage of the cardiac impulse through the atrioventricular bundle. *See also* E.C.G.

heartburn. Burning sensation at lower end of the oesophagus, due to acid regurgitation from the stomach.

heart-lung machine. Machine used in cardiac surgery to oxygenate the blood.

heat exhaustion (*ek-saws-tyon*). Condition caused by great heat when patient has rapid pulse, dyspnoea and abdominal cramp due to excessive sweating and loss of sodium chloride.

heatstroke. Hyperpyrexia due to failure of temperature-regulating mechanisms of the body.

hebephrenia (*he-bĕ-frē-ni-a*). A form of schizophrenia sometimes found in young adults.

Heberden's disease (*he-ber-dens*). Generalized form of osteo-arthritis in which there is symmetrical involvement of joints of the hands, knees,

jaw and spine. It occurs in postmenopausal women and is characterized by osteophytes on the dorsal surface of the terminal phalanges (Heberden's nodes).

Heberden's nodes. Small bony nodules which form at the sides of the finger joints in osteo-arthritis.

hedonism (*hē-do-nism*). Excessive devotion to pleasure.

Hegar's dilators (*hā'-garz*). A series of graduated metal bougies for dilating the cervix and uterus.

Hegar's sign (*hā'-garz*). Spongy feel of the cervix in pregnancy.

heliotherapy (*hē-li-o-the'-ra-pi*). Treatment by exposure to sunlight.

helium (*hē'-lē-um*). An inert gas used in certain respiratory tests.

helix (*hē'-liks*). Literally twisted. Used to describe the configuration of certain molecules, *e.g.* D.N.A. and also the outer rim of the external ear.

hellebore (*hel-le-bor*). A poisonous drug, used as a depressant. Antidote for overdose: stimulants. Green hellebore is used in the treatment of hypertension. *See* VERATRUM VIRIDE.

Heller's operation. Division of muscle between stomach and oesophagus in cases of dysphagia in cardiospasm.

helminthagogue (*hel-min'-tha-gog*). Medicine to expel worms.

helminthiasis (*hel-min-thī-a-sis*). Infestation with worms.

helminthology (*hel-min-tho'-lo-ji*). The study of worms.

hemeralopia (*he-me-ra-lō'-pi-a*). Partial blindness; patient can only see in broad daylight.

hemi. Prefix meaning half.

hemianopia (*he-mi-an-ō'-pi-a*). Loss of sight in half of the visual field.

hemiatrophy (*hem-ē-at'-ro-fi*). Atrophy of one side of the body only.

hemiballismus (*he-mi-ba-lis-mus*). Violent, flinging sort of involuntary movement due to disease of the basal ganglia.

hemicolectomy (*he-mi-kō-lek-to-mi*). Surgical removal of half the colon, thus right or left hemicolectomy.

hemicrania (*he-mi-krā-ni-a*). Headache on one side of the head. Migraine, *q.v.*

hemiparesis (*he-mē-pa-rē-sis*). Paralysis of one side of the body.

hemiplegia (*hem-i-plē'-ji-a*). Paralysis of one side of the body. The lesion is in the opposite side of the brain.

hemispheres (*hem'-i-sfārs*). Usually cerebral hemispheres, the two sides of the forebrain.

henbane (*hen-bān*). Hyoscyamus, *q.v.*

Henoch's purpura (*he-noks per-pū-ra*). A form of syndrome caused by sensitivity reaction of the vascular endothelium. Blood leaks out of the damaged vessels causing purpuric spots in the skin and other variable symptoms according to which organs are affected. In the *Henoch type* there is abdominal pain; the *Schönlein type* is associated with joint involvement. Often both types co-exist.

hepar. The liver.

heparin (*hep'-ar-in*). An anticoagulant derived from liver tissue. Given by intravenous injection in doses based on laboratory determinations of patient's blood-clotting time.

hepatectomy (*he-pa-tek-to-mi*). Excision of the whole (in animals) or part of the liver.

hepatic (*he-pat'-ik*). Relating to the liver.

hepatic flexure. The right bend of the colon, under the liver.

hepaticostomy (*he-pa-ti-kos-to-mi*). Operation to make a fistula in the hepatic duct.

hepatitis (*hep-a-tī'-tis*). Inflammation of the liver.

hepatization (*hep-at-īz-ā'-shon*). Conversion into a liver-like substance. A term used to describe the lungs in lobar pneumonia.

hepatocele (*hep'-at-ō-sēl*). Hernia containing hepatic tissue.

hepatoma (*hep-at-ō'-ma*). Neoplasm of liver cells.

hepatomegaly (*he-pa-tō-me-ga-li*). An enlarged liver.

hereditary (*he-red'-i-ta-ri*). Transmitted from one's ancestors.

heredity (*he-re-di-ti*). The transmission of genetic characteristics.

hermaphrodite (*her-maf'-rō-dīt*). Abnormality of development in which an individual has tissue capable of producing both male and female gametes. It is associated with ambiguity of secondary sexual characteristics and the individual is generally sterile.

hernia (*her'-nē-a*). Protrusion of an organ from its normal position, most common in the case of the bowels. *Inguinal hernia* is through the inguinal canal. *Femoral* through the femoral ring. *Strangulated*, so tightly constricted that gangrene results if operation does not relieve. *Scrotal* is hernia descending into the scrotum, and *umbilical* is hernia at the navel.

DIAGRAM OF HERNIA

A hernia not amenable to manipulation is termed *irreducible*. If the blood supply to this is interfered with it is termed strangulated. *Hernia Cerebri* is protrusion of the brain through a wound in the skull. *Ventral H.*, of the ventral surface of the body such as an umbilical or incisional H., the latter is through an old scar.

hernioplasty (*her-nē-ō-plas-ti*). Operation for hernia when the weak structures are repaired.

herniorrhaphy (*her-ni-or-ra-fi*). Operation to repair a hernia.

herniotomy (*her-ni-ot'-o-mĭ*). Dividing the constricting band of a strangulated hernia and returning the protruding part.

heroin (*her'-ō-in*). Synonym for DIAMORPHINE, *q.v.*

herpes (*her'-pēz*). Vesicular eruption due to infection by a virus. *H. simplex* virus may reside in epidermal cells without causing any reaction, but under certain circumstances, *e.g.* associated with a cold, an immunological reaction to the virus occurs with blistering and ulceration of the skin known as 'cold sores'. *H. zoster* virus is closely related to, if not identical with, the chickenpox virus and attacks sensory nerves producing pain and vesiculation in the distribution of the nerves (shingles).

Herxheimer reaction (*herks-hī-mer re-ak-shon*). Exacerbation of syphilitic lesions for a short period following the commencement of penicillin therapy.

hetero-. Prefix meaning unlike.

heterogeneous (*het-er-ō-jē'-ne-us*). Differing in kind or in nature.

heterogeneous vaccine. Made from some source other than the patient's own organisms; usually from a stock laboratory culture. Opposite to *autogenous*.

heterologous (*he-te-ro'-lo-gus*). Derived from a different species.

heterophoria (*he-te-rō-fo'-ri-a*). Latent squint. A squint which develops only when the patient is tired or in ill health.

heteroplasty (*he-te-rō-plas'-ti*). In plastic surgery when the graft is taken from another person and not from another part of the patient's body.

heterosexual (*he-te-rō-sek-sū-al*). Normal relationship between male and female.

heterotropia (*he-te-rō-trō'-pi-a*). Squint.

hexachlorophane (*hek-sa-klo-rō-fān*). Non-irritant bactericide which can be used in soaps and creams.

hexamethonium bromide. A ganglionic blocking agent used in hypertension.

hexamine (*hek-sa-mēn'*). Urinary antiseptic—formerly known as urotropine.

hexobarbitone (*hek-so-bar'-bi-tōn*). The official name for Evipan, *q.v.*

Hg. Chemical symbol for mercury.

hiatus (*hī-ā-tus*). An opening or space. *H. Hernia.* Hernia of the stomach through the diaphragm at the oesophageal opening.

hibernation (*hī-ber-nā-shon*). To pass the winter in a sleeping state as *e.g.* the tortoise. *Artificial H.* The body temperature is lowered by applying cold externally, to reduce oxygen requirements and to aid as an anaesthetic. *See* HYPOTHERMIA.

Hibitane (*hi-bi-tān*). Proprietary preparation of chlorhexidine diacetate.

hiccup, hiccough (*hi'-kup*). Repeated spasmodic inspiration associated with sudden closure of the glottis which gives rise to the characteristic 'hic' sound. It may be produced by irritation of the diaphragm but in most cases the cause is unknown.

hidradenitis (*hī-drad-en-ī'-tis*). A staphylococcal infection of the skin, occurring usually in the axillae.

hidrosis (*hī-drō'-sis*). Sweating.

Higginson's syringe. The ordinary india-rubber syringe, consisting of two tubes, a bulb and valves to maintain flow in one direction only.

hilar (*hī-la*). Relating to the hilum.

hilum (*hī-lum*). Site at which the pedicle of an organ is attached.

hindbrain (*hīnd-brān*). Embryological component which becomes the medulla and cerebellum.

hip. Upper part of thigh where it joins the pelvis.

hip joint. Ball and socket joint between the head of the femur and the acetabulum. *Congenital Dislocation of H.J.* Abnormality of development in which the head of the femur does not articulate with the acetabulum. The condition is almost always preventible if recognised within a few days of birth. The nurse should know the simple routine tests and how to apply early splintage if necessary. *See* BARLOW'S SIGN.

HIP JOINT

Hippocrates (*hip-pok'-ra-tēz*). A Greek physician who lived about 400 B.C. He is the father of modern medicine.

Hirschsprung's disease (*her-sproongz di-zēz*). Developmental abnormality in which there is a defect in the nerve supply to part of the terminal colon which acts as an obstruction and results in dilation and hypertrophy of the more proximal segment (congenital megacolon).

hirsute (*her-sūt*). Hairy.

hirsuties (*her-sū-tēs*). Abnormal growth of hair.

hirudin (*hi-roo-din*). Extract of leech's secretion which prevents clotting of blood.

hirudo (*hi-roo-dō*). Leech.

His, bundle of. *See* ATRIO-VENTRICULAR BUNDLE.

histamine (*his'-tam-ēn*). An organic base which is released from tissues, esp. mast cells, following injury. It increases the permeability of blood cells and thus initiates the inflammatory reaction.

histidine. *See* AMINO-ACIDS.

histiocyte (*his-ti-ō-sīt*). Connective tissue cell.

histology (*his-tol'-o-ji*). The morphological study of tissues.

histolysis (*his-to-li-sis*). Disintegration of organic tissue.

hives (*hīvs*). Urticaria.

hobnail liver. A liver whose surface is rendered irregular by cirrhosis. A form of CIRRHOSIS, *q.v.*

Hodge. *See* PESSARY.

Hodgkin's disease. *See* LYMPHADENOMA.

Hogben's test (*hog-bens test*). A pregnancy test in which the patient's urine is injected into a toad.

Holger Nielsen method. Method of artificial respiration. *See* p. 434.

Homan's sign (*hō-mans sīn*). Physical sign of deep vein thrombosis in the leg. Pain is felt in the calf when the toes are dorsiflexed.

homatropine (*ho-mat'-rō-pēn*). A drug derived from belladonna. Drops of 1 or 2 per cent solution are used to dilate the pupil for the purpose of examining the eye. It acts quicker and more transitorily than atropine.

homeo (*ho-mē-ō*). Prefix meaning similar.

homeostasis (*ho-mē-ō-stā'-sis*). Maintenance of a stable system.

homeothermic (*hō-mē-o-ther-mik*). Term applied to animal when body heat is kept constant regardless of the environment.

homicide (*hom-i'-sīd*). Killing a person.

homo (*hō-mō*). Prefix meaning the same.

homoeopathy (*hō-mē-op'-a-thi*). Medicine worked on the system of cures such as those started by Hahnemann. Homoeopathic medicines are mostly given in infinitesimal doses.

homogeneous (*hō-mō-jē'-ne-us*). Having the same nature.

homogenized (*hō-mo-je-nīzd*). Term applied to substance made into the same consistency throughout *e.g.* milk which has its fat evenly distributed.

homolateral (*hō-mō-la'-ter-al*). Relating to the same side.

homologous (*ho-mo'-lō-gus*). Of the same type. Identical in structure.

homosexuality (*ho-mō-sek-sū-a'-li-ti*). A sexual attraction existing between two persons of the same sex.

hookworm. See ANKYLOSTO-MA.

hordeolum (*hor-dē-ō'-lum*). A stye on the eyelid.

hormone (*hor'-mōn*). A substance produced in one organ, which excites functional activity in another organ.

Horner's syndrome (*sin'-drōm*). Unilateral small pupil, ptosis and vasodilation of the cheek with absence of sweating, due to damage to the sympathetic nerves in the neck.

horseshoe kidney. The most important of all serious forms of congenital abnormality of the kidney. The two kidneys are united at their lower poles and form a horseshoe mass. This is generally at a lower level than normal.

Horton's syndrome (*haw-tons sin-drōm*). Release of histamine in the body causing severe headache.

host (*hōst*). Organism on which a parasite lives.

hourglass contraction. A complication of the third stage of labour, seen especially after prolonged and difficult first and second stages. Postpartum haemorrhage is not uncommonly the result of this condition.

HOURGLASS CONTRACTION OF UTERUS

humerus (*hū'-me-rus*). The bone of the upper arm.

RIGHT HUMERUS, ANTERIOR VIEW

hourglass stomach. A stomach divided by a constriction or spasm into two separate cavities seen after a barium meal X-ray. It may be due to a temporary spasm or the result of fibrosis of a gastric ulcer.

house fly (*hows flī*). The common fly. Latin name, Musca domestica.

housemaid's knee. Inflammation of the bursa patellae, caused by constant kneeling on hard substances. *See* PATELLAR BURSAE.

Houston's folds (*hoos-tonz*). Three oblique folds in the mucous membrane of the rectum.

humanized milk. Cow's milk with reduced fat and increased sugar.

humidity (*hū-mid'-it-i*). Moisture. State of being moist.

humour (*hū'-mur*). Any fluid of the body other than blood. *See* VITREOUS HUMOUR.

hunger pain. A symptom of peptic or duodenal ulcer. The pain is relieved on eating.

Huntington's chorea (*ko-rē'-a*). Chronic, progressive chorea. The disease is hereditary.

Hurler's syndrome (*her-lers sin-drōm*). *See* GARGOYLISM.

Hutchinson's teeth. A condition of the upper central permanent incisors: the cutting edge is smaller than the base, and therefore the teeth are peg-shaped. The edge is deeply notched, a sign of congenital syphilis.

hyaline (*hī'-a-lin*). Transparent like glass. Hyaline cartilage is smooth and pearly. It covers the articular surfaces of bones.

hyaline membrane. Eosinophilic material found in the air passages of the new-born. It is probably derived from amniotic fluid and may cause collapse of the lungs in the so-called 'pulmonary syndrome of the new born'. The primary cause, however, is failure of the pulmonary circulation.

hyalitis (*hī-al-ī-tis*). Inflammation of the vitreous humour or the hyaloid membrane of the eye.

hyaloid membrane (*hī'-a-loyd mem'-brān*). The glassy membrane which encloses the vitreous humour of the eye.

hyaluronidase (*hī-al-yŭr-on-i-dāz*). A spreading factor that promotes absorption: in an injection, 500 units aid absorption of 500 ml injection solution.

hybrid (*hī-brid*). Offspring resulting from gametes which are genetically unlike.

hydatid (*hī-dat'-id*). Cyst formed by the larvae of certain tapeworms.

hydatidiform mole (*hī-dat-id'-if-orm*). *See* MOLE.

hydnocarpus oil (*hīd-nō-kar'-pus*). Obtained from the seeds of Hydnocarpus wightiana. Formerly used in the treatment of leprosy.

hydragogue (*hī'-dra-gog*). Substance which attracts water, *i.e.* it is osmotically active.

hydramnios (*hī-dram'-nē-os*). Excess of amniotic fluid.

hydrargyrum (*hī-drar'-ji-rum*). Mercury, *q.v.*

hydrarthrosis (*hī-drar-thrō'-sis*). Accumulation of fluid in a joint, most common in the knee.

hydrate (*hī-drāt*). A chemical compound of a base with water.

hydro (*hī-drō*). Prefix referring to water or hydrogen.

hydroa (*hī-drō-a*). A skin disease causing watery blisters to arise.

hydrocarbon (*hī-drō-kar'-bon*). A compound formed of hydrogen and carbon.

hydrocele (*hī'-drō-sēl*). Swelling containing clear fluid. Most often applied to watery swelling of scrotum.

hydrocephalus (*hī-drō-kef'-a-lus*). A rare disease seen in children. The sutures of the skull do not unite, the cerebrospinal fluid increases, causing the head to swell to an enormous size; often mental symptoms. *Acute H.* Distension of the ventricles, due to a cerebral tumour or meningitis.

hydrochloric acid (*hī-drō-klo'-rik as-id*). Normal constituent of gastric juice: therefore a dilute solution is given when there is a deficiency.

hydrocortisone (*hī-drō-kor'-ti-zōn*). One of the adrenocortical hormones, similar in action to, but more powerful than, cortisone.

hydrocyanic acid (*hī-drō-sī-an'-ik*). A gastric sedative, when diluted. Also antispasmodic. Poison. *See* PRUSSIC ACID.

hydrogen (*hī'-drō-jen*). A colourless inflammable gas combined with oxygen in the proportions of H_2O forms water.

hydrogen peroxide. H_2O_2. A valuable non-irritating and non-poisonous antiseptic. It effervesces in the presence of pus due to the liberation of oxygen. Usual strength 10 volumes, *i.e.* it contains ten times its volume of available oxygen.

hydrolysis (*hī-drol'-i-sis*). Breakdown of complex substance(s) with the addition of water to give simpler substances.

hydroma (*hī-drō'-ma*). Watery swelling of a limb.

hydrometer (*hī-drom'-e-ter*). An instrument for determining the specific gravities of liquids.

hydrometria (*hī-drō-mē-tri-a*). Abnormal collection of mucus or watery fluid in the uterus.

hydronephrosis (*hī-drō-nef-rō'-sis*). Distension of the pelvis and calyces of the kidney due to obstruction to the ureter. Prolonged back-pressure results in atrophy of the renal substance.

hydropathic (*hī-drō-path'-ik*). Relating to cure by means of water; as by baths.

hydropericardium (*hī-drō-pe-ri-kar'-dē-um*). Fluid in the pericardial sac, *i.e.* pericardial effusion.

hydroperitoneum (*hī-drō-pe-ri-tō-nē'-um*). Peritoneal effusion, *i.e.* ascites.

hydrophobia (*hī-drō-fō'-bi-a*). Rabies. An acute infectious disease contracted from the bite of a rabid dog and accompanied by peculiar mental disturbance. The saliva of a hydrophobia patient is capable of conveying infection.

hydropneumothorax (*hī-drō-nū'-mō-tho-raks*). Fluid and air in the pleural cavity.

hydrops (*hī-drops*). Oedema. *H. foetalis.* Generalized oedema associated with severe haemolytic anaemia in the foetus due to rhesus incompatibility.

hydrorrhachis (*hī-dror'-a-kis*). Abnormal accumulation of cerebrospinal fluid in the spinal canal.

hydrosalpinx (*hī-drō-sal'-pinx*). Distension of the Fallopian tube by clear fluid.

hydrotherapy. Treatment of disease by the use of water.

hydrothorax (*hī-drō-thaw'-rax*). Fluid in the cavity of the chest.

hydroxyl (*hī-drok-sil*). OH group. The chemical group of one hydrogen atom and one oxygen atom.

hygiene (*hī'-jēn*). The science of the preservation of health.

hygroma (*hī-grō'-ma*). Cyst in the neck resulting from abnormal development of the lymphatic system.

hygrometer (*hī-grom'-et-er*). An instrument for measuring the moisture in the atmosphere.

hygroscopic (*hī-gro-skop'-ik*). Having the property of absorbing moisture from the air, *e.g.* salt.

hymen (*hī'-men*). A fold of membrane at the entrance to the vagina.

hymenotomy (*hī-me-no-to-mi*). Incision of the hymen to increase size of vaginal opening.

hyoid (*hī'-oyd*). Shaped like a V; the name of a bone at the root of the tongue.

hyoscine (*hī-ō-sēn*). Synonym, Scopolamine. One of the alkaloids of hyoscyamus. Used as a hypnotic in cases of acute mania, combined with morphia (twilight sleep) it is used to reduce labour pains.

hyoscyamus (*hī-o-si'-a-mus*). Henbane, a poisonous antispasmodic and narcotic. Specially used to reduce spasm of the bladder. Enlarges the pupil of the eye. *Antidotes*, emetic of sulphate of zinc, ammonia and stimulants.

hypaemia (*hī-pē'-mi-a*). Lack of blood in a part.

hyper (*hī-per*). A prefix denoting excessive, above, or increased.

hyperacidity (*hī-per-as-id'-it-i*). Undue concentration of acid, as in the gastric juice in some cases of ulcer of the stomach (*hyperchlorhydria*).

hyperactivity (*hī-per-ak-ti-vi-ti*). Over-activity.

hyperaemia (*hī-per-ē'-mi-a*). Excess of blood in a part.

hyperaesthesia (*hī-per-es-thē'-zi-a*). Excess of sensitiveness in a part.

hyperalgesia (*hī-per-al-jē'-si-a*). Excessive sensibility to pain.

hyperasthenia (*hī-pe-ras-thē-ni-a*). Great weakness.

hyperbaric (*hī-per-ba-rik*). Term applied to a gas at greater pressure than normal, *e.g.* H. Oxygen chamber.

hypercalcaemia (*hī-per-kal-sē'-mi-a*). Increase of calcium in the blood.

hypercapnia (*hī-per-kap'-ni-a*). Excess of carbon dioxide in the blood.

hyperchlorhydria (*hī-per-klor-hī'-dri-a*). Excess of hydrochloric acid in the gastric juice.'

hyperchromia (*hī-per-krō-mi-a*). Excessively coloured.

hyperemesis (*hī-per-em'-e-sis*). Excessive vomiting. H. *Gravidarum*, of pregnancy.

hyperextension (*hī-per-eks-ten-shon*). Over-extension, *e.g.* of a joint.

hyperflexion (*hī-per-flek-shon*). Over-flexion.

hyperglycaemia (*hī-per-glī-sē-mi-a*). Excessive sugar in the blood; occurs in diabetes mellitus.

hyperhidrosis (*hī-per-hī-drō'-sis*). Excess of perspiration.

hyperkeratoses (*hī-per-ke-ra-tō'-sēz*). Callosities and corns of the skin.

hyperkinesis (*hī-per-kī-nē-sis*). Excessive movement.

hypermetropia (*hī-per-me-trō'-pi-a*). Long-sight, a visual affection. The opposite of myopia. Corrected by wearing a biconvex lens.

hypermnesia (*hī-perm-nē'-zi-a*). An exaggeration of memory involving minute details of a past experience. It may occur in mentally unstable individuals after a shock.

hypermotility (*hī-per-mō-ti-li-ti*). Increased motor activity.

hypermyotonia (*hī-per-mī-ō-tō-ni-a*). Increase in muscle tone.

hypernephroma (*hī-per-ne-frō'-ma*). Malignant tumour of kidney also called Grawitz's tumour.

hyperonychia (*hī-per-ō-ni-ki-a*). Thickening of the nails.

hyperostosis (*hī-per-os-tō'-sis*). Hypertrophy of bony tissue.

hyperparathyroidism (*hī-per-par-a-thī'-royd-izm*). Excessive secretion of the parathyroid glands.

hyperphagia (*hī-per-fā-ji-a*). Eating to excess.

hyperphoria (*hī-per-fo-ri-a*). Elevation of one visual axis above the other.

hyperpiesis (*hī-per-pī-ēs'-is*). Abnormally high blood pressure. *See* HYPERTENSION.

hyperpituitarism (*hī-per-pit-ū'-it-ar-izm*). Over-activity of the pituitary gland. Occurring in childhood the patient becomes a giant; in adult life, acromegaly develops, *q.v.*

hyperplasia (*hī-per-plā'-sē-a*). Excessive growth of tissue.

hyperpnoea (*hī-per-pnē'-a*). Respirations increased in rate and depth: a symptom of uraemia.

hyperpyrexia (*hī-per-pī-rek'-si-a*). High fever, arbitrarily above 105° F. or 40.56° C.

hypersecretion (*hī-per-se-krē'-shon*). Excessive secretion.

hypersensitive (*hī-per-sen-si-tiv*). Abnormally sensitive, *e.g.* to certain foodstuffs.

hypertensin (*hī-per-ten-sin*). Angiotensin, *q.v.*

hypertension (*hī-per-ten-'shon*). Blood pressure above the normal limits, *i.e.* above 140/95 resting B.P. Hypertension may be *primary* or *essential*, *i.e.* cause unknown, or *secondary* to artery obstruction, renal disease, endocrine disturbances and other factors.

hyperthermia(*hī-per-ther-mi-a*). Raised body temperature.

hyperthymia (*hī-per-thī-mi-a*). An overactive state of mind with a tendency to perform impulsive actions.

hyperthyroidism (*hī-per-thī'-roy-dism*). Excessive secretion of thyroid hormones.

hypertonia (*hī-per-tō'-ni-a*). Excessive tonicity, as in a muscle or an artery.

hypertonic (*hĭ-per-to'-nĭk*). High tone. (1) Increased tone of muscle. (1) Having a higher osmotic pressure than body fluids, *cf.* isotonic, hypotonic saline.

hypertrichosis (*hĭ-per-trĭk-ō'-sĭs*). Excessive growth of hair, or growth of hair in unusual places.

hypertrophy (*hĭ-per'-tro-fĭ*). Increase in size in response to demand on the structure, *cf.* hyperplasia.

hyperventilation (*hĭ-per-ven-tĭ-lā-shon*). Overbreathing.

hypnosis (*hip-nō'-sĭs*). Condition resembling sleep in which conscious control of behaviour is reduced. The state is brought about voluntarily in the subject by suggestion.

hypnotic (*hip-not'-ĭk*). (1) Relating to hypnotism. (2) Drug producing sleep.

hypnotism (*hip-nō'-tism*). Practice of hypnosis.

hypo (*hĭ-pō*). Prefix denoting below.

hypoaesthesia (*hĭ-pō-ēs-thē-sĭ-a*). Diminished sense of feeling in a part.

hypocalcaemia (*hĭ-pō-kal-sē-mĭ-a*). Diminished amount of blood calcium.

hypochlorhydria (*hĭ-pō-klor-hī'-drĭ-a*). Deficiency of hydrochloric acid in the gastric juice.

hypochlorite (*hĭ-pō-klo'-rīt*). A salt of hypochlorous acid, Sodium hypochlorite is used in the treatment of wounds, burns, and the disinfection of food utensils. Sensitive to ultra-violet light, therefore store in brown bottles.

hypochondria (*hĭ-pō-kon'-dri-a*). An anxiety state about health, the patient suffering from many imaginary ills.

hypochondriac (*hĭ-pō-kon'-dri-ak*). Person suffering from hypochondria.

hypochondrium (*hĭ-pō-kon'-drē-um*). Surface anatomy nomenclature relating to the region of the anterior abdominal wall beneath the ribs.

hypochromic (*hĭ-pō-krō'-mĭk*). With decreased pigmentation.

hypodermic (*hĭ-pō-der'-mĭk*). Strictly: below the skin, but in general (incorrect) usage means intradermal.

hypodermoclysis (*hĭ-pō-der'mo-klī'-sĭs*). Continuous infusion of saline fluid under the skin.

hypogastric (*hĭ-pō-gas'-trĭk*). Pertaining to the hypogastrium.

hypogastrium (*hĭp-ō-gas'-trĭum*). Term applied to the region of the abdomen just below the umbilicus. *See* ABDOMEN.

hypoglossal (*hĭ-pō-glos'-al*). Situated under the tongue. The motor nerve of the tongue, situated under it towards the back.

hypoglycaemia (*hĭ-pō-glī-sē-mĭ-a*). Deficiency of sugar in the blood.

hypokalaemia (*hī-pō-ka-lē-mi-a*). Deficiency of potassium in the blood.

hypomania (*hī-pō-mā-ni-a*). Mild form of the affective disorder, mania, in which there is abnormal elation of mood and great energy.

hypomotility (*hī-pō-mō-ti-li-ti*). Decreased movement.

hypoparathyroidism (*hī-pō-pa-ra-thī-roy-dism*). Diminished function of parathyroid glands.

hypophoria (*hī-pō-fo'-ri-a*). Depression of one visual axis below the other.

hypophosphatasia (*hī-pō-fos-fa-tā-si-a*). Inherited deficiency of alkaline phosphatase in the bone cells. As a result there is a failure of the bones to calcify adequately and the serum calcium concentration may rise and there may be anorexia, vomiting and wasting. The amount of alkaline phosphatase in the serum is greatly reduced.

hypophosphite (*hī-pō-fos'-fīt*). Any salt of hypophosphorous acid. Hypophosphites of lime and soda are given as nerve tonics.

hypophysectomy (*hī-pō-fis-ek-to-mi*). Operation to remove the pituitary gland.

hypophysis cerebri (*hī-po-fi-sis se-re-brē*). Pituitary gland, *q.v.*

hypopiesis (*hī-po-pī-ē'-sis*). See HYPOTENSION

hypopituitarism (*hī-pō-pi-tū'-it-a-rism*). Condition result-

ing from insufficiency of pituitary secretion.

hypoplasia (*hī-pō-plā'-zi-a*). Tendency to grow to a size smaller than normal.

hypoproteinaemia (*hī-pō-prō-ti-nē-mi-a*). Too little protein in the blood.

hypopyon (*hī-pō'-pi-on*). Pus in the anterior chamber of the eye.

hyposecretion (*hī-pō-se-krē'-shon*). Too little secretion.

hypospadias (*hī-pō-spā'-dē-as*). Malformation of lower wall of the urethra, so that the urethra opens on the under-surface of the penis.

hypostasis (*hī-po-stā-sis*). Deposit: passive congestion.

hypostatic pneumonia (*hī-pō-stat'-ik*). Due to congestion at bases of lungs, often caused by allowing elderly patients to lie flat on their backs for long periods.

hypotension (*hī-pō-ten-shon*). Low blood pressure.

hypotensive (*hī-pō-ten-siv*). Term applied to drug which lowers the blood pressure.

hypothalamus (*hī-pō-thal-a-mus*). A special area of grey matter in the floor of the third ventricle of the brain. Linked with the pituitary gland and also with the thalamus and the autonomic nervous system.

hypothenar eminence. Prominence on the palm below the little finger.

hypothermia (*hī-pō-ther-mi-a*). State of being abnormally cold. *Artificial H.* Technique used in conjunction with major heart surgery, etc., in which the blood is cooled by passing it through a heat exchanger. The body temperature is lowered to about 85° F (29·44° C) at which level the oxygen requirements of tissues, especially the brain cells, are greatly reduced. This enables the circulation to be stopped for a time.

hypothesis (*hī-po'-the-sis*). A suggested explanation of some happening.

hypothrombinaemia (*hī-pō-throm-bi-nē-mi-a*). Deficiency of thrombin in the blood.

hypothyroidism (*hī-pō-thī'-roy-dism*). Insufficiency of thyroid secretion.

hypotonia. Deficient tone.

hypotonic (*hī-pō-to-nik*). (1) Lacking in tone. (2) Of salt solution: having an osmotic pressure less than that of physiological saline (0·9 per cent NaCl). *Cf.* hypertonic.

hypovitaminosis (*hī-pō-vi-ta-mi-nō-sis*). Suffering from lack of vitamins in food intake.

hypoxia (*hī-pok-si-a*). Lacking oxygen.

hystera (*his'-te-ra*). The uterus or womb.

hysterectomy (*his-ter-ek'-to-mi*). Removal of the womb by operation. *Sub-total Hysterectomy* is removal of all the womb except the cervix. *Pan H.,* total hysterectomy.

Vaginal H., womb removed per vaginam.

hysteria (*his-tā'-ri-a*). A functional neurosis in which there is a reaction, never fully conscious on the part of the patient, to obtain relief from stress by the exhibition and experience of symptoms of illness.

hysterical (*his-te-ri-kal*). Relating to hysteria.

hysterocele (*his'-ter-ō-sēl*). Hernia involving the uterus.

hysteromyoma (*his-te-rō-mī-ō-ma*). Uterine fibroid.

hysteromyomectomy (*his-te-rō-mī-ō-mek-to-mi*). Surgical removal of a uterine fibroid.

hysteropexy (*his-te-ro-pek'-si*). Suturing of the uterus to the abdominal wall to prevent prolapse.

hysteroptosis (*his-ter-op-tō'-sis*). Uterine prolapse.

hysterosalpingography (*his-te-rō-sal-pin-gō-gra-fi*). X-ray examination of the uterus and the Fallopian tubes.

hysterotomy (*his-ter-ot'-o-mi*). Incision into the uterus. The term usually excludes Caesarian section.

hysterotrachelorrhaphy (*his-ter-o-trak-el-or'-raf-fi*). Repair of a lacerated cervix uteri.

I. Symbol for iodine.

iasis. Suffix used to denote a resulting condition, *e.g.* ankylostomiasis as a result of infection with Ankylostoma duodenale.

ice (*īs*). The solid state of water when temperature is lowered to 0° C (32° F). As the water freezes it expands. *I. compress* and *I. poultice* may be used to treat bruises and arrest haemorrhage.

ichthyol (*ik'-the-ol*). Viscid brown substance with a fishy odour, used for skin infections. It is an antiseptic. Also called ichthammol.

ichthyosis (*ik-thi-ō'-sis*). Inherited defect of keratinization in which the skin is dry and scaly. The so-called acquired ichthyosis is similar in appearance but due to defective nutrition.

icterus (*ik'-ter-us*). Jaundice, *q.v.*

icterus neonatorum (*ik'-ter-us nē-ō-nā-tor'-um*). Jaundice of the new-born child. A slight degree of jaundice is not uncommon a few days after birth, and has no special significance; but serious and fatal cases also arise from umbilical sepsis, haemolytic disease of the newborn, and other causes. See JAUNDICE.

id. Deep unconscious part of personality containing the instinctive impulses.

idea (*i-dēr*). A mental image.

ideation (*i-dē-ā-shon*). Capacity to form and grasp ideas.

idée fixe (*ē-dā fiks*). One idea dominates all others; a delusion.

identical twins. Twins of the same sex and originating from the same ovum.

identification (*ī-den-ti-fi-kā-shon*). (1) Recognition. (2) Psychiatric emotional attachment to an individual resulting in transposition of behaviour characteristics.

ideo-motor (*i-de-o-mō'-tor*). The association of movement with an idea. Psychologically it is rather like an obsession: an idea that leads to action against the will of the person.

idiocy (*id'-i-o-sē*). Before the Mental Health Act, 1959, idiots were officially categorized as having an intelligence quotient of less than 20. The present official legal term is *severely subnormal* which covers mental defectives with an I.Q. of less than 50 who were imbeciles and idiots in the old classification. High grade defectives with I.Q.s of 50 to 75 are classed as *subnormal* and were previously termed feeble minded. In psychiatric terminology all cases with an I.Q. of less than 75 are termed cases of *amentia*.

idiopathic (*id-i-ō-path'-ik*). Without apparent cause.

idiosyncrasy (*id-i-ō-sin'-kra-si*). Individual character or property. Generally used in connection with unusual or unexpected response to drugs.

idiot (*i'-dē-ot*). See IDIOCY.

ileectomy (*i-lē-ek-tom-i*). Excision of the ileum.

ileitis (*ĭ-lē-ĭ-tis*). Inflammation of the ileum. *Regional i.* Crohn's disease. Characterized by localized regions of non-specific chronic inflammation of the terminal portion of the ileum. Occasionally other parts of the intestine are also affected. The cause is not known.

ileocaecal valve (*il'-e-ō-sē'-kal*). Valve at the junction of the large and small intestines.

ileocolitis (*il-ē-ō-ko-lī-tis*). Inflammation of the ileum and colon. A condition not uncommon in children.

ileocolostomy (*il-ē-ō-ko-los'-to-mi*). Surgical anastomosis between the ileum and the colon.

ileoproctostomy (*ĭ-lē-ō-prok-tos-to-mi*). Operation when the ileum is joined to the rectum.

ileo-rectal (*ĭ'-lē-ō-rek'-tal*). Relating to the ileum and the rectum.

ileosigmoidostomy (*il-ē-ō-sig-moy-dos'-to-mi*). Implantation of the small intestine into the sigmoid flexure.

ileostomy (*ĭ-lē-os-to-mi*). An opening is made into the ileum, and if necessary a permanent artificial anus may be made in the abdominal wall.

ileum (*il'-e-um*). The lower portion of the small intestine between the jejunum and caecum. *See* BOWEL.

ileus (*īl'-e-us*). Obstruction of the bowel. Paralytic ileus caused by paralysis of the muscle. It may be a complication of abdominal operations, particularly if the bowel has been extensively handled. It may be due to peritonitis.

iliac crest. The highest portion of the ilium. The greatest width from one iliac crest to the other of a normal female adult pelvis should be 27·9 to 29·2 cm, and should be at least 2·5 cm greater than that between the iliac spines.

iliac region. The regions of the abdomen in the neighbourhood of the iliac bones.

iliac spine. The tubercle at the anterior end of the iliac crest. *See above.*

iliococcygeal (*ĭ-li-ō-kok-si-jē-al*). Relating to the ilium and the coccyx, *e.g.* iliococcygeal ligament: ligament passing between the ilium and coccyx.

iliopsoas (*i-li-ō-sō-as*). The psoas and iliacus muscles.

ilium (*il'-i-um*). The upper part of the innominate bone, *q.v.*

illegitimacy (*i-lej-it-i-ma-si*). Born out of wedlock.

illusion (*il-lū'-zhon*). A deceptive appearance. The misinterpretation of a sensory image.

image. A mental picture of an external object.

imago (*i-mah-gō*). Fantasy woven around someone loved in childhood.

imbalance (*im-ba-lans*). Lack of balance.

imbecility (*im-be-si'-li-ti*). A marked degree of mental incapacity.

imipramine (*i-mi-pra-mēn*). Anti-depressant drug.

immiscible (*i-mi-ski-bel*). Cannot be mixed together.

immobility (*im-ō-bil'-it-i*). The state of being fixed.

immune (*i-mūn*). Protected against a particular disease as by inoculation.

immunity. State of resistance to infection due to the presence of antibodies capable of combining with antigen(s) carried by the infecting organism and thus damaging the invader or neutralizing enzymes or toxins released by the organism. As well as viruses, bacteria and other parasites the body regards cells from a different individual, *i.e.* different genotype, as infecting organisms. Hence the difficulties of homografting kidneys. In a wider, and less common, usage of the term, immunity applies to all mechanisms, such as impermeability of the skin, antiseptic properties of sebum, disinfection of food by stomach acid, etc., which enable the body to resist infection.

immunization (*im-mū-nī-zā-shon*). Process of increasing the state of immunity, either by contact with the infecting organism or some variant of it which is *Active i.* In *passive i.* there is receipt of

an antibody. Active immunization is the principle behind vaccination against smallpox, inoculation against diphtheria, tetanus etc. Passive immunization is temporary. The fetus is passively immunized by antibodies from the maternal blood enabling the new-born baby to resist infection for about six weeks after birth.

immunology (*i-mū-no-lo-ji*). The study of immunity.

immunosuppression (*i-mū-nō-su-pre'-shon*). Deliberate inhibition of normal immune response, especially to permit successful organ grafting.

impaction (*im-pak'-shon*). Wedging or jamming together, *e.g.* impacted *fracture* where the bony fragments are jammed together.

impalpable (*im-pal'-pa-bl*). Not capable of being felt.

imperforate (*im-per-'fo-rāt*). Completely closed. *See* ANUS.

impetigo (*im-pe-tī'-gō*). A skin rash of an acute kind, generally a streptococcal and staphylococcal infection. It is contagious.

implantation. The act of setting in; grafting.

implants (*im-plunz*). Pellets of drugs such as testosterone which are inserted under the skin from where they are slowly absorbed.

impotence (*im'-pō-tens*). Absence of power or desire for sexual intercourse.

impregnation (*im-preg-nā'-shon*). The fertilization of an ovum by a spermatozoon. Also the process of saturation.

impulse (*im-puls*). A sudden driving force.

impulse of the heart. Sensation of a stroke felt on placing the hand on the cardiac region, occurring as the ventricles contract.

inaccessible (*in-ak-se-sibl*). Term applied to a patient with whose mind no contact can be made.

inactivate (*i-nak-ti-vāt*). To destroy activity.

inanition (*in-a-nish'-un*). Exhaustion from want of food.

inarticulate (*in-ar-tik'-ū-lāt*). (1) Without joints. (2) Unable to speak clearly.

incarcerated (*in-kar-se-rā-ted*). Imprisoned. Term applied to a hernia which cannot be reduced, or to a gravid uterus which cannot rise from the pelvis.

incest (*in'-sest*). Sexual intercourse between near relatives.

incidence (*in-si-denz*). Occurrence, such as of a disease.

incipient (*in-si'-pi-ent*). Beginning.

incision (*in-si-zhon*). Act of cutting into with a sharp instrument.

incisors (*in-sī'-sers*). Chisel-shaped cutting teeth at the front of the mouth.

inclusion bodies (*in-klus-yon bo-dis*). Intracellular bodies found esp. in affected tissues in virus diseases.

incoherent (*in-kō-hā-rent*). Disconnected. Inconsequent.

incompatible (*in-kom-pa'-tibl*). Not capable of association. Especially applied to drugs which cannot be compounded in the same mixture.

incompetence (*in-kom'-petenz*). Incapable of natural function, *e.g.* aortic incompetence in which the aortic valve of the heart does not close adequately with the result that blood leaks back into the left ventricle.

incontinence (*in-kon'-ti-nens*). Absence of voluntary control over the passing of urine or faeces.

inco-ordination (*in-kō-or-din-ā'-shon*). Inability to perform harmonious muscular movements.

incrustation (*in-krus-tā'-shon*). Forming of a scab on a wound.

incubation (*in'-kū-bā'-shon*). Literally to hatch. *I. period.* Time between infection and the appearance of symptoms when it is assumed the infecting organisms multiply.

incubator (*in'-kū-bā-tor*). Apparatus used to provide optimum conditions for incubation.

incus (*in'-kus*). A small anvil-shaped bone of the middle ear. *See* EAR.

index. (1) The forefinger. (2) The ratio of measurement of any quantity in comparison with a fixed standard.

Indian hemp. Cannabis indica, *q.v.* Also called marihuana.

indicanuria (*in-di-ka-nū'-ri-a*). Excess of indican in the urine.

indication (*in-di-kā'-shon*). Circumstances determining a particular form of treatment.

indicator (*in-di-kā'-tor*). Substance showing a chemical reaction by its change in colour.

indigenous (*in-di'-je-nus*). Native to a particular place.

indigestion (*in-di-jest'-chon*). Failure of the digestive powers; dyspepsia.

indigo-carmine. A dye chiefly used in medicine to test the functional capacity of the kidney, 10 ml of a 0·4 per cent solution are injected intravenously into the arm. If the kidneys are normal, blue should appear in seven minutes in the urine.

indol. A constituent of faeces formed by the putrefaction of protein. In cases of chronic constipation it is absorbed and excreted in urine as indican.

indolent (*in'-do-lent*). A term applied to a painless sore which is slow to heal.

induced current (*in-dūst' kur-rent*). A secondary electrical current developed in a conductor by proximity to a primary current.

induction (*in-duk'-shon*). In ob-

stetrics, the artificial production of labour. In electricity, the production of currents in a closed circuit upon the appearance and disappearance of a magnetic or electric field in its neighbourhood.

induration (*in-dū-rā'-shon*). The process of hardening; also, the state of being hardened, as in the early stage of inflammation.

industrial disease. A disease due to a person's occupation, such as silicosis found among silica workers, etc.

inebriety (*in-e-brī'-et-i*). Habitual drunkenness.

inertia (*in-er'-sha*). Sluggishness; (1) Resistance to change in motion. (2) In psychiatry, extreme apathy. (3) *Uterine I.* Sluggish contraction of the uterus during labour.

inevitable haemorrhage. Bleeding due to placenta praevia, *q.v.*

in extremis (*in eks-trā-mis*). At the point of death.

infant (*in'-fant*). A newly born child: A full-term infant should be 50 to 53 cm in length. In English law, a person under 18 years of age. *I. mortality. See* MORTALITY.

infanticide (*in-fan'-ti-sīd*). Murder of an infant.

infantile eczema (*in'-fan-tīl ek-se-ma*). Type of eczema affecting infants and children.

infantile paralysis. Anterior poliomyelitis, *q.v.*

infantilism (*in-fan-ti-lism*). Persistence of childish ways in an adult.

infarct. A wedge-shaped area of dead tissue in an organ. The result of the clogging of an artery by an embolus. *See* EMBOLISM.

infection (*in-fek'-shon*). The communication of a disease from one patient to another. *Droplet I.* In the fine spray which is ejected from the mouth on talking, sneezing, coughing.

infectious disease (*in-fek-shus*). A communicable disease.

infectious mononucleosis (*in-fek-shus mo-nō-nū-kle-ō-sis*). Glandular fever. Probably a virus infection and characterized by malaise, pyrexia, muscle pains, sore throat, enlargement of lymph glands and the spleen and an increase in the numbers of mononuclear white blood cells. Occasionally there is enlargement of the liver, jaundice and rash.

inferior (*in-fē-ri-or*). Lower.

inferior maxilla (*mak-sil'-la*). The mandible. *See* MAXILLA.

inferior vena cava. The chief vein of the lower part of the trunk of the body.

inferiority complex (*in-fē-ri-o-ri-ti kom-pleks*). Aggressive, extrovert behaviour compensating for feeling of inferiority.

infertility (*in-fer-ti-li-ti*). Inability to reproduce. It may affect either the male or the female.

infestation (*in-fes-tā-shon*). The invasion of the body by parasites such as lice.

infiltration (*in-fil-trā'-shon*). An effusion of fluid into the connective tissue.

inflammation (*in-flam-mā'-shon*). The response of the tissues to an injury. The signs are heat, redness, swelling, pain, loss of function.

inflation (*in-flā'-shon*). Blown out and expanded by air or gas.

influenza (*in-floo-en'-za*). Virus infection affecting the epithelium of the respiratory tract.

infra (*in-fra*). Below.

infra-red (*in-fra-red*). Electromagnetic waves with longer wave length than visible red light, *i.e.* photons with a lesser frequency than the lower end of the visible spectrum. Because it is easily absorbed infra-red radiation transfers heat to the absorbing material and is used therapeutically for this purpose.

infundibulum (*in-fun-dib'ū-lum*). (1) A funnel-shaped orifice or passage. (2) Outgrowth of floor of brain forming part of the pituitary gland.

infusion (*in-fū'-zhon*). (1) Fluid allowed to flow into a vein (intravenous infusion) or a muscle (intramuscular infusion) by a gravity feed. (2) Crude extract of material using boiling water, *e.g.* tea is an infusion of tea leaves.

ingestion (*in-jes-tyon*). The taking in of food or other substances into the body.

ingrowing toe-nail. Lateral extension of the nail bed.

inguinal (*in'-gwi-nal*). Pertaining to the groin. *Inguinal Canal*, about $1\frac{1}{2}$ in. in length, lies in groin, and is occupied in the male by the spermatic cord, and in the female by the round ligament, with their corresponding vessels and nerves. The exit from the abdomen of these structures is at the internal abdominal ring or upper extremity of the inguinal canal. This is a potential source of weakness, and may be the point of exit of a hernia which, pushing its way below the muscles roofing over the canal, appears at the external abdominal ring as a tender swelling.

inhalation (*in-ha-lā'-shon*). Act of breathing in vapour or fumes by the mouth or nose, a form of treatment frequently ordered in disorders of the throat or chest.

inhaler (*in-hā'-ler*). *See illustration.* The drug and boiling water are put into the container and the patient inhales through the mouthpiece.

inherent (*in-hār'-ent*). Inborn.

inhibition (*in-hi-bish'-on*). Literally to restrain. The term is used ubiquitously to imply the prevention of some activity; thus psych-

ological inhibition, enzymatic inhibition, nerve inhibition, etc.

initial (*in-i'-shal*). Pertaining to the beginning.

injected (*in-jek'-ted*). Congested.

INHALER

injection (*in-jek'-shon*). Introduced material under pressure into tissues.

innate (*i-nāt*). Congenital, inborn.

innervation (*in-ner-vā'-shon*). The supply of nerves or the conveyance of nervous impulses to or from a part. *Reciprocal I.* One set of muscles contracts whilst those opposing it relax.

innocent (*i-nō-sent*). Not malignant.

innocuous (*i-no'-kū-us*). Harmless.

innominate artery (*in-om'-in-āt*). The large artery which arises from the arch of the aorta and divides into the right common carotid and right subclavian arteries.

innominate bone. Bone forming anterior walls and sides of the pelvic cavity.

innoxious (*i-nok-sē-us*). Not harmful.

inoculation (*in-ok-ū-lā'-shon*). Introduction of microorganisms into tissue or culture media etc.

inorganic (*in-or-ga'-nik*). Mineral as opposed to living material or its products. The distinction at a refined level is not obvious.

inositol (*i-no-si-tol*). Substance in vitamin B complex found in muscle and other animal tissue and also in seeds.

inquest (*in-kwest*). A judicial inquiry into the cause of death.

insanity (*in-san'-i-ti*). Madness, disease of the brain causing loss of reason.

insecticide (*in-sek-ti-sīd*). A preparation for destroying insects.

insemination (*in-se-mi-nā'-shon*). Introduction of semen into the vagina. *Artificial I.* Injection of semen into vagina or uterus.

insertion (*in-ser'-shon*). The attachment of a muscle to the part it moves.

insidious (*in-sid'-ē-us*). Literally cunning. Usually applies to onset of disease in which there are no perceptible signs or symptoms.

insight (*in-sīt*). An awareness of one's own mental state and behaviour.

in situ. In position.

insolation (*in-so-lā'-shon*). Exposure to the sun's rays.

insomnia (*in-som'-ni-a*). Sleeplessness; often a troublesome complication during convalescence.

inspiration (*in-spir-rā'-shon*). Drawing air into the lungs, the act of breathing.

inspissated (*in-spi-sā'-ted*). Thickened by evaporation.

instep. Arch on the dorsal surface of the foot.

instillation (*in-stil-lā'-shon*). Pouring in drop by drop.

instinct. An inherited organization of perception, feeling and action, *e.g.* the sight of something which threatens life arouses the emotion of fear and the instinct of flight.

instruments. *See* Appendix VII, page 444.

insufflation (*in-sūf-flā'-shon*). Blowing powder into a cavity of the body. The instrument used has a long tube or nozzle with a rubber bulb attached to the distal end.

insula (*in'-sū-la*). Small part of the cerebral cortex lying deeply in the lateral sulcus.

insulation (*in-sū-lā'-shon*). Material preventing loss of or access to internally situated structure of heat, light, electrical current, water, etc.

insulator (*in-sū-lā'-tor*). A substance which does not conduct electricity.

insulin. Secretion of the islets of Langerhans in the pancreas which exerts control over the metabolism of glucose in the body. Used as a subcutaneous injection for reduction of blood sugar in diabetes. *Protamine I.*, insulin combined with an amino-acid, protamine. The effect lasts much longer than insulin alone. It may also be combined with zinc. *Zinc Protamine Insulin*, prolongs the action of the insulin still further.

insulinase (*in-sū-li-nās*). Enzyme which inactivates insulin.

insulinoma (*in-sū-li-nō-ma*). An adenoma of the islet cells of the pancreas.

integument (*in-teg'-ū-ment*). The skin.

intellect (*in-te-lekt*). Reasoning power whereby we can think logically.

intelligence (*in-tel-li-jentz*). Certain mental ability involving reasoning and recognition of pattern, etc., as distinct from memorization of information or other mental functions.

intelligence quotient. Divide the mental age, as ascertained by tests, by the actual age and multiply by 100. The divisor must not exceed 16.

intelligence tests. Tests not based on a person's knowledge but on his ability to learn. *See* INTELLIGENCE.

intention tremor. Tremor which occurs only during active movement.

inter (*in'-ter*). A Latin prefix meaning 'between' and used

with many medical terms, such as *intercostal*, between the ribs; *intermittent* fevers, in which there are regular pauses between the attacks.

interarticular (*in-ter-ar-tik'-ū-la*). Between the joints.

intercellular (*in-ter-se-lū-la*). Between cells, *e.g.* inter-cellular fluid.

intercostal. Between the ribs.

intercourse (*in-ter-kors*). Communication. *Sexual I.* Coitus.

intercurrent (*in-ter-ku'-rent*). Occurring between. *I. infection.* Another infection occurring in a patient already suffering from some other one.

intermenstrual (*in-ter-men-strū-al*). Between the monthly periods.

intermittent. Occurring at intervals. When applied to the pulse, signifies that some of the beats of the heart fail to reach the wrist. *I. claudication.* Literally intermittent limping due to ischaemia of the muscles of the legs.

internal (*in-ter'-nal*). Inside.

internal os. The junction of the cavity of the cervix uteri with that of the body of the uterus. *See also* UTERUS.

internal version. Version by inserting one hand completely into the uterus, and so changing the presentation or lie of the foetus.

interosseous (*in-ter-os-sē-us*). Between two bones.

intersex (*in-ter-seks*). Imperfect sexual differentiation of an individual into either male or female.

interstitial (*in-ter-sti'-shal*). Between parts, *i.e.* in connective tissue.

interstitial keratitis (*ke-ra-tī'-tis*). Manifestation of syphilis consisting of inflammation of the cornea.

intertrigo (*in-ter-trī'-gō*). Eczematous condition of deep crevices or folds of skin, due to retention of perspiration.

intertrochanteric (*in-ter-trō-kan-te-rik*). Between the trochanters.

interventricular (*in-ter-ven-tri-kū-la*). Between the ventricles.

intervertebral (*in-ter-ver-te-bral*). Between the vertebrae.

intestinal malabsorption. Malabsorption syndrome. Failure to absorb certain foodstuffs. There are numerous causes. Usually there is failure to absorb fats and fat-soluble vitamins.

intestinal obstruction. Obstruction to the passage of food or faeces through the intestine. Either due to physical blockage or absence of peristalsis.

intestines (*in-tes'-tinz*). The alimentary canal from the stomach to the anus.

intima (*in'-ti-ma*). Inner coat of arteries consisting of endothelium and its elastic fibre attachment to the connective tissue of the media.

intolerance (*in-tol'-er-ans*). Constitutional incapacity to endure or benefit by a remedial agent.

intoxication (*in-tok-si-kā-shon*). Poisoning; drunkenness.

intra. Within.

intra-abdominal (*in-tra-ab-do-mi-nal*). Within the abdominal cavity.

intra-articular. Within the capsule of a joint.

intracellular (*in-tra-sel-lū-la*). Within a cell.

intracerebral (*in-tra-se-re-bral*). Between the two cerebral hemispheres.

intracranial (*in-tra-krā-ni-al*). Within the skull.

intradermal (*in-tra-der-mal*). Within the skin.

intradural (*in-tra-dū'-ral*). Within the dura mater.

intragastric (*in-tra-gas-trik*). Within the stomach.

intrahepatic (*in-tra-he-pa'-tik*). Within the liver.

intralobular (*in-tra-lo'-bū-la*). Within a lobule.

intramedullary (*in-tra-me-du-la-ri*). Within the bone marrow.

intramuscular (*in-tra-mus'-kū-la*). Pertaining to the interior substance of a muscle. The buttock is the site often chosen for an intramuscular injection. On a line drawn from the crest of the ilium to the coccyx at the junction of the outer and middle third.

intranasal (*in-tra-nā'-sal*). Within the nasal cavity.

intraocular (*in-tra-o-kū-la*). Within the globe of the eye.

intra-osseous (*in-tra-os-sē-us*). Within a bone.

intraperitoneal (*in-tra-pe-ri-to-nē-al*). Pertaining to the peritoneal cavity.

intrathecal (*in-tra-thē'-kal*). Pertaining to the lumen of a sheath or canal, usually meaning the spinal canal.

intratracheal (*in'-tra-trak-ē'-al*). Inside the trachea. Thus *intratracheal cannula*. Those used for the administration of anaesthetic are known as *endotracheal* tubes.

intra-uterine (*in'-tra-ū'-ter-īn*). Within the uterus. *I. contraceptive device* (I.U.C.D.). A small device of plastic or stainless steel placed in the uterus by the doctor to prevent pregnancy.

INTRA-UTERINE
DOUCHE NOZZLE

intravenous (*in-tra-vē-nus*). Pertaining to the lumen of a vein.

intrinsic (*in-trin-sik*). Inherent, peculiar to a part.

intrinsic factor. Castle's antipernicious anaemia substance. Factor present in normal gastric juice which enables the absorption of cyanocobalamin (B_{12}) to take place. It is probable that it is an enzyme.

introitus (*in-trō'-it-us*). An entrance, applied to the inlets of the pelvis and vagina.

introspection (*in-tro-spek-shon*). State of mental self-examination.

introvert (*in-trō-vert'*). An individual whose attention centres on himself rather than on outside things. Opposite to an extrovert, *q.v.*

intubation (*in-tū-bā'-shon*). Insertion of a tube into a passage or organ, esp. tracheal intubation.

INTUBATION

intumescence (*in-tū-mes'-sens*). Swelling, increase.

intussusception (*in-tus-sus-sep'-shon*). The reception of one part of the intestine (the intussusceptum) into another (the intussuscipiens); common in children, and causing intestinal obstruction, with the passage of blood and mucus per anum and frequent vomiting. The treatment is immediate laparotomy. (*See* p. 200.)

**DIAGRAM OF
INTUSSUSCEPTION**

inunction (*in-ungk'-shon*). Rubbing in of medicines or nourishment. The skin should first be briskly washed with warm water.

in utero (*in ū-te-rō*). Within the uterus.

invagination (*in-vaj-i-nā'-shon*). Forming a pouch.

invasion (*in-vā-zhon*). Onset, esp. of a disease.

inverse (*in-vers*). Inverted in position, etc. The direct opposite.

inversion (*in-ver-shon*). Turning upside down or inside out.

invertase (*in-ver-tās*). Enzyme in intestinal juice converting cane sugar into glucose and laevulose.

in vitro (*in-vē-trō*). Literally in glass, *i.e.* in the test-tube as opposed to in life, *cf.* IN VIVO.

in vivo (*in vē-vō*). In the living body.

involucrum (*in-vo-lū-krum*). Layer of new bone ensheathing a sequestrum.

involuntary (*in-vo-lun-ta-rĭ*). Independent of the will. *I. muscles* are innervated by the autonomic nervous system.

involute (*in'-vo-lūt*). Rolled inward from the edges; becoming smaller.

involution (*in-vo-lū'-shon*). (1) A turning in. (2) The shrinking of the uterus and surrounding structures after labour. The uterus, from weighing 1 kg at labour, shrinks in six weeks to the weight of 50 g. Arrest of this process is called subinvolution, *q.v.*

involutional melancholia (*in-vo-lū-sho-nal me-lan-kō-li-a*). Depression due to hormonal changes at the menopause. A similar syndrome occurs in males.

iodides (*ĭ-ō-dīdz*). Combinations of iodine with metals, prescribed for tertiary syphilis and for promoting absorption of fluid, or chronic inflammatory matter due to other causes, *e.g.* in bronchitis. The common combination used is potassium iodide.

iodine (*ĭ'-ō-dēn*). A poisonous element obtained from the ashes of seaweed. A useful antiseptic for the skin.

iodised oil (*ĭ-ō-dīz'd oyl*). Contrast medium especially used in X-ray of the bronchial tract.

iodism. Iodine poisoning. Symptoms are those of a cold in the head with a pustular rash.

iodoform. A compound containing iodine and consisting of yellow crystals or a primrose-coloured powder. It is an antiseptic and deodorant.

iodoxyl. An iodine-containing compound used in pyelography, *q.v.* Also known as Pyelectan and Uropac.

ion (*i'-on*). Atom, molecule or radical carrying an electrical charge.

ionizing radiation (*i-o-ni-zing rā-di-ā-shon*). High energy radiation capable of producing ions in materials exposed to it.

ionization (*i-on'-i-zā-shon*). The process of producing ions in a substance.

iopanoic acid (*i-ō-pa-noy-ik*). Drug given orally as a cholecystographic agent. As well as the gall bladder it shows up the cystic, common and hepatic ducts on X-ray.

ipecacuanha (*ip-e-ka-kū-an'-na*). Expectorant and emetic secured from the root of a Brazilian plant. Used chiefly as an expectorant; an ingredient in Dover's powder.

ipsilateral (*ip-si-la-te-ral*). On the same side.

I.Q. Abbreviation for intelligence quotient, *q.v.*

iridectomy (*ir-i-dek'-to-mi*). Cutting off a piece of the edge of the iris to make an artificial pupil to the eye.

iridocele (*i-ri-dō-sēl*). Protrusion of a portion of iris through a wound in the cornea.

iridocyclitis (*ir'-id-ō-si-klī'-tis*). Inflammation of the iris and uveal tract.

iridodialysis (*i-ri-dō-di-a-li-sis*). The ciliary border of the iris is separated from its attachment.

iridoplegia (*i-ri-dō-plē'-ji-a*). Paralysis of the muscle which constricts or dilates the pupil.

iridotomy (*i-ri-do-to-mi*). An incision into the iris.

iris (*i'-ris*). The coloured circle surrounding the pupil of the eye. *See* EYE.

iritis (*i-rī'-tis*). Inflammation of the iris.

iron (*i-rn*). When ordered as a tonic, should be given after food. Dialysed iron does not injure teeth. Iron causes black stools.

irradiation (*i-rā-di-ā-shon*). Exposure to electro-magnetic waves or charged particles (α and β rays)

irreducible (*ir-re-dū'-si-bl*). Incapable of being returned to its proper place by manipulation; usually term applied to a hernia.

irrigation (*ir-ri-gā'-shon*). Washing out.

irritant (*ir'-ri-tant*). Agent causing irritation, *i.e.* resulting in a response.

ischaemia (*is-kē'-mi-a*). Diminished supply of blood to a part.

ischaemic contracture (*is-kē-mik con-trak-tūr*). Volkmann's contracture. Permanent shortening of muscle due to fibrosis resulting from impairment of blood supply.

ischio-rectal abscess (*is'-kē-ō*). A collection of pus in the fatty cavity on one or other side of the rectum. May burst externally through the skin or internally into rectum when a fistula-in-ano results.

ischium (*is'-kē-um*). The lower and hind part of the inno-minate bone, *q.v.*

Ishihara test (*i-shi-hah-ra*). Colour charts used to test for colour blindness.

Islets of Langerhans. *See* LANGERHANS' ISLETS.

isolation (*i-sō-lā'-shon*). The act of setting apart; an isolation room or ward is one kept for contagious or infectious diseases, and the nurse has to follow strict rules to prevent the spread of the disease.

isomers (*i-sō-mers*). Compounds made up of the same elements in the same proportions but having different arrangements of their atoms which gives them differing physical or chemical properties.

isometric (*i-sō-me-trik*). Of equal measure.

isonicotinic acid hydrazide. Isoniazid. Synthetic drug widely used in the treatment of tuberculosis; usually given in association with other anti-tubercular drugs.

isoprenaline sulphate (*i-zō-pre-na-lēn sul-fāt*). Drug having a powerful stimulating action on the heart. Causes peripheral vasodilation and produces a fall in blood pressure. Given in bronchial asthma, etc.

isotonic (*i-sō-ton'-ik*). Having the same tendency to pass through a living membrane. Thus a solution which is isotonic with blood serum neither attracts fluid from the vessels nor itself tends to pass through into them.

isotopes (*i-zō-tōps*). Differing forms of the same element with different atomic weights but the same chemical properties. *Radioactive I.* Isotopes with radioactive properties, emitting beta rays and sometimes gamma rays. Used to diagnose and treat disease.

isthmus (*is'-mus*). The neck or constricted part of an organ.

itching. Sensation, probably due to sub-threshold pain stimuli, which is characterized by the *scratch* reaction.

-itis (*i'-tis*). Suffix meaning inflamed, *e.g.* dermatitis, inflammation of the skin.

I.U.C.D. *See* INTRA-UTERINE.

J

Jacksonian epilepsy. *See* EPILEPSY.

Jacquemier's sign (*jak-mē-āz sin*). Blueness of the vaginal walls seen in early pregnancy.

jaundice (*jawn'-dis*). A syndrome characterized by increased levels of bile pigments in the blood and tissue fluids. These pigments are taken up by the tissues giving rise to a yellow colour of the sclera, skin and mucous membranes. The cause of jaundice may be obstructive hepato-cellular and haemolytic. Excessive destruction of red blood cells (haemolysis) may be secondary to inherited abnormalities in their metabolism (spherocytosis) or infection, *e.g.* malaria or lysis in antigen-antibody reactions, *e.g.* Rhesus incompatibility or other causes. Hepato-cellular jaundice includes conditions such as infective hepatitis, a virus disease affecting the liver; toxic damage to the liver cells, *e.g.* acute yellow atrophy and other conditions which reduce the efficiency of the liver in excreting bile pigments. Obstruction to any portion of the biliary tree may result in jaundice. The commonest cause of obstruction is gall stones.

jaw-bone. *See* MAXILLA.

jejunectomy (*je-jŭ-nek-to-mi*). Excision of part of the jejunum.

jejunostomy (*je-jū-nos'-to-mi*). Making an artificial opening into the jejunum.

jejunum (*je-jū'-num*). That portion of the small intestine which lies between the duodenum and the ileum. *See* BOWEL.

jerk. A sudden contraction of muscle.

jigger. A tropical sand flea (*Dermatophilus penetrans*) which is parasitic in man, burrowing into the toes. Another name is chigoe.

joint (*joynt*). Point of contact of two or more bones. An articulation.

HINGE
movement in one direction only
eg. inter-phalangeal

CONDYLOID
all movements except axial rotation
eg. radio-carpal

SADDLE
all movements except axial rotation
eg. carpo-metacarpal of thumb

PIVOT
annular lig.
ulna
radius
axial rotation
eg. superior radio-ulnar

BALL AND SOCKET
all movements
eg. hip

PLANE
gliding movements only
eg. inter-carpal and inter-tarsal

VARIOUS TYPES OF JOINTS

jugular (*jug'-ū-lar*). Relating to the neck.

jugular veins. Two large veins in the neck which convey most of the blood from the head.

Jung's method (*yoongs*). Psychoanalysis.

jurisprudence, medical. See MEDICAL J.

justo minor pelvis. Form of CONTRACTED PELVIS, *q.v.*

juxtaposition (*juks'-ta-po-si-shon*). Placed alongside or next to.

K

K. Chemical symbol for potassium.

Kahn test (*karn*). A method of investigating the serum of patients suspected of syphilis. It is more convenient, simpler, and quicker than the Wassermann Reaction, but should confirm rather than supplant it, the W.R. on the whole being more reliable.

kala-azar (*ka-la-ā'-za*). A tropical disease transmitted from man to man by sand-flies. There is enlargement of the spleen and anaemia. It is caused by the Leishman-Donovan parasite.

kanamycin (*ka-na-mī-sin*). Antibiotic with action similar to neomycin.

kangaroo ligature. Suture material from the tendons of a kangaroo's tail.

kaolin (*kā-ō-lin*). China clay; a hydrated silicate of alu-

minium. It is an ingredient of cataplasma kaolini. It may be given internally as an astringent for diarrhoea.

Kapilon. Acetomenaphthone, *q.v.*

karyokinesis (*ka-re-ō-kīn-ē'-sis*). Indirect cell-division, *i.e.* division preceded by complicated changes in the nucleus of the cell.

katabolism (*kat-ab'-ol-ism*). See METABOLISM.

katathermometer. A wet and dry bulb thermometer for measuring the cooling and drying powers of the atmosphere, thus it is a test of the efficiency of the ventilation.

katatonia (*ka-ta-tō'-ni-a*). See CATATONIA.

kathode (*ka-thōd*). See CATH-ODE.

kation (*ka-ti-on*). See CATION.

Katonium (*ka-tō-ni-um*). Diuretic drug.

Kayser Fleischer rings (*kā-ser fli-sher*). Brownish pigmented rings seen in the cornea of patients with Wilson's disease.

Keller's operation. Operation to correct hallux valgus, *q.v.*

keloid (*kē'-loyd*). A connective tissue growth of the skin, arising always in a scar of some previous injury.

keratectasia (*ke-ra-tek-tā'-si-a*). Protrusion of the cornea.

keratectomy (*ke-ra-tek'-to-mi*). Surgical removal of part of the cornea.

keratin (*ke-ra-tin*). Fibrillar protein. It is produced by epithelial cells and is found in horns, hooves, hair and the protective covering of the skin.

keratitis (*ker-a-tī'-tis*). Inflammation of the cornea.

keratolytics (*ke-ra-tō-li-tiks*). Agent such as salicylic acid which breaks down keratin.

keratoma (*ke-ra-tō'-ma*). A callosity or horny overgrowth.

keratomalacia (*ker-at-ō-malā'-ki-a*). Softening of the cornea which may lead to ulceration and blindness. Occurs in association with vitamin A deficiency.

keratome (*ker'-at-ōm*). Surgical knife used for incisions of the cornea.

KERATOMES

keratometer (*ke-ra-to-me-ter*). Ophthalmometer, for measuring corneal astigmatism.

keratoplasty (*ke-ra-tō-pla-sti*). Corneal graft, *q.v.*

keratosis (*ke-ra-tō-sis*). Skin disease with excess of horny tissue.

kerion (*ke'-ri-on*). A term for crusted ringworm.

kernicterus (*ker-nik'-te-rus*). Many areas of the brain, particularly the basal ganglia, central cerebellar nuclei, the medulla and hippocampus are stained yellow with bilirubin. The brain cells are damaged. A complication of haemolytic jaundice of the new born.

Kernig's sign. A sign of meningitis. It consists of an inability to extend the knee joint when the thigh is flexed to a right angle with the trunk.

ketogenic diet (*kē-tō-je-nik dī-et*). Diet with high fat producing ketosis.

ketonaemia (*kē-tō-nē-mi-a*). Ketone bodies in the blood.

ketone (*kē-tōn*). Acetone. K. bodies. Oxybutyric acid, aceto-acetic acid and acetone, the last two being products of incomplete fat metabolism in the body as a result of insufficient catabolism of carbohydrates.

ketonuria (*kē-to-nū-ri-a*). Ketone bodies in the urine.

ketosis (*kē-tō-sis*). Acidosis, *q.v.*

ketosteroids (*kē-tō-ste-royds*). Androgens, *q.v.*, secreted in the adrenals and testes, whose presence in the urine is an indication of the activity of these glands.

kettle. A bronchitis or croup kettle has a long spout coming out of the lid, so that the steam can be directed well out into the room. A roll of brown paper added to the spout of an ordinary kettle does in an emergency.

kidneys. Two organs in the region of the hollow of the back which secrete the urine. *Artificial k.* Apparatus through which blood is passed and allowed to dialyse, across a membrane, usually a coiled tube, placed in a warm bath of saline. This process allows waste products and other materials to be removed from the blood and simulates the function of the kidneys.

Inferior Vena Cava

Left Kidney

Right Kidney

Aorta

Ureter

L. Common Iliac art.

Interior of bladder

Ureteric orifices

Urethra

URINARY ORGANS
FROM IN FRONT

Killian's operation. For suppuration in the frontal sinus. Removal of part of frontal

bone to allow of complete drainage.

kilogram (*kil'-lō-gram*). A thousand grams, equivalent to 2⅕ lb.

Kimmelstiel-Wilson disease (*ki-mel-stēl wil-son di-sēz*). Disease with glycosuria, nephrotic symptoms, albuminuria and oedema.

kinaesthesis (*kin-ēs-thē'-sis*). The sense of muscular movement.

kinase (*kī-nāz*). Substances in the tissues which make proenzymes become enzymes.

kinematics (*kī-ne-ma-tiks*). The study of motion.

kineplasty (*kin'-e-plas-ti*). A plastic amputation with the object of making the stump useful for locomotion.

kinesis (*kī-nē-sis*). Movement.

kinetics (*kī-ne-tiks*). The study of movement or change.

Kirschner wire (*ker-shner*). Wire used in orthopaedic surgery to apply skeletal traction to a fractured bone.

kiss of life. Mouth-to-mouth artificial respiration (*see* p. 430).

Klebs-Loeffler bacillus (*lef'-ler*). The bacillus of diphtheria. Also known as corynebacterium diphtheriae.

Klebsiella (*kleb-si-e-la*). Genus of bacteria which may cause respiratory infections.

kleptomania (*klep-tō-mǎ'-ni-a*). Obsessional neurosis manifested by compulsive stealing.

Klinefelter's syndrome (*klīn-fel-ters sin-drōm*). Infertility in the male due to congenital malformation of gonads.

Klumpke's paralysis (*kloomp-kers pa-ra-li-sis*). Paralysis of the flexor muscles to the wrist and fingers caused by injury to the eighth cervical and first dorsal nerves.

knee (*nē*). The joint between the femur and the tibia. (*See below.*)

knee-cap. Patella, *q.v.*

KNEE-JOINT

knee-elbow position. *See* Ge-NU-PECTORAL.

knee-jerk. A jerk of the leg elicited by tapping on the patellar tendon when the knee is flexed. May be absent or exaggerated in diseases of the nervous system.

knock-knee. Genu valgum, *q.v.*

knuckle (*nukl*). Dorsal aspect of a phalangeal joint.

Koch's bacillus (*koks ba-si-lus*). Mycobacterium tuberculosis.

Koch-Weeks bacillus (*kok-wēks ba-si-lus*). Micro-organism causing acute conjunctivitis.

Köhler's disease (*ker-lers di-sēz*). Osteochondritis affecting the scaphoid bone in the foot which becomes compressed and sclerotic. Occurs in children.

koilonychia (*koy-lō-ni-ki-a*). Spoon-shaped nails found in iron deficiency anaemia.

Koplik's spots. Small white spots to be found on the inner surface of the cheeks in measles, often before the skin rash appears.

Korsakow's syndrome (*kor'-sa-kovs sin'-drōm*). A confusional state especially as to recent events due to brain injury or toxic causes such as chronic alcoholism.

kraurosis vulvae (*kraw-rō'-sis*). Senile degeneration of the skin of the vulva. *See* Leu-KOPLAKIA.

Kretschmer's types (*kret-ch-mers tīps*). Classification of potential psychopathic tendencies in relation to physical characteristics, *e.g.* pyknic type is short and fat with a tendency to manic-depressive psychosis. Aesthenic type is tall and thin with a tendency to schizophrenia.

Krukenberg's tumour (*kroo-ken-bergs tū-mer*). A secondary carcinoma in the ovary, the primary usually occurring in the stomach.

Küntscher nail (*koon-cher*). An intramedullary nail used to fix fragments of fractured long bone in alignment.

Kupffer's cells (*koop-fers sels*). Star-shaped cells in the liver. Part of the reticulo-endothelial system.

kwashiorkor (*kwa-shi-aw-kor*). Disease with wasting, oedema, anaemia and enlargement of the liver due to lack of protein in the diet.

kyphoscoliosis (*kī-fō-skō-li-ō'-sis*). Combined anteroposterior deformity (kyphosis) and lateral curvature (scoliosis) of the spine.

kyphosis (*kī-fō-sis*). Humpback, angular deformity of the spine. May be caused by Pott's disease, *q.v.*

KYPHOSIS

L

labia majora (*lā-bi-a ma-jo-ra*). (*Sing.* labium). Two large folds at the mouth of the pudendum; called also the *labia pudendi*.

labia minora (*lā-bi-a mi-nor'-a*). Two smaller folds within the majora. Syn. nymphae.

THE LABIA MAJORA
AND MINORA

labial (*lā-bi-al*). Relating to the lips or to the labia.

labile (*lā-bīl*). Unstable.

laboratory (*lab-or'-a-to-ri*). A place where scientific experiments and investigations are carried on.

labour (*lā'-ber*). The progress of the birth of a child. There are three stages. (1) The dilatation of the cervix. (2) The passage of the fetus through the canal and its birth. (3) From the birth of the child to the expulsion of the placenta.

labyrinth (*lab'-i-rinth*). The internal ear. *See* EAR.

labyrinthitis (*lab'-i-rin-thī'-tis*). Inflammation of the labyrinth.

laceration (*las'-er-ā-shon*). A lacerated wound with torn or irregular edges; not clean cut.

lachesine chloride (*la-che-sēn klo-rīd*). Mydriatic used if there is sensitivity to atropine.

lacrimal (*lak'-ri-mal*). Relating to tears and the glands which secrete them.

lacrimal apparatus. *See below.*

lacrimation (*lak-ri-mā'-shon*). Flow of tears.

DIAGRAM OF TEAR APPARATUS

lactagogue (*lak'-ta-gog*). *See* GALACTAGOGUE.

lactalbumin (*lak-tal-bū'-min*). The albumin of milk. A protein.

lactase (*lak'-tāz*). An enzyme of the succus entericus which converts lactose into glucose.

lactate. A salt of lactic acid.

lactation (*lak-tā'-shon*). The process or period of suckling.

lacteals (*lak'-te-als*). The lymphatic vessels, which convey the chyle from the intestinal canal.

lactic acid. An acid produced by the fermentation of lactose. The souring of milk is accompanied by the formation of this acid.

lactiferous ducts (*lak-tif'-er-us dukts*). The canals of the mammary glands.

lactifuge (*lak-ti-fūj*). Lessening the secretion of milk.

lactobacillus (*lak-tō-ba-si-lus*). A non-pathogenic Gram-positive bacterium.

lactogenic (*lak-tō-jē'-nik*). Promoting the flow of milk. *L. hormone.* Prolactin. A hormone released from the anterior pituitary which causes milk production following parturition.

lactose (*lak-tōz*). A disaccharide sugar, composed of glucose and galactose, which occurs in milk.

lacuna (*la-kū'-na*). A space.

Laennec's cirrhosis (*la-neks si-rō-sis*). The commonest type of cirrhosis of liver commonly attributable to damage to the liver by high consumption of alcohol.

laevulose. *See* LEVULOSE.

laked (*lākt*). Describes haemolysed blood.

lalling. Baby talk when the letter 'l' is used instead of the letter 'r'.

lambdoid (*lam-'doyd*). Like Greek letter λ, chiefly applied to the suture between the occipital and parietal bones.

lambliasis (*lam-blī-a-sis*). Also called giardiasis. Parasitic infection of small intestine.

lamellae (*la-mel'-lē*). Thin sheets of tissue, *e.g.* bone.

lamina (*lam'-i-na*). A thin layer.

laminectomy (*lam-in-ek'-to-mi*). Excision of some of the vertebral laminae to gain access to the spinal cord.

lancet (*lan'-set*). A sharp pointed two-edged surgical knife.

Lancefield's groups (*larnts-fēlds groops*). A classification of streptococci into groups of which Group A includes the common pathogenic hae-molytic streptococcus.

lancinating (*lan-si-nā-ting*). Cutting or tearing, often applied to pain.

lanette wax. A self-emulsifying wax used in water-miscible ointment bases.

Langerhans' islets. Small areas of special cells in the pancreas. They secrete insulin. *See* INSULIN and DIABETES.

lanolin (*lan'-ō-lin*). Purified wool-fat. Used as the basis for various ointments.

Lansing virus. A strain of polio-myelitis virus.

lanugo (*lan-ū'-gō*). The downy growth which covers an infant from the fourth month of gestation, but has mostly disappeared by term.

laparoscope (*la-pa-ros-kōp*). Endoscope for examining the abdominal cavity.

laparotomy (*lap-ar-ot'-o-mi*). Opening the abdominal cavity. Usually for investigation.

lardaceous disease (*lar-dā'-she-us*). Degeneration of the tissues till they resemble wax. Same as amyloid disease, *q.v.*

Largactil (*lar-gak-til*). *See* CHLORPROMAZINE.

laryngeal (*la-rin'-je-al*). Relating to the larynx. *L. stridor.* Gasping respiration due to spasm of the glottis.

laryngectomy (*lar-in-jek'-to-mi*). Removal of the larynx.

laryngismus stridulus (*la-rin-jis-mus stri-dū-lus*). Laryngeal spasm due to tetany in an infant. There is apnoea and then a crowing sound.

laryngitis (*lar-in-ji'-tis*). Inflammation of the larynx, causing loss of voice, and in acute cases, with much oedema, threatening suffocation.

laryngology (*la-rin-go-lo-ji*). Science of anatomy and diseases of the larynx.

laryngopharynx (*la-rin-gō-fa-rinks*). The lower part of the pharynx.

laryngoscope (*la-rin'-go-skōp*). Instrument for examining a larynx.

laryngostenosis (*la-rin'-gō-ste-nō'-sis*). Stricture of the larynx.

laryngotomy (*la-rin-go-to-mi*). *See* TRACHEOSTOMY.

laryngo-tracheo-bronchitis (*la-rin-gō-tra-kē-ō-bron-kī-tis*). Acute viral inflammatory disease affecting the respiratory tract. Often occurs during influenza epidemic and affects principally young children.

larynx (*lar'-rinks*). The upper part of the windpipe from which the voice-sounds proceed.

laser (*lā-zer*). A very narrow and intense beam of light that will cut through metals.

Lassar's paste. Ointment containing zinc oxide, starch, salicylic acid, soft paraffin. Used for skin eruptions.

lassitude (*la-si-tūd*). Feeling of weakness, a frequent feature of debilitating diseases such as anaemia.

latent (*lā'-tent*). Not visible, lying hidden for a time. *L. heat.* The heat absorbed or released in a change of state without an alteration in temperature, e.g. water into steam and vice versa. *L. Period.* Incubation time.

lateral (*lat-er-al*). On the side. For *lateral sinus, see* SINUS.

laudanum (*lod'-an-um*). Tincture of opium, poison.

laughing gas. Nitrous-oxide gas. An anaesthetic.

lavage (*lav-ahj*). Washing out.

laxative (*laks'-a-tiv*). A mild purgative.

lead (*led*). A soft heavy metal whose salts are poisonous. *L. Lotion* is a solution of subacetate of lead and is

(a)

(b)

THE LARYNX
(a) laryngoscopic view.
(b) sagittal section.

used for external application to bruises and other superficial injuries. Used in the form of diachylon to protect abrasions. *Lead Poisoning* usually occurs in children due to chewing cots and toys covered with paint containing lead. The symptoms and signs include malaise, colic, peripheral neuropathy and sometimes encephalitis. Pallor is often marked and a blue line on the gums is characteristic.

leather-bottle stomach. Loss of elasticity in the stomach wall resulting from infiltration by neoplastic cells.

lecithin (*les'-i-thin*). A phospholipid, *q.v.*

leech (*lētsh*). Aquatic worm which is able to suck blood from the skin.

leg. Anatomically the part of the lower limb from knee to ankle. *White L.* Condition caused by venous thrombosis in the lower limb. Sometimes seen after childbirth. *See* PHLEGMASIA.

legumin (*le-gū-min*). A globulin derived from the seeds of various plants such as peas and beans.

Leishman-Donovan body. Eosinophilic bodies representing rounded forms of leishmania donovani found in the cells parasitized by kala-azar.

Leishmaniasis (*lēsh-ma-nī-a-sis*). Infection with organisms of the type which cause kala-azar and oriental sore.

Lembert's suture. Special suture used in stitching up the peritoneal coat of the intestine or other abdominal organs after any incision or injury.

LEMBERT'S SUTURE

Lennander's incision. An abdominal incision to the right or left of the middle line down to the rectus; the inner edge of this muscle is then retracted and the posterior layer of its sheath incised as well as the peritoneum.

lens (*lenz*). Transparent refractile tissue of the eye (*see* EYE), which focuses the image on the retina.

lente insulin (*len-tā in-sū-lin*). Insulin chemically modified so as to delay absorption and so reduce the need for frequent doses.

lenticular. Pertaining to a lens.

lentigo (*len-tī-go*). A freckle.

Leon virus. A strain of poliomyelitis virus.

leontiasis ossea (*lē-on-tī'-a-sis os'-se-a*). A disease in which the bones of the face are deformed and greatly increased in size; sometimes found in leprosy.

leproma (*le-prō-ma*) (plu. lepromata). Swelling in the skin found in certain cases of leprosy.

leprosy (*lep'-ro-si*). An infective disease, cutaneous in its earlier stages, but afterwards involving both soft tissue and bone. The first stage may last days or months; there are pains in the limbs, lassitude, and feverish attacks. The second stage is eruptive, and the blotches on the skin come and go. In the third stage the disease becomes either nodular (*lepra tuberculosa*) or blotched (*lepra maculosa*); if the blotches become white and anaesthesia sets in, it is called white leprosy. Leprosy, also called Hansen's disease, was formerly treated with chaulmugra oil. Modern treatment is sulphone therapy, which can cure leprosy in its early stages.

leptazol (*lep'-ta-zol*). The official name for Cardiazol, *q.v.* Stimulates the central nervous system and counteracts the depressant action of barbiturate drugs. Large doses produce convulsions. It has therefore been used in the treatment of schizophrenia.

leptomeningitis (*lep-tō-men-in-jī-tis*). Inflammation of the pia mater and arachnoid coverings of the brain, distinguished from pachymeningitis, in which the dura mater is the seat of inflammation.

leptospira (*lep-tō-spī'-ra*). Type of spirochaete. Notably *L. Icterohaemorrhagiae* which causes Weil's disease, *q.v.*

Leriche syndrome (*le-rēsh sin-drōm*). Obstruction to the flow of blood at the lower end of the aorta giving rise to intermittent claudication.

lesbianism (*les-bi-a-nism*). A female homosexual relationship.

lesion (*lē-'zhon*). Any injury or morbid change in the function or structure of an organ.

lethal (*lē-thal*). Deadly, fatal.

lethargy (*le'-tha-ji*). Drowsiness.

Lethidrone (*le-thi-drōn*). Nalorphine, *q.v.*

leucin (*lū'-sin*). An aminoacid.

leucocyte. A white blood corpuscle. See BLOOD COUNT.

leucocythaemia (*lū-kō-sī'-thē'-mi-a*). Morbid increase of the white corpuscles of the blood. Same as leukaemia.

leucocytolysis (*lū-kō-sī-tol'-is-is*). Destruction of leucocytes.

leucocytosis (*lū-kō-sī-tō'-sis*). An increase of white corpuscles of the blood; usually occurs in sepsis and is then a defensive mechanism.

leucoderma. A condition in which there are patches of skin which are defectively pigmented, and consequently pale in colour.

leuco-erythroblastic anaemia *lū-ko-e-ri-thrō-blas-tik a-nē-mi-a*). Descriptive term applied to the appearance of nucleated red cells and primitive white cells in the circulation. It is due to neoplastic infiltration of bone marrow.

leuconychia (*lū-ko-nik'-i-a*). Curved white lines on the finger-nails showing interrupted nutrition.

leucopenia (*lū-kō-pē'-ni-a*). Diminution of the number of white corpuscles in the blood.

leucopoiesis (*lū-kō-poy-ē-sis*). Formation of white blood cells.

leucorrhoea (*lū-kor-re'-a*). A whitish mucoid discharge from the vagina.

leucotomy (*lū-ko-to-mi*). Transection of nerve fibres passing to and from a lobe of the brain. Usually *Prefrontal leucotomy*, an operation undertaken to relieve certain types of mental disorder in which the prefrontal lobes are surgically isolated from the rest of the brain.

leukaemia (*lū-kē'-mi-a*). A disease of blood-forming organs, characterized by increase of white corpuscles of the blood. *Lymphatic L.*: that in which large numbers of primitive lymphocytes appear in the blood. *Myeloid L.* That in which primitive polymorphonuclear leucocytes appear in large numbers. *Monocytic L.*, *Eosinophilic L.*, as for the other forms, but exhibiting monocytes and eosinophils respectively. *See* BLOOD.

leukoplakia (*lū-kō-plā-ki-a*). A smooth glazed white state of the tongue which may precede cancer of that organ. A similar condition of the vulva is also found in women.

levallorphan (*le-val-or-fan*). Morphine antagonist and a respiratory stimulant.

levator (*le-vā'-tur*). A muscle which lifts up a part. *Levator Ani*: muscle of the pelvis which plays an important part in keeping pelvic viscera in position. *Levator Palpebrae Superioris*: muscle which raises the upper eyelid.

Levophed (*le-vō-fed*). Noradrenaline, *q.v.*

levorphanol tartrate (*le-vor-fa-nol tar-trāt*). Analgesic similar to morphine but less hypnotic.

levulose (*lev'-ū-lōs*). Fruit sugar or fructose. *L. Tolerance Test*. In the normal individual there is little or no rise in the blood sugar taken 1 hour after 100 grams of levulose. In hepatic insufficiency the blood sugar will show an increase of 30 mg per 100 ml in the first half-hour and may later rise much higher.

libido (*li-bi-dō*). The drive to obtain satisfaction through the senses. Term sometimes used for sexual desire.

lice (*līs*). Plural of louse, *q.v.*

lichen (*li-'ken*). A term for skin diseases of which the striking feature is chronic inflammatory papules. *Lichen planus*: showing papules, which are angular, lilac in colour, often with a depression in their centre and in some lights shiny. Usually affects flexor aspects of forearms, back of neck, and inner side of thighs.

lie of fetus. The position of the fetus in the uterus is termed its **lie,** *i.e.* transverse lie, vertical lie.

Lieberkühn's glands (*lē'-ber-kūn*). Tubular glands of the small intestine, which secrete the intestinal juice.

lien (*lē-en*). The spleen.

lienculus (*lē-en'-kū-lus*). An accessory spleen.

ligament (*lig'-a-ment*). A tough band of fibrous tissue connecting together the bones at the joints.

ligation (*lig-ā'-shon*). The application of a ligature.

ligatures (*lig'-a-tūrs*). Threads of silk, wire, catgut, fascia, nylon, etc., used to tie arteries, stitch tissue, etc.

light adaptation. The adaptation of the pupil of the eye to light incident on the retina. Also termed light reflex.

lightening (*lī-te-ning*). Relief of pressure in upper part of abdomen during last few weeks of pregnancy when fetal head enters the pelvis.

lightning pains (*līt'-ning pānz*). Shooting, cutting pains felt in some cases of tabes dorsalis.

lignocaine (*lig'-nō-kān*). Local anaesthetic similar to Procaine but with more intense action.

limbus. A border. Junction of cornea and sclera.

lime (*līm*). Calcium oxide. Lime salts increase the coagulability of the blood; they take part in the formation of bone, and are a compo-

nent part of many tonic medicines.

lime water (*līm'-wor'-ter*). A solution of calcium hydrate in distilled water. Used as a diluent for milk, and generally to counteract acidity.

liminal (*li-mi-nal*). The lowest threshold at which stimuli can be perceived.

linctus (*link'-tus*). A syrup, usually applied to a cough mixture to be taken in small doses.

linea alba (*lin-e-a al'-ba*). The white line down the centre front of the abdomen. It is formed by the tendons of the abdominal muscles.

lineae albicantes (*lin'-e-ē al-bik-an'-tēz*). *See* STRIAE GRAVIDARUM.

linea nigra (*lin'-e-a nē-gra*). A pigmented line seen in pregnant women running in midline from above the umbilicus to the symphysis pubis.

lingual (*ling'-gwal*). Relating to the tongue.

liniment (*lin'-i-ment*). A liquid preparation for application to the skin with friction.

linolenic acid (*li-nō-le-nik*). A constituent of vegetable fats, essential for health.

linseed (*lin-sēd*). Seeds of the flax plant.

lint. Loosely woven cotton material, having one side smooth and the other rough. The smooth side is applied next to the skin.

lipaemia (*lip-ē'-mi-a*). Presence of excess of fat in the blood.

lipase (*lī-pāz*). An enzyme in the pancreatic secretion which splits fat into glycerin and a fatty acid. Synonym, steapsin.

Lipiodol (*lip'-ī-od-ol*). Official name Oleum Iodisatum. A compound of iodine and oil, which is opaque to X-rays, and therefore is used for diagnostic examination. It is injected into the respiratory tract and other cavities of the body.

lipo-atrophy (*lī-pō-a-trō-fi*). Loss of subcutaneous fat. A complication which may arise in sites of insulin injections.

lipochondrodystrophy (*lī-pō-kon-drō-dis-tro-fi*). Term sometimes used to describe gargoylism or Hurler's syndrome.

lipodystrophy (*li-po-dis-tro-fi*). A disorder of fat metabolism which most commonly affects women who show little fat above the waist but are obese around the buttocks and legs.

lipoidosis (*li-poy-dō-sis*). Disturbance in metabolism of lipoids.

lipoids (*li-poyds*). Substances (*e.g.* lecithin) which resemble fats, in being dissolved by organic solvents such as alcohol and ether. They occur in living cells.

lipoma (*li-pō'-ma*). Tumour of fat cells.

lipotrophic substances (*li-pō-trō'-fik*). Factors such as choline and methionine, found in the diet and preventing excess of fat being deposited in the liver.

liquefaction (*li-kwe-fak-shon*). Being converted into a liquid.

liquor amnii (*lī-kwor am-nē-ē*). The watery fluid by which the fetus is surrounded.

liquor folliculi (*lī-kwor fo-li-kū-lē*). Fluid in a Graafian follicle.

liquores (*lī-kwor-ēz*). Solutions of active substances in water. *Liquor calcis saccharatus*, lime-water.

liquorice (*lik'-o-ris*). See GLYCYRRHIZA.

liquorice powder (*lik'or-is powder*). Contains senna; a purge for children.

Listerine (*lis'-ter-ēn*). A proprietary preparation containing many ingredients, of which the chief is boric acid. It is used as an antiseptic mouthwash.

Listerism. The principles of antiseptic surgery.

Liston's splint (*lis'-tonz splint*). To immobilize the hip; made of wood. Little used now.

LISTON'S SPLINT

lithagogues (*lith-'a-gogs*). Drugs which expel or dissolve stones.

lithiasis (*lith-ī'-a-sis*). Formation of stone.

litholapaxy (*li-thō-la-paks'-ē*). Operation for crushing a stone in the bladder and removing the fragments at the same time.

lithopaedion (*lith-ō-pĕd'-ion*). A calcified fetus in the abdominal cavity.

lithotomy (*li-tho-to-mi*). Operation of cutting into a bladder to remove a stone.

lithotomy position. Patient supine with thighs and knees flexed. The hips must be abducted.

LITHOTOMY POSITION

lithotrite (*lith'-ō-trīt*). An instrument for crushing stones in the bladder. It is passed through the urethra.

lithotrity (*lith-ot'-ri-ti*). Operation of crushing a stone in the bladder.

lithuria (*lith-ū-ri-a*). Passing gravel or crystals of uric acid with the urine.

litmus (*lit'-mus*). A blue pigment turned red by acids. *L. Paper.* Paper impregnated with litmus; used for testing urine and gastric secretion. A red litmus paper is turned blue by an alkali.

litre (*lē-ter*). Metric measure of volume. The volume of 1 kg water at 4° C; approximately 1¾ pint.

Little's disease. Spastic paraplegia or diplegia of infants due to birth injury or faulty development of the brain.

Littré's hernia (*lē-trā*). A diverticular hernia.

liver (*liv'-er*). Large organ occupying the upper right portion of the abdomen. It has many important functions including the secretion of bile, the manufacture of serum albumin and the storage of glycogen, etc.

UNDER SIDE OF LIVER

livid (*li'-vid*). Blue-grey in colour.

Loa Loa. One of the parasites causing filariasis.

lobar (*lō'-ba*). Pertaining to a lobe.

lobe (*lōb*). Rounded division of an organ.

lobectomy (*lō-bek'-to-mi*). Excision of a lobe.

lobule (*lo-būl*). Small lobe.

localized *lō-kal-īzd*). Limited to a certain area; not widespread.

lochia (*lo'-ki-a*). The vaginal discharge following delivery. For the first day or two is almost pure blood, but in normal cases becomes rapidly brown and then paler and ceases in a few weeks.

lock-jaw. *See* TETANUS.

locked twins. The condition of twins when some part of one absolutely prevents the birth of the other by causing complete impaction.

locomotor ataxia (*lō-kō-mō-tor a-tak'-sia*). Impaired gait in walking. A chronic disease due to degeneration of parts of the spinal cord and nerves. *See* TABES DORSALIS.

loculated (*lok'-ū-lā-ted*). Divided into many cavities.

locum tenens (*lō-kum tē'-nens*). A practitioner who temporarily takes the place of another.

loin (*loyn*). The lateral portion of the back between the thorax and pelvis.

longevity (*lon-gev'-i-ti*). Long life.

long-sight. Hypermetropia, *q.v.*

lordosis (*lor-dō'-sis*). Undue curvature of the spine with the convexity forwards; an exaggeration of the normal curve of the lumbar part of the spine.

←*lordosis*

Loreta's operation (*lo-ret-az*). Forcible dilatation of the pylorus for stricture.

lotio rubra (*lō'-ti-ō ru'-brah*). *See* RED LOTION.

lotion. A medicinal solution for external use.

loupe (*loop*). Magnifying lens used in ophthalmology.

louse (*lows*). *See* PEDICULUS.

Lovset's manoeuvre (*luv-sets ma-noo-ver*). An obstetrical manoeuvre used to deliver breech presentations with extended arms.

lower motor neurone disease. Disease affecting the lower motor neurone fibres. They arise from cell bodies in the anterior horns of the spinal cord and pass to the motor end plates of the muscles which they innervate. Lesions of the lower motor neurones result in paralysis and wasting of the muscles.

lower uterine segment (*lō-wer ū'-te-rĭn seg'-ment*). That portion of the uterus, consisting of the cervix and the lower end of the body, which undergoes dilatation during labour.

L.S.D. Lysergic acid. One of the hallucinogenic group of drugs.

lubricant (*loo-bri-kant*). Any substance, such as an oil, which makes a surface slippery.

'lubb-dupp'. The heart sounds. The first is heard when the atrio-ventricular valves close, the second on closure of the semilunar valves.

lucid (*loo'-sid*). Clear.

Ludwig's angina (*lood'-vig's an-jī'-na*). An acute inflammatory condition in the sublingual and submaxillary regions.

Lugol's solution (*loo'-gōl*). 5 per cent iodine in a 10 per cent aqueous solution of potassium iodide. The usual dose is 10 minims daily, prescribed in cases of exophthalmic goitre.

lumbago (*lum-bā'-gō*). Painful condition of the lumbar muscles, due to inflammation of their fibrous sheaths. May be caused by a displaced intervertebral disc.

lumbar (*lum'-ba*). Pertaining to the region of the loins.

lumbar puncture (*pungk-cher*) is the operation of tapping the cerebrospinal fluid in the lumbar region.

lumbar sympathectomy (*lumba sim-pa-thek-to-mi*). Operation to remove the sympathetic chain in the lumbar region.

lumen (*lū-men*). The cavity inside a tube.

Luminal. Phenobarbitone, *q.v.*

lunar caustic (*lū-na kors'-tik*). Nitrate of silver, used to cauterize wounds, or arrest the growth of exuberant granulations.

lungs. The two organs of respiration, situated in the right and left sides of the cavity of the chest.

Upper lobe

Upper lobe

Middle lobe

Lower lobes

ANTERIOR VIEW OF LUNGS

lunula (*lū'-nū-la*). White crescent at the root of the nail.

lupus erythematosus (*e-rith-em-a-tō-sus*). A disorder classed with the so-called collagen diseases. A localized form may affect the skin of exposed regions. The generalized form is known as systemic lupus erythematosus. The clinical manifestations of the disease are very varied. The criterion of diagnosis is the presence of L.E. cells in peripheral blood. L.E. cells are white cells which have ingested nuclear material.

lupus vulgaris (*loo-pus vul-ga-ris*). Tuberculosis affecting the skin.

luteinizing hormone (*lū-ti-nī-zing*). Hormone of the anterior pituitary gland stimulating the formation of corpus luteum (*q.v.*) in the ovary.

luteotrophin (*lū-tē-ō-trō-fin*). Pituitary hormone responsible for subsequent growth and development of the corpus luteum, after its formation by the follicle-stimulating hormone and the luteinizing hormone.

luteus (*loo'-tē-us*). Latin word for yellow. *See* MACULA LUTEA and CORPUS LUTEUM.

luxation (*luk-sā'-shon*). Dislocation of a joint.

lying-in (*lī-ing in'*). The puerperium.

lymph (*limf*). That part of the blood plasma which has passed through the walls of the capillaries, bathing the tissue cells, giving them nourishment and taking away waste products. It is also found in the lymphatic vessels and serous cavities.

lymphadenitis (*lim-fad-en-ī'-tis*). Inflammation of the lymphatic glands.

lymphadenoid goitre (*lim-fa-de-noyd goy-ter*). *See* HASHIMOTO'S DISEASE.

lymphadenoma (*lim-fa-de-nō'-ma*). Also called Hodgkin's disease. Serious disease characterized by enlargement of the lymphatic glands, and progressive anaemia, usually with enlargement of the spleen. There are often remissions, and it can be checked for a time by chemotherapy, X-rays, and surgical removal of localized groups of glands.

lymphangiectasis (*lim-fan-jē-ek'-ta-sis*). Dilated state of lymphatic vessels.

lymphangiogram (*lim-fan'-jē-ō-gram*). X-ray showing the lymph vessels by means of a dye.

lymphangioma (*lim-fan-jē-ō'-ma*). Tumour composed of lymphatic vessels.

lymphangioplasty (*lim-fan-jē-ō-pla'-sti*). An operation for the relief of lymphatic obstruction.

lymphangitis (*lim-fan-jī-tis*). Inflammation of lymphatic vessels.

lymphatic leukaemia (*lim-fat-ik lū-kēm-ia*). *See* LEUKAEMIA.

lymphatics (*lim-fat'-iks*). Small vessels pervading the body, and containing lymph.

lymphocytes (*lim'-fō-sīts*). One of the normal varieties of white blood corpuscles. *Lymphocytosis*, excess of these cells in the blood; found in leukaemia, whooping cough, tuberculosis and lymphadenoma. *Lymphopenia*, deficiency of lymphocytes.

lymphocythaemia (*lim-fō-sī-tē'-mea*). Increase of lymphocytes in the bloodstream.

lymphocytosis (*lim-fō-sī-tō'-sis*). Lymphocythaemia, *q.v.*

lymphogranuloma inguinale (*lim-fō-gra-nū-lō-ma in-gwi-na-lā*). A venereal disease found esp. in the tropics.

lymphoid (*limf-oyd*). Having the character of lymph. *L. Tissue*, adenoid tissue.

lymphoma (*lim-fō'-ma*). Tumour of lymphatic tissue.

lymphosarcoma (*lim-fō-sar-kō'-ma*). A sarcoma originating in lymphatic tissue.

lysergic acid (*lī-ser-jik*). See L.S.D.

lysine (*lī-sēn*). See AMINO-ACIDS.

lysins (*lī'-sins*). Antibodies able to dissolve cells. *Haemolysins*, those able to dissolve red blood cells. *Bacteriolysins*, those able to dissolve bacteria.

lysis (*lī-sis*). Dissolution. Decline of a fever.

Lysol (*lī'-sol*). A powerful antiseptic, being a solution of cresol in soap solution. Usual strength, ½ to 1 drachm in a pint of water. It has a solvent action on grease and mucus. *See also* SUDOL.

lysozyme (*lī-sō-zīm*). Bactericide found in tears, nasal mucus and other secretions.

M

m. Abbreviation for metre; minim.

M. and B. 693, M. and B. 760. *See* SULPHONAMIDE DRUGS.

McBurney's point. On line from umbilicus to anterior superior iliac spine, at outer edge of rectus muscle; corresponds to base of the appendix, and pressure here will give rise to pain when appendix is inflamed.

maceration (*mas-e-rā'-shon*). The softening of a solid by soaking it in a liquid; or of a foetus which has died some time before delivery.

Mackenrodt's ligaments (*ma-ken-rōtz li-ga-mens*). Also called transverse cervical or cardinal ligaments. One of the chief supports of the uterus.

McNaghten rules. Provisions necessary to establish diminished criminal responsibility on the grounds of insanity.

macro (*mak-rō*). Prefix meaning large.

macrocephalous (*mak-rō-kef'-a-lus*). Having a large head.

macrocheilia (*ma-krō-kī-li-a*). Excessively large lips.

macrocytes (*mak'-ro-sīts*). Abnormally large corpuscles, present in the blood in certain types of anaemia.

macrodactyly (*mak-rō-dak'-ti-li*). Enlargement of the fingers.

macroglossia (*mak-rō-glos'-ia*). Hypertrophy of the tongue.

macromastia (*mak-rō-mas'-ti-a*). Abnormally developed breasts.

macrophage (*ma-krō-fāj*). Wandering scavenger cells which form part of the reticulo-endothelial system, *q.v.* Their function is to engulf tissue debris and foreign particles. In connective tissue they are termed *histiocytes* and in the blood they are known as *monocytes*. The engulfment of material is termed phagocytosis, *q.v.*

macroscopic (*mak-rō-skop'-ik*). Visible to the naked eye.

macula (*mak'-ū-la*). A spot discolouring the skin. *M. Lutea*, central spot of the posterior surface of the retina, just lateral to the optic disc marked by a small depression, and where vision is most acute.

maculopapular (*ma-kū-lō-pa'-pū-la*). A rash having both macules and papules.

Madura foot (*mad-ū-ra*). *See* MYCETOMA.

Magendie, foramen of (*maj-en-di*). An opening in the roof of the fourth ventricle through which the cerebrospinal fluid passes into the subarachnoid space.

magnesium carbonate (*mag-nē-sē-um kar-bo-nāt*). An antacid and mild laxative.

magnesium hydroxide (*hī-drok-sīd*). An antacid and mild laxative but does not give off carbon dioxide as *m. carbonate* does. The hydroxide is used as an antidote in poisoning from mineral acids or arsenic.

magnesium sulphate (*sul-fāt*). Saline purgative and used externally to treat boils.

magnesium trisilicate (*trī-si-li-kāt*). An antacid used in treatment of gastric ulcer. Has a laxative effect.

mal. Sickness. Mal de mer, sea sickness. Grand mal, major epilepsy. Petit mal, minor epilepsy.

malabsorption (*ma-lab-sorp-shon*). Reduced ability to absorb substances in the food from causes such as intestinal hurry, loss of absorbing surface as in extensive bowel resections, and diseases affecting the bowel including tropical sprue, coeliac disease and idiopathic steatorrhoea.

malacia (*mal-ā'-ki-a*). Pathological softening.

maladjustment (*mal-a-just'-ment*). Not in line, as with a badly set bone. In psychology, poorly adapted to circumstances.

malaise (*mal'-āz*). A general feeling of illness or discomfort.

malar (*mā'-lar*). Relating to the cheekbone. *See illustration,* p. 225.

malaria (*ma-lār-ia*). A disease due to a parasite introduced into the blood by certain mosquitoes. *See* ANOPHELES.

male fern. Filix mas, *q.v.*

malformation *mal-faw-mā-shon*). Congenital deformity.

malignant (*ma-lig'-nant*). Virulent, fatal. A *malignant tumour* or *growth* is one which if not totally removed will spread and cause similar growths in other parts of the body until the patient dies, *e.g.* carcinoma, sarcoma.

malignant hypertension. Hypertension associated with papilloedema and evidence of renal failure.

malignant pustule. Anthrax contracted from cattle, causing gangrenous carbuncle.

malingering (*ma-ling'-ger-ing*). Shamming sickness.

malleolus (*mal-le'-ō-lus*). The projection of the ankle-bone. The inner malleolus is at the lower extremity of the tibia. The outer one at the lower extremity of the fibula.

mallet finger. Deformed finger with flexion of distal phalanx.

malleus (*mal'-le-us*). A hammer-shaped bone of the middle ear. *See* EAR.

malnutrition (*mal-nū-tri'-shon*). A state of undernourishment or imperfect nutrition.

malocclusion (*ma-lo-kloo-zhon*). Bad contact between the masticating surfaces of the upper and lower teeth.

Malpighian corpuscle (*mal-pig-ian kor-pusl*). Mesh of capillaries which act as a filtering coil for blood passing through the kidneys.

malpresentation (*mal-prez-en-tā'-shon*). Any presentation, other than the vertex, of the fetus at birth.

malt (*mawlt*). Grain of barley which has begun to sprout and has then been dried. It contains a ferment (malt diastase) which converts starch into sugar.

Malta fever. *See* UNDULANT FEVER.

maltase (*mawl-tāz'*). An enzyme of the succus entericus which converts maltose into glucose.

maltose (*mawl-tōz*). A disaccharide composed of two molecules of glucose.

malunion (*mal-ū'-ni-on*). Faulty union of divided tissues, as of the fragments of a broken bone.

mamilla (*ma-mil'-la*). The nipple.

mammae (*mam'-mē*). The breasts, or milk-supplying glands.

mammaplasty (*ma-ma-pla'-sti*). Plastic surgery on the breasts such as that done to reduce the size of very heavy breasts.

mammary (*mam'-ma-ri*). Relating to the breasts.

Manchester repair. A type of gynaecological operation for uterovaginal prolapse.

mandelic acid (*man-dē-lik*). Urinary antiseptic given as ammonium mandelate.

mandible (*man'-di-bl*). The lower jaw. (*See illustration*, p. 225.)

Mandl's paint (*man'-dlz pānt*). An antiseptic paint containing tincture of iodine, used in tonsillitis.

mania (*mā'-nia*). Pathological combination of elation and energy. The patient is uncontrollably excited.

manic depressive psychosis (*sī-kō-sis*). A mental illness when intense excitement alternates with depression.

manipulation (*ma-nip-ū-lā'-shon*). Handling, rubbing and working with the hands to procure some healing result.

mannerism (*ma'-ne-rizm*). Habitual expression or actions of an individual which are characteristic of him. Under stress they may become exaggerated.

manoeuvre (*ma-noo'-ver*). Special movement by the hand or with an instrument.

manometer (*man-om'-e-ter*). An instrument for measuring the pressure of gases and liquids.

Mantoux test (*man-too'*). Test of the body's reaction to antigenic material prepared from tubercle bacilli. This material called tuberculin is injected intradermally in serial dilutions (1 in 10,000; 1 in 1,000; 1 in 100). A localized inflammatory reaction within 48 hours signifies a positive response.

manual (*man'-nū-al*) (adjective). Done by hand.

manubrium sterni (*man-ū'-bri-um ster'-nē*). The uppermost part of the sternum, *q.v.*

manus (*ma-nus*). Latin for hand.

marasmus (*ma-ras'-mus*). Progressive emaciation.

marble bone disease. Disease which may be familial, with osteosclerosis of the entire skeleton, the spongy part of the bone becoming compact. There is also anaemia.

Marfan's syndrome (*mar-fans sin-drōm*). *See* ARACHNODACTYLY.

marihuana (*ma-roo-ah-na*). *See* CANNABIS INDICA.

Marmite (*mar'-mīt*). A proprietary preparation of dried yeast rich in vitamin B. Can be used for soups or sandwiches.

marrow (*ma'-rō*). The soft substance which fills the medullary canal of a long bone and the small spaces in cancellous bone. The red cells of the blood are formed in the red bone marrow.

marrow puncture (*ma-rō pung-cher*). Investigative procedure involving the aspiration of marrow cells, usually by puncturing the sternum with a needle.

masochism (*ma'-zo-kism*). A delight in being tortured or humiliated from which a sexual pleasure may be derived.

Mason's gag (*mā'-sonz*). A mouth gag.

MASON'S GAG

massage (*ma'-sahj*). Manipulation and rubbing of body designed to promote blood flow.

masseter (*mas-sē'-ter*). A strong facial muscle which moves the lower jaw. (*See below.*)

THE MASSETER MUSCLE

masseur (*mas-ser'*). A male physiotherapist.

masseuse (*mas-ser'z*). A female physiotherapist.

mastalgia (*mas-tal-ji-a*). Pain in the breast.

mast-cells. The basophile cells of the blood and tissues.

mastectomy (*mas-tek-to-mi*). Surgical removal of the breast. *Radical M.* The breast is removed together with the lymph glands of the axilla and the pectoral muscle.

mastication (*mas-tik-ā'-shon*). Chewing.

mastitis (*mas-tī'-tis*). Inflammation of the breast.

mastodynia (*mas-tō-di-ni-a*). Pain in the breasts often in the premenstrual phase.

mastoid (*mas'-toyd*). Literally, breastlike. The *mastoid process* is the projecting portion of the temporal bone behind the ear; it contains numerous air spaces including the *mastoid antrum.*

mastoidectomy (*mas-toy-dek'-to-mi*). Excision of the inflamed mastoid cells.

mastoiditis (*mas-toyd-ī'-tis*). Inflammation of the mastoid antrum and cells.

mastoidotomy (*mas-toy-do-to-mi*). Incision of cells of mastoid process.

masturbation (*mas-ter-bā'-shon*). Excitation of one's own genitals to produce an orgasm.

materia medica (*mat-er-ia-med'-ik-a*). Branch of medical study dealing with the nature and use of drugs, *i.e.* pharmacology and therapeutics.

matrix (*mā-triks*). Continuous medium in which structures are embedded.

matter. Any substance. Pus is sometimes referred to as matter. *Grey M.* The nerve cells or non-medulled nerve fibres. *White M.* Medullated nerve fibres which are enveloped by a white sheath.

mattress suture. A continuous stitch through both the skin edges.

maturation (*mat-ū-rā'-shon*). Ripening: the process of becoming fully developed.

maxilla (*mak-si'-la*). The upper jaw-bone. *See illustration.*

THE MAXILLA

maxillary (*mak-sil'-a-ri*). Pertaining to the maxilla.

mean (*mēn*). The average.

measles, morbilli (*mē-zels*). An infectious disease common in children. Incubation period 10 to 12 days. Early symptoms are those of a cold, sore throat, cough and rise in temperature, Koplik's spots. The rash appears on the fourth day, about the neck and behind the ears, gradually spreading to the rest of the body and extremities. The normal is reached about the seventh or ninth day. Most infectious period is before

the rash appears. *German measles*, Rubella, *q.v.*

meatus (*mē-ā'-tus*). An opening into a passage.

mecamylamine hydrochloride (*me-ka-mi-la-mīn hī-drō-klaw-rīd*). A ganglion-blocking agent used to treat high blood pressure.

mechanism of labour (*mek'-an-izm*). The series of forces which act upon the foetus while it is being driven through the birth canal, with the resistances to those forces, and the resulting effects of both upon the attitude and movements of the foetus.

Meckel's diverticulum (*me-kels dī-ver-tik'-ū-lum*). A small blind protrusion occasionally found in the lower portion of the ileum. In rare cases it produces acute intestinal obstruction by strangulating an adjacent coil of gut.

meconium (*me-kō'-ne-um*). A black, sticky substance voided from the bowels of an infant during the first day or two after its birth.

medial (*mē-di-al*). The middle.

median (*mē-di-an*). In the middle. *M. Line*, an imaginary longitudinal line dividing the body down the centre. *M. Nerve*, one of the nerves of the arm.

mediastinum (*mē-di-as-tī'-num*). The space in the chest between the two lungs. It contains the heart, glands and important vessels.

medical jurisprudence (*jūris-prū'-dens*). Medicine as it is connected with the law; for instance, in case of suicide or murder.

medicament (*med-ik'-a-ment*). Any medicinal drug or application.

medicated (*me-di-kā-ted*). Impregnated with a medicament.

medication (*me-di-kā'-shon*). Giving a medicine to a patient. *Pre-operative M.* One given before an operation as a basal anaesthetic.

medicinal (*me-di'-si-nal*). Pertaining to the science of medicine or to a drug.

medicine (*me'-di-sin*). The treatment of disease. A drug used to prevent or treat disease. Term often used for diseases for which surgery is not required.

medico-chirurgical (*me-di-kō-ki-rur-ji-kal*). Relating to both medicine and surgery.

medico-social worker. Specially trained worker in hospital concerned with the patient in the community. Formerly called hospital almoner.

Medinal. Barbitone sodium. A hypnotic drug.

Mediterranean fever (*med-it-e-rān-ian*). *Same as* UNDULANT FEVER, MALTA FEVER.

medium (*mē'-di-um*). Material used to nourish cultures of tissues, cells and micro-organisms.

Medresco. Hearing aid provided under the National Health Service.

medulla (*med-ul'-a*). Latin for marrow.

medulla oblongata. The lowest part of the brain where it passes through the foramen magnum and becomes the spinal cord. It contains the vital centres which govern circulation and respiration. *See* BRAIN.

medullary (*me-dul'-la-ri*). Relating to the marrow.

medullated (*mē'-du-lā-ted*). With an enveloping medulla or marrow.

medullated nerve fibre. Nerve fibre surrounded by a myelin, *q.v.*, sheath.

medulloblastoma (*me-du-lō-bla-stō'-ma*). Malignant tumour, from embryonic cells of neuro-epithelial origin, occurring in the cerebellum.

megacephaly (*me-ga-ke'-fa-li*). An abnormally large head.

megacolon (*meg-a-kō'-lon*). Hirschsprung's disease, *q.v.*

megakaryocytes (*me-ga-ka-ri-ō-sīts*). Large bone marrow cells which produce the blood platelets, *q.v.*

megalo (*me-ga-lō*). Prefix meaning large.

megaloblast (*meg-alō'-blast*). An abnormally large nucleated blood cell. Megaloblasts occur in the blood in pernicious anaemia. Also known as macrocytes.

megalokaryocytes (*me-ga-lō-ka'-ri-ō-sīts*). *See* MEGAKARYOCYTES.

megalomania (*meg-al-ō-mā'-nia*). Insanity with delusional ideas of personal greatness.

Megimide (*me-ji-mīd*). Proprietary preparation of bemegride, *q.v.*

Meibomian glands (*mī-bō'mian*). Sebaceous glands of the eyelids, M. Cyst, Chalazion, *q.v.*

Meigs' syndrome (*mīgs sindrōm*). Ascites and hydrothorax associated with ovarian fibroma.

meiosis (*mī-ō-sis*). (1) Successive divisions of diploid cell to yield haploid gametes. The gametes (spermatozoa, ova) must have their chromosome number reduced by half in order to compensate for the doubling which occurs by fertilization. (2) Contraction of pupil of eye.

mel. Honey.

melaena (*mel-ē'-na*). Black tarlike stools, due to the presence of blood which has undergone changes in the alimentary tract. The blood is often from a gastric or duodenal ulcer.

melancholia (*mel-an-kō'-li-a*). Morbid depression, a form of insanity. There is often obstinate constipation and a strong suicidal tendency.

melanin. A name for the dark pigments found in the eye, skin, hair, Addison's disease, etc.

melanoma (*mel-an-ō'-ma*). A tumour containing black pigment, melanin. May start as innocent pigmented wart, but possesses tendency to malignancy. (Malignant melanoma or melanotic carcinoma.)

melanosis (*mel-an-ō'-sis*). Black spots in the tissues.

membrane (*mem-brān*). A thin layer of tissue.

menaphthonum. Vitamin K.

menarche (*me-nar-kā*). The beginning of menstruation.

Mendel's law (*men'-delz lor*). A theory that the offspring do not inherit the characteristics of the parents in equal or intermediate proportions, but that certain characteristics of each parent are predominant, and are therefore transmitted to the offspring in full measure.

Ménière's disease (*mā-nē-ārs*). Giddiness resulting from disease of the internal ear or the equilibrating mechanism of the brain.

meningeal (or *men-in-jē'-al*). Pertaining to the meninges.

meninges (*me-nin'-jēz*). The membranes surrounding and covering the brain and spinal cord. They are, from without: the dura mater, the arachnoid, the pia mater.

meningioma (*me-nin-jē-ō'-ma*). Tumour derived from the meninges.

meningism (*men-in-jis'-m*). Syndrome characterized by symptoms and signs of meningitis but occurring in the absence of any causative organism. Probably a non-specific inflammatory reaction of the meninges to circulating toxins or some other trauma.

meningitis (*men-in-jī'-tis*). Inflammation of the meninges due to infection by organisms. Acute bacterial or viral meningitis is characterized by fever, headache, vomiting, backache and development of a stiff neck. Stupor, coma, convulsions may follow. A more insidious onset is sometimes seen in tuberculous meningitis.

meningocele (*men-in'-jō-sēl*). Protrusion of meninges from a bony defect usually in the spine, *e.g.* spina bifida.

meningococcus (*men-in'-jō-kok'-us*). A micro-organism, the cause of cerebrospinal fever.

meniscectomy (*me-nisk-ek-to-mi*). Removal of a semilunar cartilage from the knee joint.

meniscus (*me-nis-kus*). (1) A semilunar cartilage. (2) A lens. (3) The crescent-like surface of a liquid in a narrow tube.

menopause (*men'-ō-pawz*). Cessation of menstruation. Ovulation stops and reproductive life ends. It usually occurs between 40 and 50 years of age and is associated with alterations in hormonal balance which sometimes produce troublesome symptoms such as hot flushes, etc.

menorrhagia (*men-o-rā-ji-a*). Excessive menstrual bleeding.

menses (*men-sēz*). The menstrual flow.

menstruation (*men-stroo-ā'-shon*). Monthly discharge of uterine mucosa with resultant bleeding which occurs in the absence of pregnancy in sexually mature women.

mental (*men'-tal*). (1) Pertaining to the mind. (2) Pertaining to the chin.

mental defective. See IDIOCY.

Mental Welfare Officer. A local authority official concerned with mental health and the care of the mentally retarded and the mentally disordered.

menthol (*men'-thol*). A local anodyne.

mento-anterior (*an-te'-rē-or*). The ordinary kind of face presentation, with the chin to the front; *i.e.* towards the maternal pubes.

mento-posterior (*pos-tār-ior*). Having the chin behind. A term applied to a variety of face presentation. See FACE PRESENTATION.

mepacrine hydrochloride (*mep-a-krin hi-drō-klor'-īd*). Used in the prophylaxis and treatment of malaria.

meprobamate (*me-prō-ba-māt*). A relaxant and tranquillizer. The drug is anticonvulsant and sedative.

mepyramine (*me-pi-ra-mēn*). An antihistamine drug used in some allergic conditions.

meralgia paraesthetica (*me-ral'-ji-a par-ēs-thet-'i-ka*). An affection of the nerves of the lumbar plexus giving rise to pain and sensory disturbances in the legs.

mercaptopurine (*mer-kap-to-pū-rin*). Cell-destroying drug used in the treatment of leukaemia.

mercurialism (*mer-kū'-ri-al-ism*). Chronic poisoning by mercury occasionally is seen as a result of continuous administration of mercury for medical purposes. Also occurs in workmen who labour with the metal, or inhale its vapours. *Symptoms:* (1) soreness of gums and loosening of teeth; (2) increased salivation; (3) foetor of breath; (4) griping and diarrhoea. Antidote, p. 389.

mercurochrome (*mer-kū'-rō-krōm*). A red compound of mercury and fluorescein used as an antiseptic, applied to the skin or mucous membrane as 1 to 2 per cent solution.

mercury (*mer'-kū-ri*). Sometimes used as a purgative when given as mercurous chloride. Some salts of mercury are antiseptic and some are parasiticides and fungicides. Its salts are poisonous in concentrated form, and the antidotes are white of egg and milk and water. *See* MERCURIALISM and CALOMEL.

mersalyl (*mer'-sal-il*). A complex mercurial compound. It is a diuretic occasionally used for oedema of cardiac and renal origin. In the latter case there are limitations to its use. Administered intravenously or intramuscularly.

mesarteritis (*mes-ar-ter-ī'-tis*). Inflammation of the middle coat of an artery.

mesencephalon (*mes-en-kef'-a-lon*). The midbrain.

mesenchyme (*me-sen-kīm*). Embryonic connective tissue which forms bone, cartilage, connective tissue and blood, etc.

mesenteric (*mes-en-ter'-ik*). Pertaining to the mesentery.

mesentery (*mes'-en-ter-i*). A large fold of the peritoneum to which the small intestines are attached.

THE MESENTERY

mesmerism (*mez'-mer-izm*). Hypnosis, *q.v.*

meso-appendix (*mes-ō-ap-en'-diks*). The mesentery of the appendix vermiformis.

mesocolon (*mes-ō-kō'-lon*). The fold of the peritoneum attached to the colon.

mesoderm (*mes'-o-derm*). Germ layer of cells which have migrated from the surface of the developing embryo during gastrulation and which is situated between the ectoderm and the endoderm. The mesoderm gives rise to muscle, blood and connective tissues, etc.

mesometrium (*mes-ō-mē'-tri-um*). The broad ligaments which attach the uterus to the sides of the pelvis.

mesosalpinx (*mes-ō-sal'-pinks*). The part of the broad ligament which lies immediately below the Fallopian tubes.

mesothelium (*me-sō-thē-li-um*). General term applied to the epithelium lining serous cavities.

mesovarium (*mes-ō-vār'-i-um*). A short peritoneal fold connecting the ovary to the posterior layer of the broad ligament.

metabolic (*met-a-bol'-ik*). Pertaining to metabolism.

metabolism (*met-a'-bol-izm*). The changes in the tissues of an animal due to the fact that it is alive; constructive or building-up processes, anabolism and destructive or breaking-down processes, katabolism, are continually going on in the cells.

metacarpals (*met-a-kar-pals*). The five bones of the hand joining the fingers to the wrist.

metacarpophalangeal (*me-ta-kar-pō-fal-an-jē-al*). Relating to the metacarpus and the phalanges.

metamorphosis (*me-ta-mor-fō'-sis*). Transformation.

METACARPALS

metaphysis (*me-ta'-fi-sis*). Part between the shaft, diaphysis, *q.v.*, and the end, epiphysis, *q.v.*, of the long bones.

metaplasia (*met-a-plā'-zi-a*). Conversion of one tissue into another.

metastasis (*me-tas'-ta-sis*). Transfer or spreading of a disease from one organ to another which is remote. A malignant growth is spread in this way.

metatarsalgia (*met'-a-tar-sal'-ji-a*). Pain in the fore part of the foot).

metatarsals (*met-a-tar'-sals*). The five bones of the foot between the tarsus and the toes. *See* p. 232.

meteorism (*mē-tē-or-ism*). Distension of the intestines by gas.

methadone hydrochloride (*me-tha-dōn hī-drō-klor-id*). Analgesic used to relieve severe pain. Also called amidone hydrochloride.

methaemoglobin (*met-hē-mō-glō-bin*). Altered haemoglobin producing cyanosis.

os calcis

metatarsals
1
2
3
4
5

proximal
middle
distal
phalanges

METATARSALS

methaemoglobinuria (*met-hē-mo-glo-bin-ū'-ri-a*). The passage of methaemoglobin in the urine.

methandienone (*me-than-di-e-nōn*). An anabolic steroid derived from testosterone.

methicillin (*me-thi-si-lin*). Antibiotic used for penicillin-resistant staphylococci.

methionine (*me-thē-ō-nīn*). An essential amino-acid containing sulphur. Used in liver damage and hepatitis.

methotrexate (*me-thō-trek-sāt*) Folic acid antagonist used in leukaemia.

methyl (*me-thil*). The chemical radical—CH₃.

methylamphetamine hydrochloride (*me-thil-am-fe-ta-mēn hī-drō-klor-īd*). Drug stimulating the central nervous system and raising blood pressure. Can be used to counteract poisoning by morphine or the barbiturates.

methylated spirit (*me-thi-lā-ted*). Ordinary ethyl alcohol to which some methyl alcohol has been added in order to give it a nauseous taste and odour.

methyldopa (*me-thil-dō-pa*). Drug used to lower the blood pressure.

methylene blue (*meth-il-ēn bloo*). A dye which is also used as an antiseptic.

methylpentynol (*me-thil-pen-ti-nol*). A sedative and tranquillizer.

methyl phenidate (*me-thil fe-ni-dāt*). An anti-depressant drug.

methyl salicylate (*me-thil sal'-is-il-āt*). The active principle of gaultheria oil (oil of wintergreen). Used as an external application for the relief of pain in the joints.

methyltestosterone (*me-thil-tes-tos-te-rōn*). Oral form of testosterone, *q.v.*

methylthiouracil (*meth-il-thī-ūr-a-sil*). A compound of sulphur and urea prescribed in thyrotoxicosis. It inhibits the secretion of thyroxine.

metra (*me'-tra*). The womb.

metre (*mē'-ter*). A measure of length, containing 100

centimetres, and equal to 39·370 in.

metric system (*met'rik sis-tem*). System of weights and measures employing the metre and the gram as standard units which are multiplied or divided by powers of ten.

metritis (*me-trī-tis*). Inflammation of the womb.

metrocolpocele (*met-rō-kol'-pō-sēl*). Protrusion of the uterus into the vagina, the wall of the vagina being pushed in advance.

metronidazole (*me-trō-ni-da-zōl*). Drug used for trichomonal infections.

metropathia haemorrhagica (*me-trō-pa'-thia hē-mō-ra'-ji-ka*). Excessive menstrual bleeding due to excess of oestrin and associated with follicular ovarian cysts.

metroptosis (*met-rop-tō-sis*) Prolapse of the womb.

metrorrhagia (*met-ro-rā'-ji-a*). Bleeding from the uterus, other than at the menstrual period. It should always be investigated, as it is usually due to some pathological condition.

Meulengracht's diet (*moy'-len-gratz*). Diet used to treat gastric ulcer.

Mg. Chemical symbol for magnesium.

Michel's clips (*mi-chels*). Small metal clips used for suturing skin wounds after surgical operations. A special forceps is necessary for their removal.

MICHEL CLIP-REMOVING FORCEPS

micro (*mī-krō*). Prefix meaning small.

microbe (*mī-krōb*). Micro-organism. *See* BACTERIA, VIRUS.

microbiology (*mī-krō-bī-o-lo-ji*). The study of micro-organisms.

microcephalic (*mī-krō-kef-al'-ik*). Having an abnormally small head.

micrococci (*mī-krō-kok'-kī*). Genus of bacteria, *q.v.*

microcyte (*mī-krō-sīt*). A small red blood corpuscle.

microcythaemia (*mī-krō-sīt-hē'-mi-a*). Circulation of abnormally small erythrocytes in the blood.

microcytic anaemia (*mī-krō-si-tik*). Due to iron deficiency. The red cells in the blood are smaller than normal. The treatment is to give large doses of iron.

microgram (*mī-kro-gram*). µg. One millionth part of a gram, *q.v.*

micrometer (*mī-krom'-e-ter*). Instrument for measuring very small distances.

micron (*mī′-kron*). A millionth part of a metre, represented by the Greek letter µ.

micro-organism (*mī-krō-or′-gan-izm*). Any microscopic plant or animal.

microphthalmos (*mī-krof-thal′-mos*). Abnormal smallness of the eyes.

microscope (*mī-kro-skōp*). An instrument which magnifies minute objects invisible to the naked eye.

lenses of eyepiece

lenses of objective

stage

condenser lenses

slide

light

adjusting screws

MICROSCOPE

microsporon (*mī-krō-spo′-ron*). A fungus causing disease of the skin and hair.

microtome (*mī′-krō-tōm*). An instrument for cutting fine sections for microscopic examination.

micturition (*mik-tū-rish′-on*). The act of passing urine.

midbrain (*mid-brān*). Small part of the brain between the forebrain and hindbrain.

midriff (*mid′-rif*). The diaphragm, *q.v.*

midwife (*mid′-wīf*). A woman who conducts the confinement of another.

midwifery (*mid′-wif-ri*). The art and science of the conduct of pregnancy, labour and the puerperium.

migraine (*mē-grān′*). Paroxysmal attacks of headache, usually with nausea and often preceded by disorders of vision. Migraine is usually unilateral.

miliaria papillosa (*mi-lē-ā-ri-a pa-pi-lō-za*). Prickly heat; an affection due to a disorder of the sweat glands. Their ducts are obstructed.

miliary (*mil-i-a-ri*). Like millet seed. Thus *miliary tuberculosis* is an acute form of infection in which the tissues are studded with small tubercles so as to resemble a mass of millet seeds.

milium (*mil′-i-um*). Small white round tumour, the size of a pin's head, which results from obstruction of the duct of a sebaceous gland. Occurs chiefly on forehead, eyelids, cheeks.

milk. The secretion of mammary glands. The average composition is:

	Human Milk		Cow's Milk	
	%		%	
Protein:—				
Lactalbumin	1·4	2	·75	4
Casein	·6		3·25	
Fat . .	4		4	
Carbohydrate	6		4	
Salt . .	·2		·7	
Water .	87·8		87·3	

Human milk is neutral or slightly alkaline. Cow's milk is usually slightly acid by the time it reaches the consumer. Specific gravity 1026 to 1036.

milk sugar. See LACTOSE.

milk teeth. The first set of teeth. See TEETH.

Miller-Abbott tube. A double-bore rubber tube which is passed via the mouth into the duodenum so that intestinal suction can be applied in obstruction of the upper intestinal tract.

milliampere (*mil-i-ahm-pār*). One thousandth part of an ampere.

millicurie (*mi-li-kū-ri*). Unit of radioactivity, one thousandth of a curie.

milligram (*mil'-i-gram*). One thousandth part of a gram.

millilitre (*mil-i-lē-tr*). One thousandth part of a litre. Abr. ml. It is taken as equivalent to a cc.

millimetre (*mi-li-mē-tr*). One thousandth part of a metre.

Millin's prostatectomy (*mil-lins pros-ta-tek-to-mi*). In this operation the bladder is not incised but the prostate gland is enucleated from around the neck of the bladder. Also called retropubic prostatectomy.

Milton (*mil'-ton*). Proprietary antiseptic containing sodium hypochlorite.

miner's nystagmus. Nystagmus, *q.v.*, due to insufficient light striking the retina.

minim (*min'-im*). The sixtieth part of a fluid drachm; practically one drop.

miosis (*mī-ō-sis*). Syn. meiosis.

miotic (*mī-o-tik*). Syn. meiotic. Term applied to a drug which contracts the pupil of the eye.

miscarriage (*mis-ka'-rāj*). See ABORTION.

Misuse of Drugs Act 1971. This Act supersedes the Dangerous Drugs Act. It controls possession and supply of certain habit-forming narcotic drugs and others producing profound effects on the central nervous system. All drugs coming under the Act and its Regulations are known as Controlled Drugs.

mitosis (*mi-tō'-sis*). A method of cell division.

mitral valve (*mī-tral val'v*). The valve of the heart between the left atrium and the left ventricle. Disease of this valve may give rise to *mitral stenosis* when there is narrowing of the orifice of the valve or *mitral regurgitation* or *incompetence* when the valve fails to close properly.

mittelschmerz (*mi-tel-shmā-rz*). Pain occurring at the time of ovulation allegedly due to peritoneal irritation by blood from the ruptured follicle.

ml. Millilitre, *q.v.*

modiolus (*mō-di-ō'-lus*). Central axis of the cochlea.

molar teeth (*mō'-lar tēth*). The grinders. See TEETH.

mole (*mōl*). (1) Hairy, pigmented raised area of skin.

(2) In obstetric practice, a tumour composed of coagulated blood, fetal membranes and the embryo; due to haemorrhage into a gestation sac, and followed sooner or later by abortion. *Carneous* or *Fleshy M.* When mole is retained in utero for some time, the fluid part of the blood-clot becomes absorbed, leaving solid fleshy masses, in the midst of which traces of the embryo may or may not be found. *Hydatidiform* or *Vesicular M.* Degeneration of the chorion in the early weeks of pregnancy, resulting in the death of the embryo and the conversion of the chorionic villi into beadlike cysts or vesicles which may attain the size of a grape. Two prominent symptoms are (*a*) undue enlargement of the uterus for the period of amenorrhoea, (*b*) a watery pink discharge which may contain vesicles. No fetal parts are felt and no fetal heart heard, and the uterus feels softer than in a normal pregnancy. As soon as diagnosed the uterus should be emptied. The villi may become malignant, and invade the wall of the uterus. It is then known as *Chorionepithelioma*.

molecule (*mol'-e-kūl*). A combination of atoms forming a definite substance. Thus one atom of sodium with one atom of chlorine forms one molecule of sodium chloride.

molluscum (*mol-us-kum*). Skin disease, either *contagiosum*, common in childhood, or *fibrosum*, involving the formation of overgrowths of fibro-cellular tissue.

Mönckeberg's arteriosclerosis (*mernk-bergs ar-tār'-ē-ō-skle-rō'-sis*). Sclerosis of the medium and small arteries with extensive degeneration of the middle muscle lining, with atrophy and calcareous deposits in the muscle cells.

mongolism (*mon-go-lism*). Down's syndrome. Due to abnormality of chromosome 21 occurring during meiosis. A chromosome pair fails to separate with the result that the child has a chromosome too many, *i.e.* 47 instead of 46. Mongols usually have slanting eyes, short head, hypotonia and a low I.Q.

Monilia (*mo-ni'-lia*). A yeast, which is liable to infect mucous membranes, giving rise to thrush.

monitoring. A recording, usually by automatic means, of the patient's blood pressure, temperature, pulse and respiration.

mono (*mo-nō*). Prefix meaning one.

mono-amine oxidase inhibitor. Drug which relieves depression by preventing breakdown of serotonin and other amines in brain tissue, *e.g.* phenelzine. During treatment, alcohol and foods rich in tyramine, *e.g.* cheese, should be avoided.

monocular (*mo-nok'-ū-lar*). Relating to one eye only.

monocyte (*mo-nō-sīt*). A cell with one nucleus.

monocytosis (*mo-nō-sī-tō-sis*). Term employed when monocytes comprise more than 8 per cent of the total white cell count.

monograph (*mon'-ō-graf*). Book on one subject only.

monomania (*mon-ō-mā'-ni-a*). A neurosis when the patient has fixed ideas on one particular subject.

mononuclear (*mo-nō-nū-klē-a*). With one nucleus.

monoplegia (*mon-ō-plē'-ji-a*). Paralysis of one limb.

monorchid, monorchis (*mon-or'-kid*). Having only one testicle.

monosaccharide (*mon-ō-sak'-ar-īd*). Simplest sugar, *e.g.* glucose.

Monro's foramen (*mun-rōz*). Interventricular foramen. The communication between the two lateral ventricles and the third ventricle of the brain.

monster (*mon'-ster*). An abnormal individual owing to fetal maldevelopment.

mons veneris (*monz ven'-e-ris*). The eminence just over the os pubis in women.

Montgomery's glands (*muntgum'-er-ēz glanz*). Small prominences about the nipple, which become more evident during pregnancy and lactation. *See also* AREOLA.

Mooren's ulcer (*moo-renz*). Basal cell carcinoma affecting the cornea.

morbid (*mor'-bid*). Diseased, disordered, pathological.

morbilli (*mor-bil-ē*). Measles, *q.v.*

morbus (*mor'-bus*). Latin for disease.

Morgagni, hydatids of (*mawga-nyi hī-da-tids*). Small translucent cysts arising from the embryonic pronephros which occur attached by pedicles to the fimbriated end of the Fallopian tubes.

morgue (*mawg*). A public mortuary.

moribund (*mor'-i-bund*). In a dying state.

morning sickness. *See* VOMITING OF PREGNANCY.

moron (*maw'-ron*). Feebleminded person.

morphine (*mor'-fin*). An alkaloid obtained from opium, used as a sedative or anodyne.

morphinism (*mor'-fin-izm*). Chronic poisoning from indulgence in the drug.

morphoea (*maw-fē-a*). Scleroderma affecting the skin only. Patches of atrophic, depigmented skin overlie connective tissue which has lost its elasticity.

morphology (*mor-fol-o-ji*). The science of form and structure of organisms.

mors (*mawz*). Latin for death.

mortality (*maw-ta'-li-ti*). Death rate. The annual death rate in this country is the no. of registered deaths × 1,000 divided by the mid-year population. The *Infant M. Rate* is the no. of deaths of infants under 1 year × 1,000 divided by the no. of registered live births. The *Maternal M. Rate* is the no. of deaths of women ascribed to pregnancy or childbearing × 1,000 divided by the no. of registered live and stillbirths.

mortuary (*mor'-tū-a-ri*). A place where dead bodies are kept.

morula stage (*mo-rū-la stāj*). Early stage found in developing ovum.

motile (*mō'-tīl*). Able to move independently.

motions (*mō'-shons*). The evacuations of the bowels. *See* FAECES.

motor end plate. An accumulation of nuclei and cytoplasm of muscle fibres at the termination of motor nerves.

motor nerves (*mō'-ter*). Those nerves which, passing *from* a nerve centre, convey an order of motion: the opposite to sensory nerves, which, passing *to* a nerve centre, convey a sensation.

motor neurone disease (*mō-ter nū-rōn di-sēz*). Disease of unknown cause characterized by degeneration of the anterior horn cells of the spinal cord, the motor nuclei of the cranial nerves and the corticospinal tracts; also called progressive muscular

atrophy and amyotrophic lateral sclerosis.

mould (*mō'-ld*). Any minute fungus.

moulding (*mōl'-ding*). The alteration in shape of the infant's head produced by the pressure it is subjected to whilst being driven through the birth canal.

mountain sickness (*mown'-tān*). Vomiting, tachycardia, breathlessness.

movements (fetal) (*moov-mentz*). *See* QUICKENING.

moving beam radiotherapy. Technique employed to increase the dose incident on the target tissue while reducing the skin dose by rotating the beam in an arc with its centre in the target.

mucilage (*mū'-sil-lāj*). Aqueous solutions of gums or starch.

mucin (*mū'-sin*). An albuminoid constituent of mucus.

mucocele (*mū'-kō-sēl*). A cyst distended with mucus, as of the gall bladder or lacrimal sac.

mucoid (*mū'-koyd*). Resembling mucus.

mucolytic (*mū-kō-li-tik*). Drug which helps to soften mucus.

mucopurulent (*mū-kō-pu-roo-lent*). With mucus and pus.

mucosa (*mū-kō'-za*). A mucous membrane.

mucous membrane (*mū'-kuss*). A surface which secretes mucus. The lining of the alimentary canal, air passages, and urinogenital organs: merges into true skin at the various orifices of these canals. *Mucous polypus*, a small outgrowth from the mucous surface of the cervix uteri or of the nose.

mucoviscidosis (*mū-kō-vis-ki-dō-sis*). Fibrocystic disease of the pancreas. A recessively inherited disorder of salt secretion in which there is an inability of secreting glands to reabsorb sodium. As a result the mucous secretions are extremely viscous and obstruction to the ducts of glands results with consequent dilation, stasis, infection and fibrosis. The extent of the involvement by the disease is variable but usually affects the pancreas and lungs.

mucus (*mū'-kus*). A viscid fluid of the body secreted by the mucous membranes. Mucus in the urine shows as a transparent, cloudy sediment, easily dispersed by shaking the vessel.

multigravida (*mul-ti-gra'-vi-da*). A pregnant woman who has previously had two or more pregnancies.

multilocular (*mul-ti-lok'-ū-lar*). Having many locules.

multipara (*mul-tip'-a-ra*). A woman who has had more than one child.

multiple myeloma (*mul-ti-pl mī-e-lō-ma*). Neoplasm of plasma cells which infiltrate and replace the bone marrow. Characteristic features are anaemia, bone pains, and large quantities of circulating globulins of an abnormal type which may be excreted in the urine. *See* BENCE JONES PROTEIN.

multiple pregnancy (*mul-ti-pl*). Twins, triplets, or any larger number of fetuses gestated together by one mother.

mumps (*mu'-mpz*). Infectious parotitis, inflammation of the parotid glands. Long incubation period, twelve to twenty-eight days, and quarantine must therefore be most carefully enforced. A complication not uncommon is acute swelling of the testes with great pain; and occasionally acute ovaritis in females.

murmur (*mer'-mer*). Abnormal sound of the heart or the lungs heard upon auscultation.

Murphy's sign. If continuous pressure is exerted over an inflamed gall bladder while the patient takes a deep breath it causes him to 'catch' the breath just before the zenith of inspiration.

Musca domestica (*mus'-ka dō'-mes-ti-ka*). The common fly.

muscae volitantes (*mus'-kē*). Spots or filaments which float in the vitreous humour of the eye and which are visible to the patient.

muscarine (*mus'-kar-in*). A poisonous alkaloid which is a product of putrefaction and is occasionally found in mushrooms.

muscle (*mus'-sl*). Specialized tissue composed of highly contractile cells. There are three varieties of muscle in the body: (1) Striated, voluntary muscle. (2) Smooth, involuntary, and (3) Cardiac muscle. *M. atrophy peroneal.* **Charcot-Marie-Tooth disease.** An inherited condition in which there is degeneration of the anterior horn cells of the peroneal nerves, *M. dystrophy.* A group of conditions also known as myopathies in which there is degeneration of groups of muscles without apparent nerve involvement.

musculo-spiral nerve (*mus-kŭ-lŏ-spī-ral nerv*). A nerve of the arm.

mustard (*mus'-tud*). Plant of which the crushed seeds are used. *M. flour* can be used as an emetic (one tablespoonful in a tumbler of warm water). Formerly mustard was used in baths for stimulating effect and as a poultice for its counter-irritant property.

mutant (*mū-tant*). A gene which has undergone a mutation, or an individual possessing characteristics due to such a gene.

mutation (*mū-tā'-shon*). Change. Also applied to a change in the germ-plasm, which may occur in one gene or be due to missing genes, producing a noticeable change in an individual's characteristics.

mute (*mūt*). Without the power of speech. Dumb.

myalgia (*mī-al'-ji-a*). Pain in the muscles. *M. epidemic.*

Bornholm disease. Characterized by sudden onset of fever and intercostal or diaphragmatic pain. It is thought to be caused by a virus.

myasthenia (*mī-as-thē'-ni-a*). Debility of the muscles.

myasthenia gravis (*mī-as-thē-ni-a grah'-vis*). A progressive loss of power in groups of muscle. Relieved by injections of prostigmine and surgical removal of the thymus gland.

myatonia (*mī-a-tō-ni-a*). Lack of muscle tone.

mycelium (*mi-sē'-li-um*). The filaments of fungus forming an interwoven mass.

mycetoma (*mī-se-tō'-ma*). Also known as Madura foot. A tropical disease due to infection with a vegetable parasite akin to that of actinomycosis. The part affected— most commonly the foot— becomes the seat of chronic inflammatory swelling with formation of ulcers and sinuses.

Mycobacterium (*mī-kō-bak-tā-rē-um*). A genus of bacteria. *M. leprae* causes leprosy and *M. tuberculosis*, tuberculosis.

mycosis (*mī-kō'-sis*). Disease caused by fungus.

mydriasis (*mid-ri'-a-sis*). Increase in the size of the pupil of the eye.

mydriatics (*mid-rē-at'-iks*). Drugs which dilate the pupil of the eye, *e.g.* atropine, homatropine.

myelin (*mī-el-in*). Medullary sheath of a nerve.

myelitis (*mī-e-lī-tis*). Inflammation of the spinal cord.

myelocele (*mī-e-lō-sēl*). A spina bifida in which the sac contains a portion of the spinal cord.

myelocyte (*mī-e-lō-sīt*). Bone marrow cell.

myelogram (*mī-el-ō-gram*). Radiograph of the spinal cord.

myeloid (*mī'-e-loyd*). Like marrow. *M. tissue.* Tissue giving rise to the cellular elements of the blood, *viz.* red cells, white cells and platelets.

myeloma (*mī'-el-ō'-ma*). Neoplasm of plasma cells.

myelomatosis (*mī-e-lō-ma-tō-sis*). Multiple myeloma which is malignant. Bence-Jones protein is found in the urine.

myelosclerosis (*mī-el-ō-skle-rō-sis*). Replacement of bone marrow by fibrous tissue.

myocardial (*mī-ō-kar'-di-al*). Pertaining to the muscle of the heart.

myocarditis (*mī-ō-kar-dī'-tis*). Inflammation of the muscular tissue of the heart. Often follows acute rheumatism.

myocardium (*mī-ō-kar'-di-um*). The heart muscle.

Myocrisin (*mī-ō-kris-in*). Sodium aurothiomalate. *See* GOLD THERAPY.

myogenic (*mī-ō-je'-nik*). Originating from muscular tissue.

myoglobin (*mī-ō-glō-bin*). A specialized haemoglobin found in muscle which has slightly different dissociation characteristics from that in the blood so that oxygen is transferred from the blood to the muscle.

myoma (*mī-ō'-ma*). Any tumour composed of muscular tissue.

myomectomy (*mī-ō-mek'-to-mi*). Removal of a myoma; usually referring to a fibroid from the uterus.

myometrium (*mī-ō-mē-tri-um*). The uterine muscle.

myopathy (*mī-op'-ath-i*). Any disease of a muscle.

myope (*mī'-ōp*). A short-sighted person. *Myopic*, pertaining to shortsightedness.

myopia (*mī-ō'-pi-a*). Short-sightedness; corrected by wearing a biconcave lens.

myosarcoma (*mī-ō-sar-kō'-ma*). A malignant tumour of muscle.

myosin (*mī-ō-sin*). Protein found in muscle.

myosis (*mī-ō'-sis*). Contraction of the pupil of the eye. *Syn.* meiosis, miosis.

myositis (*mī-ō-sī'-tis*). Inflammation of a muscle. *M. Ossificans.* May follow stretching of an injured muscle. Its fibres and haematoma are replaced by cancellous bone. The condition can be prevented by resting the injured muscle.

myotics (*mī-ot'-iks*). Drugs which cause the pupil to contract, *e.g.* eserine. Syn. meiotics, miotics.

myotomy (*mī-ot'-o-mi*). Cutting through a muscle.

myotonia (*mī-o-tō'-ni-a*). (1) Tonic muscular spasm. (2) Muscle stretching.

myringa (*mir-in'-ga*). The tympanic membrane of the ear.

myringitis (*mir-in-jī'-tis*). Inflammation of the tympanic membrane of the ear.

myringotome (*mir-in-go-tōm'*). Knife used for myringotomy, *q.v.*

myringotomy (*mir-in-got'-o-mi*). Incision of the tympanic membrane of the ear, performed when the presence of pus is suspected in the middle ear.

myrrh (*mer*). An astringent gum-resin of pleasant odour, used in mouthwashes.

myxoedema (*miks-e-dē'-ma*). Syndrome due to hypothyroidism and characterized by dry atrophic skin, swelling of the limbs and face and retardation both physical and mental. The metabolic rate is diminished and the patient dislikes the cold intensely.

myxoma (*miks-ō'-ma*). Tumour of connective tissue containing mucoid material.

myxosarcoma (*miks-ō-sar-kō'-ma*). A malignant myxoma.

N

N. Chemical symbol for nitrogen.

Na. Chemical symbol for sodium.

N.A.B. *See* NEOARSPHENAMINE.

Naboth's follicles (*nah'-bŏt*). Small cystic bodies resulting from infection of *N. Glands*.

Naboth's glands. Small glandular bodies situated in the neck of the uterus.

NaCl. Chemical symbol for sodium chloride, *i.e.* common salt. It is present in all the body fluids.

Naegele's obliquity (*nā'-gēl-e*). Tilting of the fetal head towards one or other shoulder as it enters the brim of the pelvis; by this attitude a slightly smaller transverse diameter of the head is presented to the brim.

naevus (*nē'-vus*). A birthmark due to a mass of dilated veins or arteries, usually very tiny ones.

nail (*nāl*). Horny plate found at the tip of finger or toe.

nalorphine hydrobromide (*na-law-fin hī-drō-brō-mīd*). Drug stimulating respiration and raising blood pressure. Used

MYRINGOTOME

as an antidote to methadone. morphine and pethidine.

nape (*nāp*). The back of the neck.

napkin rash. Inflammation of the 'napkin area' in a baby. Caused by alkalis, dampness, friction or infection. The nappies should not be washed in detergents as this is a frequent cause of the rash.

narcissism (*nar-sis'-izm*). An abnormal love for oneself: named after Narcissus, who fell in love with the reflection of himself.

narco-analysis (*nar-kō-a-na'-li-sis*). In psychotherapy, the patient is made to talk freely, bringing repressed matter to consciousness after having had an injection of one of the barbiturates.

narcolepsy (*nar-ko-lep-si*). A condition characterized by sudden attacks of sleep occurring repeatedly during the day.

narcosis (*nar-kōs'-is*). A state of unconsciousness produced by the use of narcotics.

narcotic (*nar-kot'-ik*). A drug which produces unconsciousness, *e.g.* paraldehyde, the barbiturates.

nares (*na'-rēz*). The nostrils.

nasal (*nā-'sal*). Relating to the nose.

nascent (*nās'-sent*). At the moment of birth.

nasogastric (*nā-zō-gas-trik*). Relating to the nose and stomach. N. tube. Used in artificial feeding.

nasolacrimal (*nā-zō-la'-kri-mal*). Relating to the nose and lacrimal apparatus.

nasopharyngeal (*nā'-zō-far-in-je'-al*). Pertaining to the nasopharynx.

nasopharynx (*nā'-zō-far'-inks*). The space between the posterior nares, the base of the skull, the soft palate, the upper end of the oesophagus, and the epiglottis.

nates (*nā'-tēz*). The buttocks.

natural childbirth. A school of opinion concerning childbirth which advocates the minimum of medical interference with the process of delivery.

nausea (*naw'-sē-a*). A feeling of sickness.

navel (*nā'-vel*). The umbilicus, the point of connection of the umbilical cord.

navicular (*na-vi-kū-la*). The boat-shaped tarsal bone.

nebula (*neb'-ū-la*). A cloud or mist. Term applied to filmy corneal opacities.

nebulae (*ne-bū-lē*). Plural of nebula. Used to describe sprays of very fine particles used, for example, to facilitate absorption of inhaled substances.

nebulizer (*neb'-ū-lī-zer*). *See* ATOMIZER.

neck (*nek*). Narrow part near the end of an organ, *Derbyshire N.* Goitre. *Wry N.* Torticollis.

necrobiosis (*ne-krō-bī-ō'-sis*). Death of tissue. *Red N.* A type of degeneration occurring in a fibroid of the uterus if pregnancy takes place. After labour, the fibroid can recover its vitality.

necropsy (*ne-crop'-si*). Examination of a body after death.

necrosis (*ne-krō'-sis*). Death of tissue.

necrotic (*ne-krot'-ik*). Relating to necrosis.

needle holder (*nē'-dl hōl-der*). Instrument for holding surgical needles. *See illustration.*

NEEDLE HOLDER

needling. Perforation with a needle especially in cataract. *See* DISCISSION.

negativism (*neg'-a-tiv-izm*). A state of mind in which the ideas and behaviour of an individual are in opposition to those of the majority and contrary to suggestion.

Neisseria (*nī-se-ri-a*). Genus of diplococci. *N. gonorrhoeae* causes gonorrhoea; *N. meningitidis* causes epidemic cerebrospinal meningitis.

Nelaton's line (*ne-la-tons*). Line from the anterior superior iliac spine to the tuberosity of the ischium.

nematodes (*ne-ma-tōds*). Worms including round worms, threadworms and eelworms. Some of these are parasitic to man, *e.g.* hookworm.

Nembutal (*nem'-bū-tal*). Pentobarbitone sodium. Hypnotic, sedative and anticonvulsant drug. Sometimes used as a basal anaesthetic and also given in obstetrics.

neoarsphenamine (*nē-ō-ars-fen-a-mīn*). An arsenic compound used in the treatment of syphilis and other infective diseases. Also known as neosalvarsan, neoarsphenolamine, novarsenol.

neoarthrosis (*nē-ō-ar-thrō-sis*). A new joint.

Neo-epinine (*nē-ō-e-pi-nin*). Isoprenaline sulphate. A powerful broncho-dilator, Used as a spray or in tablet form.

neologism (*nē-o-lo-jism*). A new word coined for the occasion.

neomycin (*nē-ō-mī-sin*). Antibiotic used in treatment of intestinal infections and for eradicating staphylococci from skin lesions.

neonatal (*nē-ō-nā-tal*). Relating to the first four weeks of life.

neonate (*nē-ō-nāt*). Term applied to a child during the first month of life.

neoplasm (*nē'-ō-plasm*). A tumour. An abnormal local multiplication of some type of cell. A neoplasm may be either *benign* if it shows no tendency to spread, or *malignant* if the growing cells infiltrate surrounding tissues and invade other parts of the body.

neostigmine (*nē-ō-stig-mēn*). Drug similar to physostigmine. Used in treatment of myasthenia gravis. Counteracts muscular relaxation produced by tubocurarine, etc. Used in solution to lower intra-ocular pressure in glaucoma.

Nepenthe (*ne-pen'-thē*). Proprietary opium preparation.

nephrectomy (*nef-rek'-tŏ-mi*). Removal of a kidney.

nephritis (*ne-fri'-tis*). Inflammation of the kidney. The term nephritis is used to describe a large number of widely differing conditions affecting this organ.

nephro- (*nef-rŏ*). Pertaining to the kidney.

nephroblastoma (*ne-fro-bla-stŏ'-ma*). Wilm's tumour. A neoplasm of the kidney which occurs in children.

nephrocalcinosis (*ne-frŏ-kal-si-nŏ'-sis*). A complication of hyperparathyroidism, *q.v.*, in which calcium becomes deposited in the renal tubes.

nephrocapsulectomy (*nef-rŏ-kap-sū-lek'-to-mi*). Operation to remove the kidney capsule.

nephrography (*nef-ro-gra-fi*). X-ray examination of the kidney.

nephrolithiasis (*nef-rŏ-lith-ī'-as-is*). Stone in the kidney.

nephrolithotomy (*nef'-rŏ-lith-ot'-o-mi*). Removal of a stone from the interior of the kidney.

nephroma (*nef-rŏ'-ma*). Tumour of the kidney.

nephron (*nef'-ron*). A unit of the kidney. It consists of a glomerulus, with the secreting part of its tubule. One kidney has about a million nephrons.

nephropexy (*nef'-rŏ-pek'-si*). Stitching a movable kidney into a firm position.

nephroptosis (*nef-rop-tŏ'-sis*). Downward displacement of the kidney.

nephrosis (*nef-rŏ'-sis*). Chronic progressive degenerative disease of the renal tubules.

nephrostomy (*nef-ros-to-mi*). Surgical opening into the kidney to drain it.

nephrotic syndrome (*nef-ro-tik sin'-drōm*). Degenerative disease of renal tubules characterized by heavy albuminuria, with reduction of plasma protein and oedema.

nephrotomy (*ne-frot'-o-mi*). Cutting into the kidney.

nephro-ureterectomy (*nef-rŏ-ū-rē-te-rek'-to-mi*). Operation to remove both kidney and ureter.

nerve (*nerv*). A bundle of fibres, conveying the impulses of movement and sensation to and from the organs. *See* MOTOR NERVES, SENSORY NERVES, VASOMOTOR.

nerve root. Each spinal nerve arises from the spinal cord by two roots; the dorsal root carries the sensory fibres and the ventral root the motor fibres.

nervous (*ner'-vus*). Pertaining to the nerves. May also mean anxious and excited.

nettle-rash. Same as urticaria.

neural (*nū-ral*). Relating to nerves.

neuralgia (*nū-ral'-ji-a*). Pain in the distribution of a nerve. *e.g. trigeminal n.* Severe pain in the distribution of the trigeminal nerve. *Sciatica* is neuralgia of the sciatic nerve distribution. The cause may be irritation of the nerve by some bony structure or a tumour, but frequently the cause cannot be ascertained. For intractable pain interruption of the sensory fibres of the nerve is often helpful.

neurapraxia (*nū-rā-prak'-si-a*). There is a temporary block to nerve conduction as after giving a local anaesthetic.

neurasthenia (*nū-ras-thē'-ni-a*). Nervous exhaustion.

neurectasis (*nū-rek-ta-sis*). Operation to stretch a nerve.

neurectomy (*nū-rek'-to-mi*). Excision of part of a nerve.

neurilemma (*nū-ri-lem'-a*). The sheath of a nerve fibre.

neurinoma (*nū-ri-nō-ma*). Tumour of a neurilemma, *q.v.*

neuritis (*nū-rī-'tis*). Inflammation of a nerve.

neuroblast (*nū-rō-blast*). Embryonic nerve cell.

neuroblastoma (*nū-rō-blas-tō'-ma*). Malignant growth of

sympathetic nerve ganglia, *esp.* adrenal medulla. Strictly a tumour of neuroblasts, *q.v.*

neurodermatitis (*nū-rō-der-ma-tī-tis*). Characteristic hyperkeratosis associated with habitual scratching.

neuroepithelium (*nū-rō-ep-i-thē'-li-um*). Specialized nerve epithelium, *e.g.* the retina, which consists of nerve endings, rod and cone-shaped cells of the optic nerve.

neurofibroma (*nū-rō-fī-brō'-ma*). Tumour arising from connective tissue surrounding peripheral nerves.

neurofibromatosis (*nū-rō-fī-brō-ma-tō-sis*). Von Recklinghausen's disease. Generalized distribution within the body of neurofibromas, *q.v.*

neuroglia (*nū-rō-glī-a*). Connective tissue cells of the central nervous system are collectively known as *glia*. Neuroglia are cells with long fibrous processes which are derived from embryonic nervous tissue and are closely related to Schwann cells; their exact supportive function is not known. *Microglia* are similar to macrophages, *q.v.*

neurolemma (*nū-rō-lem-ma*). See NEURILEMMA.

neuroleptic (*nū-rō-lep-tik*). Drug affecting the nervous system.

neurologist (*nū-ro'-lo-jist*). Physician who specializes in neurology.

neurology (*nū-ro'-lo-ji*). Medical science of diseases of the nervous system.

neuroma (*nū-rō'-ma*). A tumour composed of nerve tissue.

neuron (*nū'-ron*). A nerve cell and its processes. (*See below.*)

MOTOR   SENSORY

Synapse
Axon
Nucleus
Cells
Dendrites
Myelin sheath
Node of Ranvier
Motor end-plate
Striped muscle fibres
Pain fibres in skin

NEURONS

neuronotmesis (*nū-ron-ot-mē-sis*). Severance of a nerve.

neuropathic (*nū-'ro-path'-ik*). Of weak or unstable nervous organization.

neuropathy (*nū-ro-pa-thi*). Disease of the nervous system.

neuroplasty (*nū-rō-plas-ti*). Operation to repair a nerve.

neurorrhaphy (*nū-ro-ra-fi*). Operation to suture a severed nerve.

neurosis (*nū-rō'-sis*). A disorder of mental function whereby patients are ab-normally emotionally vulnerable but retain external reality; *cf.* psychosis. Neuroses include behaviour disorders such as hysterical and obsessive compulsive reactions and disturbances of 'affect', as, for example, in anxiety states.

neurosurgery (*nū-rō-ser'-je-ri*). Surgery of peripheral and central nervous system.

neurosyphilis (*nū-rō-si'-fi-lis*). Involvement of the central nervous system by syphilis.

neurotic (*nū-ro-tik*). Relating to a neurosis.

neurotmesis (*nū-rot-mē'-sis*). The nerve trunk is severed or crushed and there can be no useful recovery without surgery.

neurotomy (*nū-ro-to-mi*). Division of a nerve.

neurotripsy (*nū-rō-trip-si*). The crushing of a nerve.

neurotropism (*nū-rō-tro-pism*). Predilection of an infecting organism for nervous tissue.

neutral (*nū'-tral*). Neither acid nor alkaline.

neutropaenia (*nū-trō-pē'-ni-a*). Insufficiency of neutrophil polymorphonuclear leucocytes in the blood.

neutrophil (*nū-trō-fil*). Predilection for neutral dyes, *i.e.* not acidophil or basophil. Term used to describe the majority of polymorphonuclear leucocytes which do not demonstrate any characteristically staining granules in their cytoplasm, *cf.* basophil, eosinophil.

nicotine poisoning. Result of over-indulgence in smoking due to an alkaloid in tobacco leaves. Cardinal features are the paralysis of autonomic ganglia and constriction of coronary arteries.

nicotinic acid (ni-kō-tin'-ik). Pellagra-preventing factor of vitamin B complex. See VITAMINS.

nictitation (nik-ti-tā'-shon). Involuntary blinking of the eyelids.

nidation (ni-dā-shon). Implantation.

Niemann-Pick's disease. A lipoid storage disease in which lecithin is deposited. An inherited defect of phospholipid metabolism which leads to widespread deposition of lecithin in the tissues. It is associated with mental retardation.

night-blindness (nīt-blind'-ness). See NYCTALOPIA.

nigrescent (ni-gres'-sent). Growing black.

nigrities (ni-grish'-i-ēz). Blackness. N. linguae, a condition in which the filiform papillae of the tongue are hypertrophied and darkly pigmented.

nihilism (ni-hi-lism). Psychiatric term denoting feeling of hopelessness in the patient.

nikethamide (nik-eth-a-mīd). Official name for Coramine. An analeptic, stimulating the vital centres in the medulla; given by injection.

nipple (nip'-pl). Small eminence in the centre of each breast.

nipple shields. Coverings of glass or india-rubber put on the nipples to protect them when they are sore.

Nissl's granules (nis-lz gran-ūlz). Granular substances found in the cell body of a neuron.

nit. The egg of the louse.

nitrate (nī'-trāt). A salt of nitric acid.

nitrate of silver (nī-trāt). Lunar caustic; used in the form of a pencil to arrest the growth of granulation tissue, also as an astringent lotion when well diluted.

nitric acid (nī'-trik as'-id). A corrosive fluid used in testing for albumin, etc.

nitrite (nī-trīt). A salt of nitrous acid.

nitrite of amyl. See AMYL NITRITE.

nitrofurantoin (nī-trō-fū-ran-toyn). Drug given to treat urinary infections, Proprietary name, Furadantin.

nitrogen (nī-trō-jen). A colourless inert gas, forming about 78 per cent of the atmosphere and acting as a diluent. Nitrogenous foods. See PROTEIN. N. Mustard. Cell-destroying drug, used in the treatment of certain malignant tumours and especially Hodgkin's disease.

nitro-glycerin (nī-trō-glis'-e-rin). An oily liquid, highly explosive, used in angina pectoris to dilate the coronary arteries. Sometimes causes headache. Called also tri-nitro-glycerin and liquor trinitrini. Poison. *See* TRINITRIN.

nitrous oxide (*nī-trus ok'-sīd*). Laughing gas; an anaesthetic.

Nobecutane (*nō-bek'-ū-tān*). Resinous spray used to form a covering over wounds.

nocturia (*nok-tū-ri-a*). Passing urine at night. May be a symptom of cardiac failure.

nocturnal (*nok-ter-nal*). At night. *N. enuresis.* Bedwetting during sleep.

nodding spasm. *See* SPASMUS NUTANS.

node (*nōd*). A swelling. *Atrioventricular N.* At the base of the interatrial septum from which impulses pass down the Bundle of His. *Heberden's Ns.* Deformity of the joints in the hands in arthritis. *Sino-atrial N.* The pacemaker of the heart, found at the opening of the superior vena cava into the right atrium. *N. of Ranvier.* The constriction in the neurilemma of a nerve fibre.

nodule (*nod-ūl*). A little knob.

non compos mentis (*non kom'-pos men'-tis*). Not sound of mind.

non-viable (*non-vī-ubl*). Unable to survive, especially as to a child of less than 28 weeks' gestation.

noradrenaline (*nor-ad-ren'-a-lēn*). Hormone of the adrenal medulla. Raises blood pressure by a general vasocon-striction so given in shock, etc.

normal (*nor'-mal*). The average or usual form.

normoblasts (*nor'-mō-blasts*). Immature nucleated red cells present in red bone marrow.

normocyte (*nor'-mō-sīt*). A normally-sized erythrocyte.

nose (*nōz*). The organ of smell and used for warming, filtering and moistening the air breathed in.

nosology (*nō-so-lo-ji*). Science of the classification of diseases.

nostalgia (*nos-tal'-ji-a*). Home sickness, or a yearning for the past.

nostrils (*nos'-trilz*). The anterior apertures of the nose.

notch (*notsh*). Indentation.

notifiable (*nō-'tif-ĭ-abl*). A term applied to certain cases of disease and other occurrences which must be made known to the Medical Officer of Health, *e.g.* smallpox, tuberculosis, typhoid fever, dysentery, food poisoning, acute poliomyelitis, diphtheria, measles, whooping cough, etc.

novarsenobenzol (*nō-var-sen-ō-ben-zol*). An arsenic preparation used in the treatment of syphilis and other infective diseases.

novobiocin (*nō-vō-bī'-ō-sin*). Antibiotic for oral administration, especially for staphylococci resistant to penicillin.

Novocain (*nō'-vo-kān*). Procaine hydrochloride. Local
anaesthetic often used with
adrenaline.

noxious (*nok-si-us*). Harmful.

nucha (*nu'-ka*). The nape, or
back of the neck.

Nuck (*nook*). *See* CANAL OF.

nucleated (*nū'-klē-ā-ted*). With
a nucleus.

nucleic acid (*nūk'-le-ik*) and its
derivatives have a stimulating
effect on bone marrow, producing an increase in the
polymorphonuclear cells in
the blood. A preparation,
Pentnucleotide, is sometimes
used.

nucleoprotein (*nū-klē-ō-prō-
tēn*). Compound of protein
and nucleic acid in nuclei.

nucleus (*nū-klē-us*). Pl. **nuclei**.
(1) Of cell, the spherical
body containing the chromosomes, *q.v. See* CELL. (2) Of
brain, demarcated mass of
cell bodies, *e.g.* basal nuclei.

nucleus pulposus (*pul-pō-zus*).
A pulpy mass in the centre
of the intervertebral discs.
May become prolapsed into
the spinal canal causing pressure on the cord and spinal
nerves.

nullipara (*nu-lip'-a-ra*). A
woman who has never had
a child.

nummulated (*num'-mū-lā-ted*).
Resembling a coin; applied
to a form of expectoration
sometimes seen in pulmonary
tuberculosis.

Nupercaine (*nū-per-kān*). Cinchocaine. Local anaesthetic
much more powerful than
cocaine.

nutation (*nū-tā'-shon*). Involuntary nodding of the head.

nutrient (*nū'-tri-ent*). Nourishing. *N. foramen*, opening in
a bone for the nourishing
vessels.

nutrition (*nū-tri-shon*). Science
of feeding.

nux vomica (*nuks vom'-i-ka*).
The drug containing strychnine.

nyctalopia (*nik-tal-ō'-pi-a*). A
state of the eyes which causes
vision to be worse at night
than during the day.

nyctophobia (*nik-tō-fō'-bi-a*).
Abnormal fear of darkness.

nymphae (*nim-fē*). Labia minora, *q.v.*

nymphomania (*nim-fō-mā'-ni-
a*). Excessive sexual desire in
females.

nystagmus (*nis-tag'-mus*). Involuntary oscillations of the
eyeball; sometimes congenital; sometimes a symptom of
brain disease, ocular affection, or lesion in the internal
ear.

O

O. Chemical symbol for oxygen.

obesity (*ō-bē'-si-ti*). Excessive
fatness.

objective (*ob-jek'-tiv*). (1) The
object glass of a microscope.
(2) Pertaining to things lying
external to one's self.

O signs. Signs seen in a patient about which he may not complain.

oblique diameters of pelvis (*ō-blĕk dī-am'-et-erz*). *See* DIAMETERS.

oblique muscles (*ō-blĕk mus'-lz*). The two external muscles of the eyeball, an upper and a lower. Also two large muscles of the abdominal wall, an internal and an external.

Oblivon (*ob-li-von*). Methylpentynol, *q.v.*

obsession (*ob-sesh'-on*). An idea of which the patient cannot rid himself. Minor obsessions are common in perfectly healthy people: but long-standing obsessions are especially frequent in the insane.

obsessive compulsive neurosis (*ob-se-siv com-pul-siv nu-rō-sis*). Mental disorder in which the outstanding feature is a feeling of compulsion to act in a way which the patient realizes to be absurd.

obsolete (*ob'-sō-lĕt*). No longer used.

obstetric (*ob-stet'-rik*). Pertaining to the practice of midwifery.

obstetrician (*ob-ste-tri-shon*). Doctor who practises obstetrics.

obturator (*ob-tūr-ā'-ter*). That which stops up a hole or cavity. The obturator of a sigmoidoscope, for example, is the blunt-ended rod which fills up the end of the instru-

ment when it is introduced into the rectum, and thus prevents any scratching of the mucous membrane. The *obturator foramen* is a hole on each side of the pelvis, closed by the powerful *obturator ligament*. The *obturator muscles* are two muscles on each side in the same region, and there are also *obturator vessels* and *nerves*.

obtusion (*ob-tū'-zhon*). A blunting, as of sensitiveness.

occipital (*ok-sip'-i-tal*). Relating to the back of the head.

occipito-anterior   } The two
occipito-posterior   } kinds of vertex presentation, according as the back of the head (occiput) is directed forwards or backwards.

occiput (*ok'-si-put*). The back of the head or skull. *See* SKULL.

occlusion (*ok-klū-zhon*). Closure.

occlusive therapy (*ok-lū-siv the-ra-pi*). The patient is encouraged to use the lazy eye by covering the good eye.

occult blood (*ok'-ult blud*). Not visible to naked eye. Term used to describe blood passed in faeces in such small amounts that no dark colour is present. This blood can only be demonstrated by the occult blood test.

Occultest. Tablets which contain reagents for the demonstration of occult blood.

occupational disease (*ok-ū-pā'-sho-nal di-zēz*). Illness induced by the patient's occupation.

occupational therapist. One who practises occupational therapy.

occupational therapy. Any occupation given to a patient to help in his recovery, both mentally and physically.

ocular (*ok'-u-lar*). Relating to the eye.

oculist (*ok'-ū-list*). An eye specialist.

oculogyric (*o-kū-lō-jī-rik*). Making the eyes roll.

oculomotor nerves (*ok-ū-lō-mō'-tor*). The third pair of cranial nerves which help to move the eyeball.

Oddi, sphincter of (*o'-di sfink-ter ov*). Muscular sphincter at the opening of the common bile duct into the duodenum.

odontalgia (*o-don-tal'-jia-*). Toothache.

odontoid (*o-don'-toyd*). Toothlike. *O. Process.* Peglike projection of second cervical vertebra.

odontolith (*o-don'-to-lith*). Calcareous matter deposited on teeth; tartar.

odontology (*ō-don-to'-lo-ji*). Dentistry.

odontoma (*od-on-tō'-ma*). Tumour arising from a tooth or a developing tooth.

oedema (*e-dē'-ma*). Abnormal amount of fluid in the tissues causing a puffy swelling. The fluid tends to collect in the dependent parts, *e.g.* oedema of the ankles.

Oedipus complex (*ēd'-i-pus*). A persistence of the normal love of a boy for his mother so that it rivals that of his father. Named after Oedipus who, according to Greek mythology, unknowingly married his mother and killed his father.

oesophageal (*ē-sof'-a-je-al*). Pertaining to the oesophagus. *O. varices.* Varicose veins in the lower part of the oesophagus resulting from hypertension in the hepatic portal system which occurs in cirrhosis of the liver.

oesophagectasis (*ē-so-fa-jek-ta-sis*). Procedure to dilate the oesophagus.

oesophagectomy (*ē-so-fa-jek-to-mi*). Resection of the oesophagus.

oesophagitis (*ē-so-fa-jī-tis*). Inflammation of the oesophagus, especially *reflex o.*, due to hiatus hernia, *q.v.*, when stomach acid regurgitates into the lower part of the oesophagus causing damage and inflammation of the wall.

oesophagoscope (*ē-sof'-a-go-skōp*). An instrument for viewing the interior of the oesophagus.

oesophagostomy (*ē-so-fa-gos-to-mi*). An artificial opening is made into the oesophagus.

oesophagotomy (*ē-sof'-a-got'-o-mi*). Cutting into the oesophagus.

oesophagus (*ē-sof'-a-gus*). The canal which runs from the pharynx into the stomach.

OESOPHAGUS

is the cause of thrush in children. *See also* SACCHAR-OMYCES.

ointment. A soft application to promote healing, usually consisting of a base impregnated with some drug.

oleandomycin (*ō-lē-an-dō-mī-sin*). Antibiotic used to treat abscesses, skin infections, pneumonia, etc. Useful for patients who are sensitive to penicillin.

olecranon (*ō-lek'-ra-non*). The bone composing the point of the elbow. The extreme upper end of the ulna, the inner of the two bones of the forearm. (*See illustration*, p. 130.)

oleum iodisatum (*ō-lē-um i-ō-dīz-atum*). Official name for Lipiodol, *q.v.*

oleum morrhuae (*ō-lē-um mor'-oo-ē*). Cod-liver oil: usual abbreviation Ol. Morrh.

oleum ricini (*ris'-ēn-i*). Castor oil: usually written Ol. Ric.

olfactory (*ol-fak'-tur-i*). Relating to the sense of smell.

oligaemia (*ol-i-gē'-mi-a*). Lack of blood.

oligo- (*ol-i'-gō*). Prefix meaning deficiency.

oligohydramnios (*ol-i-gō-hi-dram'-ni-os*). Deficiency of amniotic fluid.

oligomenorrhoea (*o-li-gō-me-nor-rēa*). Sparse menstrual flow.

oligospermia (*o-li-gō-sper-mēa*). Insufficient secretion of semen or deficiency of sperms in the semen.

oestradiol (*ē-strā'-dē-ol*). Hormone contained in Graafian follicles. Administered in oestrogen deficiency. *See* OESTROGENIC HORMONE.

oestrogen (*ēs-tro-jen*), or **oestrogenic substance** or **hormone.** Any substance, usually a steroid, capable of producing genital tract changes characteristic of the follicular phase of the menstrual cycle: an oestrogen is secreted by the ovaries. Oestrogens are also produced by the placenta during pregnancy and by the adrenal cortex. The female secondary sexual characteristics are under the influence of oestrogens.

ohm (*ōm*). Unit of electrical resistance.

oidium albicans (*oyd'-i-um*). Syn. *Candida albicans*. A microscopic fungus which

oligotrophia (*ol-ig-ō-trŏf'-i-a*). Lack of nourishment.

oliguria (*ol-i-gūr'-i-a*). A diminution in the amount of urine passed.

olivary body (*ol-iv-ar-i bo-di*). An oval mass of grey matter behind the anterior pyramid of the medulla oblongata.

olive oil. An oil obtained from olives. Used as a demulcent.

omentocele (*ō-men-tō-sēl*). Hernial sac containing omentum.

omentopexy (*o-men-tō-pek-si*). Fixation of the omentum.

omentum (*ō-men-tum*). A fold of the peritoneum. The *Great O.* is suspended from the greater curvature of the stomach and hangs in front of the gut. The *Lesser O.* passes from the lesser curvature of the stomach to the transverse fissure of the liver.

THE OMENTUM

Omnopon (*om-nō-pon*). Official name papaveretum (B.P.C.), *q.v.*

omphalitis (*om-fal-ī'-tis*). Inflammation of the umbilicus.

omphalocele (*om'-fal-ō-sēl*). An umbilical hernia.

omphaloproptosis (*om-fa-lō-prop-tō-sis*). Protrusion of the umbilicus.

oncoma (*on-kō'-ma*). A swelling or tumour.

onychia (*ō-nik'-i-a*). Inflammation of the matrix of a nail.

onychogryphosis (*o-ni-kō-gri-fō-sis*). Bizarre overgrowth of the nails, often the nail of the big toe.

onychomycosis (*o-ni-kō-mi-kō'-sis*). Infection of the nails by fungi.

oocyte (*o'-ō-sīt*). An ovum before it has left the Graafian follicle.

oogenesis (*o-o-jen'-e-sis*). The production of ova in the ovary.

oophorectomy (*o-o-fo-rek-to-mi*). Removal of an ovary. See OVARIECTOMY.

oophoritis (*o-of-o-rī'-tis*). Inflammation of an ovary.

oophoron (*o-of'-or-on*). That portion of the ovary which produces the ova. Or the ovary itself.

oophorosalpingectomy (*sal-pin-jek-to-mi*). Removal of the ovary and its associated Fallopian tube.

opacity (*ō-pas'-i-ti*). Want of transparency, cloudiness.

opaque (*ō-pāk*). Not transparent.

opening snap. Adventitious heart sound which often precedes the mid-diastolic murmur of mitral stenosis.

ophthalmia (*of-thal'-mi-a*). Inflammation of the eye. The term is applied especially to severe inflammations of the conjunctiva. There is an acute infectious form which occurs in epidemics, especially in schools and military camps.

ophthalmia neonatorum (*of-thal-mi-a nē-ō-nā-tor'-um*). Severe inflammation of the eyes in the newly born, due to gonorrhoeal or septic infection of the conjunctiva during the passage of the head through the vagina. When due to the gonococcus it responds to intensive treatment with penicillin, locally and by injection.

ophthalmic (*of-thal'-mik*). Pertaining to the eye.

ophthalmitis (*of-thal-mī'-tis*). Inflammation of the eye.

ophthalmologist (*of-thal-mo-lo-jist*). A surgeon specializing in diseases of the eye.

ophthalmology. The study of diseases of the eye.

ophthalmoplegia (*of-thal-mo-plē'-ji-a*). Paralysis of the muscles of the eye.

ophthalmoscope (*of-thal'-mo-skōp*). A small instrument, fitted with a lens, used to examine the interior of the eye.

OPHTHALMOSCOPE

ophthalmotonometer (*of-thal'-mō-tō-no-me-ter*). Instrument to measure the intraocular tension of the eye.

opiate (*o'-pē-āt*). An opium preparation. A hypnotic.

opisthotonos (*op-is-thot'-o-nōs*). Backward retraction of the head and lower limbs with arched back; seen in severe cases of tetanus, meningitis and in strychnine poisoning.

opium (*ō'-pi-um*). A preparation of poppy juice, much used to induce sleep and to allay pain. It contains the alkaloids, morphine, codeine, papaverine and narcotine. Can cause addiction.

opponens (*op-pō'-nens*). Opposing. Applied to muscles, *e.g.* *opponens pollicis* which brings the thumb towards the little finger.

opsonins (*op-so'-ninz*). Chemical substances found in the blood serum that are said to prepare the bacteria for phagocytosis.

optic (*op'-tik*). Relating to the sight. *O. Atrophy.* Degeneration of the optic nerve.

optic chiasma (*kī-as'-ma*). The crossing of the fibres of the optic tract.

optic disc (*op-tik dī'-sk*). The point where the optic nerve enters the eye. This point is insensitive to light and is known as the blind spot.

optician (*op-ti'-shan*). Maker of optical instruments.

optics (*op'-tiks*). The study of the properties of light.

optimum (*op'-ti-mum*). The best possible in the particular circumstances.

optometry (*op-to'-me-tri*). Measurement of visual powers.

oral (*aw'-ral*). Pertaining to the mouth.

orbicularis (*or-bik-u-la'-ris*). A name given to a muscle which encircles an orifice, *e.g. O. Oris,* around the mouth.

orbit (*or'-bit*). The bony cavity in the skull which holds the eye.

orbital (*or'-bi-tal*). Pertaining to the orbit.

orchidectomy (*or-kid'-ek'-to-mi*). Removal of one or both testicles. Castration.

orchidopexy (*or-kid'-o-pek-si*). The bringing down of an imperfectly descended testicle into the scrotum and fixing it there by sutures.

orchiepididymitis (*or-ki-e-pi-di-di-mī-tis*). An inflamed epididymis and testicle.

orchis (*or'-kis*). Testicle.

orchitis (*or-kī'-tis*). Inflammation of the testicles.

organ (*or'-gan*). A part constructed to exercise a special function.

organic (*or-gan'-ik*). Relating to the organs; thus, organic disease of the heart means that the structure itself is affected. *O. Chemistry.* Chemistry relating to the carbon compounds.

organism (*or'-ga-nism*). A living cell or cells.

orgasm (*or'-gazm*). Highest point of excitement in sexual intercourse.

Oriental sore (*or'-i-en-tal saw*). Delhi boil, *q.v.*

orientation (*or-i-ent-ā'-shon*). The location of one's position and attitude in relation to surrounding objects.

orifice (*o'-ri-fis*). An opening.

ornithosis (*or-ni-thō'-sis*). Respiratory disease of birds, transmissible to man.

oropharynx (*o-rō-fā-rinks*). That part of the throat which lies between the mouth and the oesophagus.

orphan viruses. *See* ADENOVIRUS.

Orr's treatment. Treatment formerly used in osteomyelitis.

orthodontics (*or-tho-don-tiks*). The correction of irregularities of the teeth.

orthopaedic (*or-thō-pē'-dik*). Surgery relating to the correction of deformities of the skeleton.

orthopnoea (*or-thop-ne'-a*). Breathlessness, the patient gaining relief only in an upright position.

orthoptics (*or-thop'-tiks*). Term applied to correcting defective vision in a squint by exercises, etc.

orthostatic. Pertaining to or caused by standing upright.

os (*os*). A bone.

os (*ōs*, but often pronounced *os*). The mouth. *External O.* The opening of the cervix into the vagina. *Internal O.* Opening of cervix into the uterine cavity.

os calcis (*kal-sis*). The bone of the heel.

—*os calcis*

oscheal (*os'-kē-al*). Pertaining to the scrotum.

oscillation (*os-si-lā'-shon*). A swinging movement.

Osgood Schlatter's disease (*os-good schla-ter*). Osteochondritis of unknown cause affecting the tibial tuberosity.

Osiander's sign. Sign appears during first three months of pregnancy when vaginal pulsation is felt.

Osler's disease (*o'-zler*). Polycythaemia, *q.v.*

Osler's nodes (*oz-lerz nōdz*). Small tender inflamed areas in the skin due to small emboli; occurs in bacterial endocarditis.

osmosis (*oz-mō'-sis*). The passage of liquids through a membrane.

osmotic fragility test. Method of determining the fragility of red blood cells.

osmotic pressure (*oz-mot'-ik*). Pressure required to prevent the passage of water by osmosis. The osmotic pressure depends on the number of solute molecules in solution.

osseous (*os'-e-us*). Like bone, bony.

ossicle (*os'-sik-al*). Literally, a small bone. Name applied to the tiny bones of the middle ear. *See* EAR.

ossification (*os-si-fi-kā'-shon*). Hardening into bone.

osteitis (*os'-tē-i'-tis*). Inflammation of bone. *O. Fibrosa,* a disease of bone caused by an adenoma of the parathyroid glands. As the result of excessive secretion calcium is absorbed from the bones into the blood.

osteitis deformans. *See* PAGET'S DISEASE.

osteoarthritis (*os-teo-ar-thrī'-tis*), or **osteoarthrosis** (*os-teo-ar-thrō-sis*). Disease due to excessive wear and tear on joint surfaces. Affecting chiefly weight-bearing joints, late in life, and resulting in pain, especially at night, deficient movement, and deformity.

osteoarthropathy (*os-tē-ō-ar-throp-ath-i*). Damage or disease affecting bones and joints.

osteoarthrotomy (*os'-tē-ō-ar-thro'-to-mi*). Excision of joint and neighbouring bone.

osteoblasts (*os'-tē-ō-blasts*). Bone cells.

osteochondritis (*os-tē-ō-kon-drī'-tis*). Combined inflammation of bone and cartilage. *O. Deformans Juvenilis*. A form occurring in children in which the head of the femur is affected. (Perthes' disease.) *O. Dissecans*. Separation of loose bodies from the joint surface.

osteochondroma (*os-tē-ō-kon-drō'-ma*). Benign tumour derived from bone and cartilage.

osteoclastoma (*os-tē-ō-klas-tō-ma*). Tumour of osteoclasts.

osteoclasts (*os'-tē-ō-klasts*). Multinucleated cells which break down the calcified bone matrix, Remodelling of bone by the combined activity of osteoclasts and osteoblasts occurs continuously during bone growth.

osteocyte (*os-tē-ō-sīt*). Osteoblasts which have become incorporated into bone.

osteogenesis (*os'-tē-ō-jen'-e-sis*). Formation of a bone. *O.*

Imperfecta. Abnormally fragile bones.

osteogenic sarcoma (*os-tē-ō-je-nik sar-kō-ma*). Sarcoma derived from osteoblasts.

osteolytic (*os-tē-ō-li-tik*). Bone destroying.

osteoma (*os-tē-ō'-ma*). A bony tumour.

osteomalacia (*os-tē-ō-ma-lā'-ki-a*). Softening of bones in adults.

osteomyelitis (*os-tē-ō-mi-e-lī'-tis*). Inflammation of the marrow of bone.

osteopath (*os-tē-ō-path*). One who practises osteopathy.

osteopathy (*os-tē-op'-ath-i*). A school of thought ascribing many diseases to structural derangement of skeletal parts and treating same by manipulation of joints. Term can also mean any bone disease.

osteopetrosis (*os-tē-ō-pe-trō'-sis*). *See* MARBLE BONE DISEASE.

osteophony (*os-tē-o'-fo-ni*). Conduction of sound by bone.

osteophyte (*os'-tē-ō-fīt*). A bony outgrowth or nodosity; occurs in osteoarthritis.

osteoplastic (*os-tē-ō-plas-tik*). Pertaining to the repair of bones.

osteoporosis (*os-tē-ō-po-rō'-sis*). Fragility of bones due to reabsorption of calcium.

osteosarcoma (*os-tē-ō-sar-kō'-ma*). A malignant tumour growing from a bone.

osteosclerosis (*os-tē-ō-skle-rō'-sis*). Increase in bone density.

osteotome (*os'-tē-ot-ōm*). A surgical instrument resembling a chisel and used for cutting through bones. The instrument is bevelled on both sides.

(chisel)

OSTEOTOME

osteotomy (*os-tē-ot'-o-mi*). The operation of cutting through a bone, usually performed for the relief or cure of bony deformities.

ostium (*os'-ti-um*). An opening. The orifice of any tubular passage.

otalgia (*ō-tal'-ji-a*). Ear-ache.

otitis (*o-tī'-tis*). Inflammation of the ear. *O. externa.* Inflammation of the skin of the external ear. *O. interna.* Inflammation of the inner ear affecting the organs of balance. *O. media.* Inflammation of the middle ear.

otologist (*ō-to-lo-jist*). Ear specialist.

otology (*ō-to-lo-ji*). Study of diseases of the ear.

otophone (*ō'-to-fōn*). Ear-trumpet.

otorrhoea (*o-tor-re'-a*). A purulent discharge from the ear.

otosclerosis (*o-tō-skler'-ō-sis*). A chronic, progressive thickening of the structures of the internal ear leading to deafness.

otoscope (*ō-tos-kōp*). Auriscope, *q.v.*

ounce (*owns*). In fluid measure, about two tablespoonfuls; or 28·4 ml. In weight, 1/16 lb. or 28·34 g.

outlet of pelvis (*owt'-let*). The space bounded by the lower edges of the pubes, ischium, sacrum and coccyx and by the sacro-sciatic ligaments.

OUTLET OF PELVIS
1–2. Antero-posterior diameter.
3–4. Transverse diameter.

ovarian cyst (*o-vā-ri-an sist*). Cyst of the ovary; may be developmental or associated with ovarian tumour.

ovaries (*ō'-va-rēz*). Two small oval bodies situated on either side of the uterus; the female organs in which ova are formed. They are also endocrine glands.

ovariectomy (*ō-vā-rē-ek-to-mi*). Oophorectomy. Surgical removal of ovary.

ovariotomy (*o-vā-ri-ot'-o-mi*). The operation of cutting into an ovary.

ovaritis (*ō-va-rī-tis*) See OOPHORITIS.

ovary. See OVARIES and p. 260.

Fallopian tube — ligament of ovary — uterus — cervix — vagina — utero-sacral ligament — broad ligament — ovary

DIAGRAM SHOWING LEFT
OVARY AND FALLOPIAN
TUBE

overcompensation. (1) Homeostasis is achieved by the body compensating for changes brought about in various circumstances. When the compensatory mechanism too far outweighs the change which it opposes, overcompensation is said to have taken place. (2) In psychiatry applies to exaggerated compensatory behaviour, *e.g.* extreme aggressiveness in response to a feeling of inadequacy.

overdosage. Excessive concentration of a drug in the blood. This may be an accumulation from repeated doses or from too high a dose.

overextension (*ō-ver-ek-sten'-shon*). Extension beyond the normal limit, *e.g.* of a joint or muscle.

oviduct (*o'-vid-ukt*). The Fallopian tube between the ovary and the womb, conveying the ova. *See* OVARIES.

ovulation (*ov-ū-lā'-shon*). The development and discharge of ova from the ovary.

ovum (*ō'-vum*). The egg cell produced in the female ovary.

oxalic acid (*ok-sal'-ik*). A poisonous acid obtained from wood sorrel; chalk and magnesium are the antidotes. *See* POISONS AND ANTIDOTES in Appendix, p. 386.

oxaluria (*ox-al-ū'-ri-a*). A disease marked by the presence of oxalic acid crystals in the urine.

oxidation (*ok-si-dā-shon*), **oxidization** (*ok-si-di-zā-shon*), The chemical combination of oxygen with a substance producing oxides, etc. and releasing energy, e.g. in burning and the break-up of carbohydrates in the body. Can also denote a reduction in the hydrogen content of a molecule, or a loss of electrons from an atom or molecule resulting in an increased ability to take up oxygen, *cf.* reduction.

oxycephaly (*ok-sē-ke-fa-li*). Abnormal development of the skull with resultant egg-shaped appearance. Most cases develop increased intracranial pressure.

oxygen (*ok'-si-jen*). A colourless, odourless gas, forming about 20 per cent of the atmosphere. It supports combustion and is indispensable to life. Inhalations are given in cases of cyanosis and shock. Applied also in the form of hydrogen peroxide to ulcers and septic wounds.

oxygen administration (*ok-si-jen ad-min-is-trā′-shon*). By (1) nasal catheters at approximately 4 litres per minute. This will raise the alveolar oxygen to approximately 30 per cent.
(2) Oxygen Tent. Rate of flow depends upon amount of disturbance for nursing care. With average care, the alveolar oxygen can be kept at 45 per cent.
(3) B.L.B. mask. Rate of flow adjusted so that a little

OXYGEN MASK

ADMINISTRATION OF OXYGEN

TUDOR-EDWARDS SPECTACLE FRAME

a.a. Connected by **Y** piece to cylinder.
b.b. Soft rubber tubing to nostrils.

gas is left in the bag at the end of inspiration; possible to raise alveolar oxygen to 90 per cent. Humidification by moisture in the bag. If any of the three holes under the rotating collar are left open, a flow-meter should be used.

oxygen debt. If the metabolic requirement for oxygen exceeds the supply, the metabolic processes are carried on under partially anaerobic conditions, *q.v.* until at a later time the 'oxygen debt' is repaid.

oxygenation (*ok-si-je-nā-shon*). To saturate with oxygen.

oxyhaemoglobin (*ok-si-hēm-o-glō'-bin*). Haemoglobin in which oxygen is in combination—as in the red corpuscles of the blood.

oxyntic (*ok-sin-tik*). Term applied to cells secreting hydrochloric acid in the stomach.

oxytetracycline (*ok-si-te-tra-sī'-klin*). See TETRACYCLINE.

oxytocics (*ok-si-tō'-siks*). Drugs used to promote uterine contractions, *e.g.* pituitrin.

oxytocin (*ok-si-tō'-sin*). The oxytocic hormone of the posterior lobe of the pituitary gland.

oxyuriasis (*ok'-si-ū-rī-a-sis*). Infection with oxyuris vermicularis.

oxyuris vermicularis (*ok-si-ūr'-is ver-mik-ū-la'-ris*). Threadworm found in the rectum and large intestine, especially in children.

OXYURIS VERMICULARIS
The worm, and head enlarged.

ozaena (*o-zē-na*). Form of atrophic rhinitis.

ozone (*ō'-zōn*). O_3. An oxidizing agent sometimes used as a disinfectant.

ozonic ether (*o-zo'-nik ē'-ther*). A solution of hydrogen peroxide in ether.

P

P. Chemical symbol for phosphorus.

Pacchioni's bodies (*pak-ī-ō-nis*). Villi from the arachnoid membrane. A path for draining cerebrospinal fluid into the venous sinuses.

pacemaker (*pās-mā-ker*). Initiator of heart impulse at sino-atrial node. An electrical stimulator can be fitted surgically.

pachy-. A prefix denoting thickness.

pachydermia (*pak-i-der'-mi-a*). Thickening of the skin.

pachymeningitis (*pak-i-men-in-jī'-tis*). Inflammation of the dura mater, with thickening of the membrane.

Pacini's corpuscles (*pa-chē-nis kor'-pusls*). Specialized sensory receptors which register pressure and to some extent vibration. They are situated in the deeper connective tissues of the skin and consist of nerve endings surrounded by concentric lamellae of fibrous tissue.

pack. Moistened material applied to a patient. A *cold pack* consists in wrapping the patient in a sheet wrung out in cold water; he is then enveloped in a dry blanket and mackintosh and left for thirty minutes, or the prescribed time. An *ice pack* consists in wringing out towels in ice water and applying them to the patient, perpetually changing them as they get warm A *hot pack* is sometimes applied to relieve the pain of muscle spasm, *e.g.* in poliomyelitis. The pack is first applied at 100° F and hotter packs applied subsequently until one of 130°F is tolerated. *Warm packs* wrung out in saline, etc., are used in operations, to cover or secure organs. Packs or swabs used in the theatre should either be attached by large rings or clamps or labelled with a radio-opaque band.

paediatrician (*pē-dē-a-tri-shon*). Specialist in diseases of children.

paediatrics (*pē-dē-at-riks*). The science or study of diseases of children.

Paget's disease. (1) Of bone, osteitis deformans, is a disorder of unknown cause which usually affects a number of bones to a greater or lesser extent. Clinical features are pain, tendency to pathological fractures and hyperdynamic circulation. (2) Of nipple. Eczema of the nipple associated with underlying duct carcinoma of the breast.

painter's colic (*pānt-erz kol-ik*). Lead poisoning.

palate (*pal'-āt*). The roof of the mouth.

palatoplegia (*pa-la-tō-plē-ji-a*). Paralysis of soft palate.

palliative (*pal'-i-a-tiv*). A medicine which relieves but does not cure.

pallidectomy (*pal-li-dek-to-mi*). Operation used in Parkinson's disease to decrease the activity of part of the lentiform nucleus in the base of the brain.

pallidotomy (*pa-li-do-to-mi*). Operation performed to relieve tremor in Parkinson's disease. Fibres from the cerebral cortex are severed.

pallor (*pal'-or*). Paleness.

palm (*parm*). The hollow or flexor surface of the hand.

palmar (*pal'-mar*). Pertaining to the palm of the hand.

palpation (*pal-pā'-shon*). Examination by the hand.

palpebra (*pal-pe'-bra*). The eyelid.

palpitation (*pal-pi-tā'-shon*). Rapid throbbing of the heart, producing consciousness of the heart's action.

palsy (*pawl'-zi*). Paralysis. *See* ERB'S PARALYSIS.

Paludrine (*pal-ū-drin*). Synthetic antimalarial drug of high potency. Proguanil, *q.v.*

pamaquin (*pa-ma-kwin*). Drug used to treat malaria.

pan. A prefix signifying all, total.

panacea (*pan-a-sē'-a*). A medicine which is claimed or advertised to cure all diseases.

panarthritis (*pan-ar-thrī-tis*). Generalized inflammation of joint structures.

pancarditis (*pan-kar-dī-tis*). Generalized inflammation of the heart.

pancreas (*pan'-krē-as*). Sweetbread. A gland situated in the mesentery in relation to the duodenum and crossing the mid-line of the body. It secretes an alkaline mixture of digestive enzymes through the pancreatic duct into the duodenum when stimulated by the hormone *secretin*. It also contains groups of cells which secrete insulin into the blood. *See* LANGERHANS, ISLETS.

pancreatectomy (*pan-krē-a-tek'-to-mi*). Excision of pancreas.

pancreatitis (*pan'-krē-a-tī'-tis*). Inflammation of the pancreas.

pandemic (*pan-dem'-ik*). A widely spread epidemic.

panhypopituitarism (*pan-hī-pō-pi-tū-i-ta-rism*). Simmonds'

disease. Deficient secretion of all of the anterior pituitary hormones with additional secondary reduction in production of hormones by the thyroid and adrenal cortex.

panhysterectomy (*his-te-rek'-to-mi*). Total removal of the uterus.

pannus (*pan'-nus*). Vascularization of the cornea; in joints the replacement of cartilage by granulation tissue.

panophthalmia, panophthalmitis (*pan-of-thal-mī'-tis*). Generalized inflammation of the eye-ball.

DIAGRAM SHOWING POSITION OF THE PANCREAS

panotitis (*pan-o-tī'-tis*). Inflammation of the middle and internal ear.

Papanicolaou stain (*pa-pa-ni-kō-law*). Stain frequently employed for the examination of vaginal smears.

papaveretum (B.P.C.) (*pa-pa-ve-rā'-tum*). Syn. Omnopon. A solution of all the alkaloids of opium.

papaverine (*pa-pav'-er-in*). An alkaloid of opium; antispasmodic and vasodilator.

papilla (*pa-pil'-la*), plu. **papillae**. (1) A small nipple-shaped eminence. (2) The optic disc. *Circumvallate Papillae*. These are found at the root of the tongue. *Filiform Papillae*. The common *P.* of the tongue and found at its tip. *Fungiform Papillae* are the broad *P.* of the tongue.

papillitis (*pap-pil-ī'-tis*). Inflammation of the optic disc.

papilloedema (*pap-il-e-dē'-ma*). Oedema of the optic nerve.

papilloma (*pap-il-lō'-ma*). Benign neoplasm of epithelial cells.

papule (*pap'-ūl*). A small solid pimple.

papyraceus (*pap-i-rā'-shus*). See FOETUS PAPYRACEUS.

para (*pa'-ra*). Prefix meaning beside or near.

para-aminobenzoic acid (*pa-ra-a-mī-nō-ben-zō-ik as-id*). A bacterial growth factor antagonized by the sulphanilamides.

para-aminosalicylic acid (*pa-ra-a-mī'-nō-sa-li-si-lik as-id*). One of the drugs given in tuberculosis. Often known as P.A.S.

para-aortic (*pa-ra-ā-or'-tik*). Near the aorta.

paracentesis (*par-a-sen-tē'-sis*). Withdrawing fluid from the body cavity. See ASPIRATION.

paracusis (*par-a-kū'-sis*). Disordered hearing.

paradoxical breathing. Part of the lung inflates during expiration and vice versa.

paraesthesia (*par-es-thēz'-i-a*). Disorder of sensation, such as tingling and pins and needles.

paraffin. Any hydrocarbon of the methane series. Liquid paraffin is refined petroleum. Soft paraffin is used as a lubricating jelly. Hard paraffin is paraffin wax.

paraformaldehyde (*pa-ra-for-mal-di-hīd*). Used to fumigate closed spaces, also for sterilization of catheters and instruments when kept in an air-tight container filled with paraformaldehyde.

paraldehyde (*par-al'-de-hīd*). A sporific, having a pungent taste. It may cause an erythematous rash. Poison. *Antidotes:* friction, strong coffee. This drug may be given per rectum as a narcotic before operation. This minimizes shock.

paralysis (*par-al'-i-sis*). Loss of power of movement or of sensation. Usually due to a lesion in the nervous system. *Spastic P.* is due to a lesion of upper motor neurones. *Flaccid P.* is the result of an injury to lower motor neurones. *Infantile paralysis* is the result of poliomyelitis.

paralysis agitans (*aj'-it-anz*). *See* PARKINSON'S DISEASE.

paralytic ileus (*pa-ra-li-tik i-lē-us*). Intestinal obstruction due to local inflammation paralysing the wave of peristalsis. *See* ILEUS.

paramedian (*pa-ra-mē'-di-an*). Close to the middle.

paramedical (*pa-ra-me'-di-kal*). Allied to medicine.

parametritis (*pa-ra-met-rī'-tis*). Inflammation of the parametrium. Also called *pelvic cellulitis*.

parametrium (*pa-ra-mēt-rium*). The connective tissue around the uterus, chiefly found round large vessels and between the layers of the broad ligament.

paramnesia (*par-am-nē'-si-a*). False memory; usually memory of events which did not occur in the connection related.

paramyotonia congenita (*pa-ra-mī-ō-tō-ni-a kon-jen-i-ta*). Form of myotonia congenita with tonic spasm esp. of face. It is aggravated by cold.

paranoia (*par-a-noy'-a*). Delusions of persecution.

paranoid (*pa-ra-noyd*). Relating to paranoia.

paraphimosis (*pa-ra-fĭ-mō'-sis*). Retraction of the prepuce behind the glans penis with inability to restore it to the natural position.

paraplegia (*par-a-plē'-ji-a*).

Paralysis of both lower limbs or both upper limbs.

parasite (*par-a-sīt*). Any living thing which lives on or in another organism.

parasiticide (*pa-ra-sī'-ti-sīd*). Substance lethal to parasites

parasympathetic system (*pa-ra-sim-pa-the-tik sis-tem*). Part of the autonomic nervous system acting in opposition to the sympathetic system, *e.g.* para-sympathetic action causes constriction of the pupil, stimulation of the gut, etc.

parathormone (*para-thor'-mōn*). A preparation of the hormone of the parathyroid glands.

parathyroid (*para-thī'-royd*). Small endocrine glands which control calcium and phosphate metabolism. They are usually four in number and they are situated in the vicinity of the thyroid gland.

paratyphoid (*pa-ra-tī'-foyd*). An infectious disease resembling typhoid fever and caused by an organism not identical with but closely allied to the bacillus of typhoid. *See* ENTERIC.

paravertebral (*pa-ra-ver'-te-bral*). To one side of the spinal column.

parenchyma (*par-en'-kī-ma*). The functional part of an organ.

parenteral treatment (*pa-ren-te-ral'*). Therapy by drugs given by routes other than the alimentary tract.

paresis (*par'-ēs-is*). A partial paralysis.

parietal (*pa-rī'-e-tal*). The two bones which form the crown and sides of the cranium. *See* SKULL and FONTANELLE.

parietes (*pa-rī-e-tēz*). The walls of any cavity of the body.

parity (*pa'-ri-ti*). The number of children a woman has borne.

Parkinson's disease (*par'-kinsonz*), also called paralysis agitans. A chronic disease of later life, showing tremors, rigidity of joints and muscles, a mask-like expression and walking with a tendency to fall forwards.

paronychia (*par-o-nik'-i-a*). Whitlow; inflammation and abscess at the end of a finger near the nail.

paroophoron (*par-o-of'-or-on*). *See* PAROVARIUM.

parosmia (*pa-ros-mi-a*). Perverted sense of smell.

parotid (*par-ot'-id*). Near the ear; applied to a salivary gland under the ear. (*See illustration.*)

parotitis (*par-o-tī'-tis*). Inflammation of the parotid gland. (1) Mumps, *q.v.* (2) Spread of infection from a septic mouth.

parovarium (*pa-ro-vā'-rium*). A vestigial structure in the broad ligaments of the uterus which occasionally gives origin to small cysts in this region.

SALIVARY GLANDS

paroxysm (*par'-oks-izm*). A sudden temporary attack.

paroxysmal nocturnal dyspnoea (*pa-rok-sis-mal nok-ter-nal dis-ne-a*). Attacks of breathlessness occurring at night due to accummulation of fluid in the lungs resulting from left ventricular failure.

paroxysmal tachycardia (*pa-rok-sis-mal ta-ki-kar-di-a*). Is due to the regular and rapid discharge of impulses from ectopic focus in the atrial walls of the heart. The focus thus replaces the sino-atrial node as the cardiac pacemaker and drives the heart at a rate of about 180 beats per minute. Attacks may last anything from a minute to several days.

Parrish's food (*pa'-rish-es*). Syrup of phosphates of iron, lime, and soda. A tonic for children. Should be given after food.

parrot disease (*pa'-rot*). Psittacosis, *q.v.*

parturient (*par-tū'-ri-ent*). In the condition of giving or being just about to give birth to a child. The *parturient canal* is the passage traversed by the fetus during birth, from the brim of the pelvis to the vulva.

parturition (*par-tū-rish'-un*). The act of giving birth to a child.

P.A.S. Para-aminosalicylic acid. Used in tuberculosis together with other antituberculous drugs.

Paschen bodies (*pash-en*). Minute bodies containing the virus of smallpox.

passive. Submissive. Not active or spontaneous. *P. Immunity.* See IMMUNITY. *Passive movements* are performed on a patient's joints by a physiotherapist to increase the mobility, prevent contractures and to improve the circulation.

Pasteurella (*pas-te-re-la*). Group of bacilli causing bubonic and pneumonic plague. Carried by rats to man.

pasteurization (*pas'-tur-ī-za'-shon*). Method of sterilization of fluids introduced by Pasteur which involves heating for 30 minutes at 70° C.

patella (*pa-tel'-la*). The knee-cap. A sesamoid bone in front of the knee joint.

patellar bursae (*ber'-sē*). The bursae around the patella. Inflammation of the prepatellar bursa used to be called housemaid's knee, as it occurs after much kneeling.

patellectomy (*pa-tel-lek-to-mi*). Operation to excise the patella.

patent (*pā'-tent*). Open. *P. ductus arteriosus.* Failure of the ductus arteriosus to close at birth. *P. foramen ovale.* Failure of closure of the foramen ovale, *q.v.*

pathogenesis (*pa-thō-jen'-e-sis*). The origin and progress of disease.

pathogenic (*path-ō-jen-ik*). Capable of causing disease.

pathognomonic (*pa-tho-nō-mon'-ik*). Characteristic of, or peculiar to, a particular disease.

pathological (*pa-tho-loj'-i-kal*). Relating to pathology. Morbid, abnormal.

pathology (*pa-thol'-o-ji*). The study of disease, particularly regarding the changes in the tissues resulting from disease.

pathophobia (*path-ō-fō'-bi-a*). Neurotic fear of disease.

patulous (*pat'-ū-lus*). Open wide.

Paul-Bragg's apparatus. A type of respirator.

Paul-Bunnell test (*porl-boo-nel*). A serological test for glandular fever (infective mononucleosis).

Paul's tube (*pawls tūb*). Glass drainage tube used to drain the bowel.

Pearson bed. Special bed for nursing fractures.

peau d'orange (*pō-dor-anj'*). Orange-skin appearance of skin overlying carcinoma of the breast which is caused by obstruction to superficial lymphatics.

pectin (*pek'-tin*). A polysaccharide found in fruit.

pectoral (*pek'-tor-al*). Relating to the chest. *P. Muscles* are on the anterior surface of chest.

pectus (*pek'-tus*). The thorax, chest.

pediatrics (*pē'-di-at'-riks*). See PAEDIATRICS.

pedicle (*ped'-ē-kl*). The stalk of an organ or tumour containing blood-vessels.

pedicle needle. An instrument for passing a ligature round the pedicle of a tumour.

PEDICLE NEEDLE

pediculosis (*ped-ik-ū-lō'-sis*). Infestation with lice.

pediculus (*pe-dik'-ū-lus*). The louse, a parasite infesting the hair and skin. *P. Capitis* infests the head; *P. Corporis*, the body and clothing; *P. Pubis*, the pubic hair. These three varieties are different in shape and size.

pedunculated (*ped-ung'-kū-lā-ted*). Possessing a pedicle.

PEDICULUS
A. Capitis. B. Corporis. C. Pubis
(Magnified)

Pel-Ebstein's fever (*pel-eb-stīns*). A regularly remitting fever which sometimes occurs in Hodgkin's disease.

pellagra (*pe-lah-gra*). A disease especially prevalent in Southern Europe and in the United States. It is marked in the initial stages by recurring redness and exfoliation—resembling sunburn—of the hands and face. There may be glossitis, diarrhoea and peripheral neuritis, and mental changes. The anti-pellagra factor is vitamin B_6.

pellet (*pel-let*). A small pill, esp. those used as implants, *q.v.*

pelletierine tannate (*pel-et'-i-er-ēn tan'-āt*). A mixture of the alkaloids obtained from the bark of the pomegranate; an anthelmintic having a specific action on the tapeworm.

pellicle (*pel'-le-kl*). A thin skin or membrane.

pelvic (*pel'-vik*). Relating to the pelvis.

pelvic cellulitis (*sel-ū-li-tis*). *See* PARAMETRITIS.

pelvic exenteration. Operative removal of organ from pelvis.

pelvimetry (*pel-vi-me-tri*). Measurement of pelvic dimensions.

pelvis (*pel'-vis*). The bony cavity composed of the hips and the lower bones of the spine and holding the bowels,

Sacrum
Illium
Coccyx
Pubic symphysis
Os pubis
Acetabulum
Ischium

FEMALE PELVIS

Sacrum
L.S
Uterus
Bladder
Rectum
Pubic symphysis
Vagina

SAGITTAL SECTION OF
FEMALE PELVIS

bladder and organs of generation.

pemphigus (*pem'-fi-gus*). Disease characterized by the formation of large blisters on the skin and mucous membranes. *P. neonatorum* is a misnomer. It is an acute staphylococcal impetigo occurring in newborn infants.

pendulous (*pen'-dū-lus*). Hanging down.

penetration (*pen-et-rā'-shon*). Entering into a surface. Focal depths of a microscope.

penicillin (*pe-ni-si-lin*). A highly potent non-toxic antibacterial substance obtained from the mould *Penicillium Notatum*. Special indications: Staphylococcal infections and gonorrhoea. Also effective against haemolytic streptococci, pneumococci, and meningococci. Ineffective against tubercle and *B. Coli.*

penicillinase (*pe-ni-si-li-nās*). Enzyme found in penicillin-resistant organisms. It inactivates penicillin.

penis (*pē'-nis*). The male organ of coition containing the urethra.

pentagastrin (*pen-tu-gas-trin*). A gastric acid stimulant used to test the secretion of the stomach.

pentobarbital sodium. A barbiturate. Official name for Nembutal, *q.v.*

Pentothal. Official name thiopentone sodium. A barbiturate drug, administered intravenously. It is valuable for producing anaesthesia of short duration.

peppermint (*pep'-per-mint*). Carminative and stimulant. Ol. menth. pip. on a lump of sugar or Aqua menth. pip.

pepsin (*pep'-sin*). An enzyme which breaks down proteins in acid solution to form peptides (*peptidase*). It is secreted in the stomach with hydrochloric acid.

peptic (*pep'-tik*). Pertaining to digestion, *P. ulcer*, a gastric, duodenal, or gastrojejunal ulcer.

peptic ulcer diet. *See* Appendix, pp. 425–428.

peptone (*pep-tōn*). Compound formed during breakdown of protein.

peptonized food (*pep'-tōn-īzed*). A partially pre-digested food. As a rule milk, beef-tea, or other simple fluid food is chosen. May be prescribed for acute gastritis.

perception (*per-sep-shon*). An awareness. Receiving impressions through the senses.

perchloride of mercury. *See* CORROSIVE SUBLIMATE.

percolation (*per-kol-ā'-shon*). The passage of a liquid through a solid but porous substance. Liquid extracts are made in this way. The drug is coarsely powdered, packed into a cylindrical vessel and the solvent trickles slowly through.

Percorten (*per-kor-ten*). Deoxycortone acetate. Used chiefly in Addison's disease.

percussion (*per-kush'-on*). Striking upon the body, the sound heard being helpful in diagnosis. The note emitted is resonant or dull according to the conditions of the organ underneath.

perforation (*per-fo-rā'-shon*). A hole in an organ caused by disease or injury. The act of perforating.

peri- (*per-i*). Prefix signifying around, near, about.

perianal (*pe-ri-ā'-nal*). Around the anus.

periarteritis (*pe-ri-ar-ter-ī-tis*). Inflammation of the outer coat of an artery.

periarthritis (*pe-ri-ar-thrī'-tis*). Inflammation of the tissues round a joint.

periarteritis nodosa. A disease of unknown cause which is characterized by the production of multiple nodules in the connective tissues surrounding the smaller arteries. The symptoms and signs associated with this disorder depend on the distribution of the lesions.

pericardial (*pe-ri-kar-dē-al*). Pertaining to the pericardium.

pericardial adhesions. Fibrosis of the pericardium which may follow pericarditis, *q.v.*, in which the two layers of the pericardium become stuck together.

pericardiotomy (*pe-ri-kar-dē-o-to-mi*). An opening made into the pericardium.

pericarditis (*per-i-kar-dī′-tis*). Inflammation of the pericardium; apt to follow on cases of acute rheumatism, typhoid, Bright's disease, pneumonia or pyaemia.

pericardium (*per-i-kar′-di-um*). The membranous sac which holds the heart. *Adherent P.* Rheumatic carditis is often followed by an adherent pericardium, especially after a pericarditis. This condition interferes with the free action of the heart.

Superior vena cava

Aorta

Right pulmonary artery

R.pulm veins

Diaphragm

Fibrous pericardium

Serous ″

potential space

Right atrium

Right ventricle

Sternum

Inferior vena cava

DIAGRAM OF
PERICARDIUM

perichondritis (*per-i-kon-drī′-tis*). Inflammation of perichondrium.

perichondrium (*per-i-kon′-drē-um*). The membranous covering of a cartilage.

pericolitis (*pe-ri-kol-ī-tis*). Inflammation round the colon.

pericolpitis or **paracolpitis** (*per-i-kol-pī′-tis*). Inflammation of the structures around the vagina.

pericranium (*per-i-krān′-i-um*). The membrane covering the bones of the skull.

perilymph (*pe-ri-limf*). Clear fluid in the osseous labyrinth of the ear.

perimeter (*pe-ri-me-ter*). (1) Circumference. (2) Instrument for measuring field of vision.

perimetritis (*per-i-me-trī′-tis*). Inflammation of the peritoneum covering the uterus.

perimetry (*pe-ri-me-tri*). Measurement of visual field.

perinatal mortality rate (*pe-ri-nā′-tal*). The number of stillbirths and deaths in the first week of life of babies weighing more than 1,000 g at birth per 1,000 births.

perineal (*pe-ri-nē-al*). Pertaining to the perineum. *P. body.* Wedge-shaped muscular body which forms the focus of the pelvic floor.

perineoplasty (*pe-rin-e-ō-plas-ti*). Same as perineorrhaphy.

perineorrhaphy (*per-i-ne-or′-raf-hē*). Operation for repairing a perineum ruptured during labour.

perinephric (*pe-ri-nef-rik*). Round about the kidney, *P. Abscess,* a collection of pus in the tissues round the kidney.

perineum (*pe-ri-nē′-um*). The region of the pelvic floor, anterior to the anus.

perineurium (*pe-ri-nū-rē-um*). A sheath investing a bundle of nerve fibres.

periodontal membrane. Ligament attaching the tooth to the walls of its socket. *P. disease.* Abnormalities of the supporting structures of the teeth.

periosteal (*pe-ri-os'-te-al*). Pertaining to periosteum. *P. Sarcoma*, sarcoma growing from periosteum.

periosteal elevator (*per-i-os'-tē-al*). See RUGINE.

periosteotome (*pe-rē-os-tē-o-tōm*). Knife used to incise the periosteum.

periosteum (*per-i-os'-tē-um*). The membrane covering a bone.

periostitis (*per-ē-os-tī-tis*). Inflammation of the periosteum.

peripheral (*pe-rif'-er-al*). Relating to the circumference or outer surface. *P. neuritis.* Inflammation of the peripheral nerves.

periproctitis (*pe-ri-prok-tī'-tis*). Inflammation of tissue around the rectum or anus.

perisalpingitis (*pe-ri-sal-pin-jī'-tis*). Inflammation of peritoneum covering the uterine tube.

peristalsis (*per-ē-stal'-sis*). The contractions and movements of the alimentary tract forcing on the contents.

peritomy (*pe-rit'-om-i*). Incision of the conjunctiva near the margin of the cornea for the cure of pannus.

peritoneal (*pe-ri-tō-nē-al*). Pertaining to peritoneum.

peritoneum (*per-i-to-nē'-um*). The membrane or sac which surrounds the intestines and most other abdominal viscera, and which also lines the abdominal cavity. It secretes a serous fluid which prevents friction.

peritonitis (*per-i-to-nī'-tis*). Inflammation of the peritoneum. *General p.* Generalized infection of the peritoneal cavity. *Pelvic p.*, of the pelvic peritoneum. *Tuberculous p.* Infection of the peritoneum by tubercles either deposited by blood-stream, or as a spread from tuberculous Fallopian tubes, or from tuberculous ulceration of the bowel. There are two types: (1) *Plastic*, when many adhesions are present and whole bowel may be matted together; (2) *Ascitic*, when abdomen is greatly distended with fluid.

peritonsillar abscess (*pe-ri-ton-sil-a*). See QUINSY.

perityphlitis (*pe-ri-tif-lī-tis*). Inflammation of the peritoneum around the caecum and appendix.

periurethral (*pe-ri-ūr-ēth'-ral*). Around the urethra.

permanent teeth (*per'-man-ent*). Teeth of the second dentition. See TEETH.

permanganate of potash (*per-man'-gan-āt of pot'-ash*). Antiseptic and disinfectant. Care should be employed in its use, as it is poisonous in crystal state.

permeable (*per'-me-abl*). Capable of being penetrated.

pernicious (*per-nish'-us*). Tending to a fatal issue. *P. Anaemia.* Anaemia resulting from cyanocobalamin (vitamin B_{12}) deficiency.

pernicious vomiting. *See* VOMITING OF PREGNANCY.

pernio (*per-nē-ō*). A chilblain.

peroneal (*pe-rō-nē-al*). Pertaining to the fibula.

peroral (*per-aw-ral*). Through the mouth.

peroxide of hydrogen. *See* HYDROGEN PEROXIDE.

perseveration (*per-sev-e-rā'-shon*). A recurring idea, feeling or way of action from which the patient finds it difficult to escape.

personality (*per-so-na-li-ti*). The make-up of a person with all his individual characteristics, both inherited and acquired, with which he faces life.

perspiration (*per-spi-rā-shon*). Sweat, which is excreted through the pores of the skin.

Perthes' disease (*per-ths*). *See* osteochondritis.

pertussis (*per-tus'-sis*). Whooping cough; an infectious spasmodic cough, common in childhood. The cough ends with a whoop and sometimes causes an attack of vomiting. The disease runs its course in four to eight weeks' time. A serious disease in young children who should be vaccinated against it. Caused by haemophilus pertussis.

perversion (*per-ver'-shon*). Turned away from the normal course. *Sexual P.*, aberrations of normal sexual behaviour.

pes (*pāz*). The foot. *Pes cavus*, a greatly exaggerated longitudinal arch of the foot, with deformity of the toes. *Pes planus*, flat foot.

pessary (*pes'-sar-i*). (1) An instrument placed in the vagina to prevent or remedy malpositions of the uterus or vaginal prolapse. The Hodge or the ring pessary are often used, usually made of plastic. Patients wearing a pessary should have a daily vaginal douche and consult a doctor every three months. (2) A medicated suppository for insertion into the vagina.

PESSARIES
Hodge Pessary and Ring Pessary

pesticide (*pes-ti-sīd*). Term used to describe a substance that kills harmful or disease carrying insects or organisms.

pestilence (*pes-ti-lens*). Virulent infectious epidemic disease.

petechiae (*pe-te'-chi-ē*). Small red spots on the skin formed by effusion of blood.

pethidine (*pe'-thi-dēn*). A synthetic drug similar in action to morphine. As it is habit-forming it has been included in the Dangerous Drugs Act.

Pethilorfan (*pe-thi-lor'-fan*). Pethidine hydrochloride and levallorphan. The combination of the latter with pethidine reduces the risk of respiratory depression.

petit mal. *See* EPILEPSY.

Petri dish (*pet-ri*). A small flat glass dish used in bacteriological laboratories.

pétrissage (*pā'-tres-saj*). A massage movement, consisting in picking up and rolling the muscles between the thumb and fingers—it is slow and continuous.

petrous (*pet'-rus*). Stony; a term given to a hard part of the temporal bone.

Peyer's patches (*pā'-yerz pa'-ches*). Small glands situated on the surface of the ileum and jejunum. Seat of ulceration in typhoid and paratyphoid fever.

pH. Scale of values denoting the hydrogen ion concentration of solutions and thus their alkalinity or acidity. Values below 7 are acid and those above 7 are alkaline.

phaeochromocyte (*fē'-ō-krō-mō-sīt*). One of two cell-types present in the adrenal medulla and in the sympathetic ganglion.

phaeochromocytoma (*fē-ō-krō-mō-sī-tō'-ma*). Tumour of phaeochromocytes usually arising in the adrenal gland and producing hypertension, hyperglycaemia and irregularity of cardiac rhythm.

phage typing (*fāj tī-ping*). Method of identifying bacteria which depends on their sensitivity to lysis by bacteriophage viruses.

phagocytes (*fag'-ō-sītz*). The polymorphonuclear white corpuscles of the blood, so called from their property of being able to ingest and destroy micro-organisms of disease which may be circulating in the blood or attacking the tissues.

phagocytosis (*fag-ō-sī-tō'-sis*). The process of enveloping and absorbing a hostile germ by a phagocyte.

PHAGOCYTOSIS

phalanges (*fal-an'-jēz*). The small bones of the fingers and toes. (*See* p. 276.)

phallus (*fa'-lus*). The penis.

PHALANGES OF FINGERS

PHALANGES OF TOES

phantasy (*fan'-ta-si*). *See* FAN-
TASY.

phantom limb (*fan'-tom lim*).
Sensation often experienced
by patient, after an amputation, that the limb is still
there.

pharmaceutical (*far-ma-sū'-
tik-al*). Pertaining to drugs.

pharmacology (*far-ma-kol'-o-
ji*). A study of drug action.

Pharmacopoeia (*far-ma-ko-
pē'-a*). An authorized hand-
book of drugs. *British P.* has
a legal status.

pharmacy (*far'-ma-sē*). The
science of preparing and
mixing medicines or drugs.

pharyngeal (*far-in'-je-al*). Pertaining to the pharynx. *P.
pouch.* Diverticulum in the
wall of the pharynx which
may form between the two
portions of the inferior con-
strictor muscle of the pharynx.

pharyngectomy (*fa-rin-jek'-to-
mi*). Excision of part of the
pharynx.

pharyngismus (*far-in-jiz-mus*).
Spasm of the pharynx.

pharyngitis (*far-in-jī'-tis*). Inflammation of the pharynx.

pharyngotympanic tube (*fa-rin-
gō-tim-pa'-nik tūb*). Eustachian tube, running from the
pharynx to the middle ear.

pharynx (*far'-inks*). The
musculo-membranous sac at
the back of the mouth leading
to the oesophagus and to the
larynx.

phemitone (*fe'-mi-tōn*). Methyl-
phenobarbitone. Is used
in epilepsy for its antispasmodic property.

phenacetin (*fen-as'-et-in*). An
analgesic.

phenazone. An analgesic similar to phenacetin. Soluble in
water, therefore quicker in
action; less well-tolerated.

Phenergan. Promethazine hydrochloride. Antihistamine
of high potency and pro-
longed activity.

phenindione (*fe-nin-dī-ōn*).
Anticoagulant with slower
action than heparin.

phenobarbitone (*fē-nō-bah'-bi-tōn*). (Luminal.) Derivative of barbituric acid. Sedative.

phenol (*fē'-nol*). Carbolic acid.

phenolphthalein (*fe-nol-tha'-le-in*). Purgative. Some of it is absorbed from the intestine, carried to the liver, excreted in the bile and so the purgative action is prolonged.

phentolamine methanesulphonate (*fen-to-la-mīn me-thăn-sul-fo-nāt*). An adrenolytic and sympatholytic drug given in phaeochromocytoma.

phenylalanine (*fē-nil-al-a-nēn*). Essential amino-acid.

phenylbutazone (*fē-nil-bū-ta-zōn*). Analgesic and antipyretic used to relieve pain in rheumatism and gout.

phenylephrine hydrochloride (*fē-nil-ef-rin hī-drō-klor-īd*). Drug producing peripheral vasoconstriction and raising blood pressure. Similar to noradrenaline but of weaker action and longer duration. Sometimes used in bronchial asthma, locally for rhinitis and in ophthalmology, given in solution to dilate the pupil. Does not paralyse accommodation.

phenylketonuria (*fē-nil-kē-tō-nū'-ri-a*). Genetically determined error of metabolism in which there is an inability of the liver to convert phenylalanine to tyrosine. Instead phenylalanine is broken down to phenylpyruvic acid which is excreted in the urine. There is associated mental deficiency.

phenytoin sodium (*fen-i-toyn sō'-dium*). An anticonvulsant used in epilepsy. Synonym, Epanutin.

phial (*fī-al*). A glass capsule or container.

phimosis (*fī-mō'-sis*). Contraction of the orifice of the prepuce; usually treated by the operation of circumcision.

phlebectomy (*fleb-ek'-to-mi*). Excision of a vein.

phlebitis (*fle-bī'-tis*). Inflammation of a vein, most commonly caused by the invasion of its coats by microorganisms. Associated with thrombosis, or coagulation of the blood in the vein.

phlebolith (*fleb'-ō-lith*). Calcified venous thrombus.

phlebothrombosis. Thrombosis in veins, particularly the veins of the legs, due to prolonged haemostasis.

Phlebotomus (*fle-bo-to-mus*). Genus of small flies bringing diseases such as kala-azar.

phlebotomy (*fle-bot'-o-mi*). Bleeding a patient by opening a vein. Venesection.

phlegm (*flem*). Mucus secreted from respiratory tract.

phlegmasia (*fleg-mā-zi-a*). Inflammation. *P. Alba dolens*, white leg; a form of phlebitis occurring sometimes after labour. The leg becomes swollen, white and tense, and is very painful.

phlegmatic (*fleg-mat'-ik*). Sluggish, dull.

phlyctenule (*flik-ten-ūl*). Red pimples met with on surface of eye. *Phlyctenular conjunctivitis*, a form of disease when phlyctenules appear upon white of eye near the cornea, each becoming the centre of a small inflamed patch. They then rupture, forming a small ulcer which readily heals. *Phlyctenular keratitis*, when cornea is similarly affected.

phobia (*fō'-bi-ah*). Abnormal fear, *e.g.* cancerophobia, claustrophobia, *q.v.*

pholcodine (*fol-ko-dēn*). Drug less toxic than codeine and used to treat non-productive cough. Often given to children.

phonation (*fō-nā'-shon*). The utterance of vocal sounds.

phonetic. Relating to the voice.

phonocardiograph (*fō-nō-kar'-dē-ō-graf*). Instrument recording heart sounds.

phosphatase (*fos-fa-tāz*). Term for enzymes concerned in phosphate metabolism.

phosphate (*fos'-fāt*). A salt of phosphoric acid. A compound of phosphoric acid and a base.

phosphaturia (*fos-fat-ū'-ri-a*). Excess of phosphates in the urine.

phospholipid (*fos-fō-li-pid*). Lipids containing phosphates, *e.g.* lecithin. They are particularly useful in living systems for forming membranes.

phosphonecrosis (*fos-fō-ne-krō'-sis*). Necrosis of the jaw, caused by inhaling phosphorus; occurs in certain trades, such as match-making, but is rare.

phosphorus (*fos'-for-us*). Poisonous non-metallic element, the salts of which are used as nerve tonics.

photalgia (*fō-tal-ji-a*). Pain caused by exposure to light.

photobiology (*fō-tō-bī-ol-o-ji*). The study of the effect of light on animal life.

photochemical (*fō-tō-ke-mi-kal*). Chemical changes caused by exposure to light.

photophobia (*fō-tō-fō'-bi-a*). Abnormal intolerance of light, a symptom of inflammation of the eyes.

photosensitization (*fō-tō-sen-si-ti-zā-shon*). Tendency of tissues to react abnormally to light usually as the result of the presence in the tissues of certain chemicals which magnify the damaging effect of the incident radiation.

phrenic (*fren'-ik*). (1) Relating to the diaphragm. (2) Relating to the mind.

phrenicotomy (*fre-ni-ko-to-mi*). Division of the phrenic nerve.

phrenoplegia (*fre-nō-plē-ji-a*). Paralysis of the diaphragm.

phrynoderma (*frī-no-der-ma*). Follicular keratosis as occurs, for example, in vitamin A deficiency.

phthalylsulphathiazole (*fthal-il-sulf-a-thī-a-zol*). Sulphonamide poorly absorbed from bowel, therefore used in intestinal infections.

Phthirus pubis (*fthī-rus pū-bis*). The pubic louse.

phthisis (*thī'-sis*). Consumption; tubercular disease of the lungs.

Physeptone (*fis'-ep-tōn*). Methadone hydrochloride, *q.v.*

physic (*fiz'-ik*). (1) The art of medicine. (2) Any medicinal preparation.

physician (*fi-si-shan*). Qualified medical practitioner.

physicist (*fis'-i-sist*). An expert in the science of physics.

physics (*fi-siks*). Sciences concerned with properties and interaction of matter and energy.

physiological saline (*fi-si-ō-lo-ji-kal sā-lin*). A 0·9 per cent solution of sodium chloride in water. Also known as 'normal saline'.

physiology (*fiz-ē-ol'-o-ji*). The study of processes occurring in living systems.

physiotherapy (*fis-ē-ō-ther-api*). Therapy by physical means, *i.e.* heat, light, electricity, massage, and exercises.

physique (*fiz-ēk*). The form and constitution of the body.

physostigmine (*fis'-os-tig'-min*). Synonym eserine. A myotic; contracts the pupil. Given hypodermically to stimulate peristalsis.

phytic acid (*fi-tik a'-sid*). Substance which prevents absorption of calcium from the gut.

pia mater (*pē-a mā-ter*). The fine membrane surrounding the brain and spinal cord.

pica (*pi'-ka*). Morbid appetite. Craving for unnatural articles of food.

Pick's disease (*piks dis-ēz*) (1) Disorder affecting serous membranes resulting in effusions in the peritoneum. pericardium and pleura. The cause is unknown. (2) Presenile dementia due to cerebral atrophy.

picric acid (*pik-rik as-id*). A yellow powder. 1 per cent. sol. in water is used for burns. 1 per cent. sol. in spirit used as an antiseptic for the skin. Idiosyncrasy to the drug is not uncommon.

picrotoxin (*pik-rō-toks'-in*). Powerful central nervous system stimulant, used as antidote in barbiturate poisoning.

pigment (*pig'-ment*). An organic colouring matter. Abnormal pigmentation of the skin occurs in certain diseases, *e.g.* Addison's disease.

piles (*pī-lz*). Enlarged veins about the anus; haemorrhoids.

pilocarpine nitrate (*pi-lo-kar'-pin nī-trāt*). A drug which causes increased salivation. and perspiration. Used in glaucoma to decrease intraocular pressure.

pilonidal (*pī-lō-nē-dal*). Containing hair as in some cysts.

pilosis (*pī-lō-sis*). Abnormal growth of hair.

pilula (*pil-ū-la*). A pill; abbreviation, *pil.*

pineal body (*pĭ'-ne-al bo-dĭ*). The so-called 'third eye'. Develops from outgrowths of the forebrain, part of which forms an eye-like structure in the lamprey. In man it is a gland-like structure whose function is not determined.

pinguecula (*pin-gwe-kū-la*). Small yellow patch of connective tissue on conjunctiva occurring in old age.

pink disease. Infantile acrodynia. A form of polyneuritis with particular involvement of the autonomic nervous system thought to be due to sensitivity to mercury from calomel containing teething powder.

pink-eye (*pink'-ī*). Infectious conjunctivitis.

pinna (*pin'-na*). The outspread part of the ear.

pint (*pĭnt*). Twenty fluid ounces.

Pipanol (*pi-pa-nol*). Benzhexol hydrochloride. Spasmolytic drug used in parkinsonism.

piperazine (*pip-er-ā-zēn*). Effective drug for expelling round worms and threadworms from the body.

pipette (*pi-pet'*). A small graduated glass tube for taking up liquids.

Piriton. A proprietary form of chlorpheniramine maleate tablets. A powerful antihistamine drug often used in hay fever. Sometimes produces drowsiness.

pisiform (*pēs'-i-form*). Pea shaped; applied to a bone of the wrist.

Pitocin (*pi-tō-sin*). Official name, Injectio Oxytocini. One of the hormones from the posterior lobe of the pituitary gland. It makes the uterus contract.

Pitressin (*pit-res-sin*). Official name, Injectio Vasopressini, A preparation of a hormone of the posterior lobe of the pituitary gland. It constricts arteries, raises the blood pressure and stimulates peristalsis.

pitting. Pits are formed in the skin on pressure, as in oedema.

pituitary extract, Pituitrin. A substance obtained from the pituitary gland; it raises the blood pressure, stimulates peristalsis, and causes uterine muscle to contract.

pituitary gland (*pit-ū'-it-a-ri*). Endocrine gland in the base of the skull; there are two lobes separated by a cleft. The *anterior lobe* secretes thyrotropic hormone (T.S. H.), corticotrophic hormone (A.C.T.H.), gonadotrophic hormones (F.S.H., L.H.), growth hormone (G.H.) and prolactin. The *posterior lobe* secretes antidiuretic hormone (A.D.H.) and oxytocin.

pityriasis rosea (*pi-ti-rī-a-sis rō-sē-a*). Skin disease characterized by scaly, erythematous macula eruption. Thought to be caused by a virus related to the measles virus.

placebo (*pla-sē'-bō*). Medicine given to please the patient.

placenta (*pla-sen'-ta*). The after-birth; a circular flesh-like substance through which the mother's blood nourishes the fetus; it is expelled from the womb after the birth of the child.

Placenta
Umbilical cord
Uterus
Foetus
Cervix
Vagina

PLACENTA

placenta praevia (*prē-vē-a*). The placenta attached partially or totally to the lower uterine segment.

placentography (*pla-sen-to-gra-fi*). Technique of examining the position of the placenta by X-rays.

plague (*plāg*). An acute epidemic infectious disease caused by Pasteurella pestis derived from infected rats and transmitted to man by fleas.

plantar (*plan-tar*). Relating to the sole of the foot. *P. response*. Reflex movement of toes when the sole of the foot is stroked.

plasma (*plaz'-ma*). The liquid in which the corpuscles of the blood are suspended.

plasmodium malariae (*plas-mo-di-um ma-lā-ri-ē*). Organism causing quartan malaria.

plaster (*pla'-ster*). Adhesive tape used for keeping dressings in position or for applying extension to a limb.

plaster of Paris. Used for preparing bandages, in making splints to immobilize part of the body. Rub the dry powder into a crinoline muslin bandage; roll loosely. The bandages are soaked for a few moments in water and applied wet.

plastic surgery. Restoration of tissue to its normal shape and appearance by operative means.

platelets (*plāt'-lets*). Blood cells concerned with the clotting of blood. Normally number 200,000–500,000 per c. mm.

platinum (*pla-ti-num*). A silver-white metal of which containers are made for radium.

Platyhelminthes (*pla-ti-hel-min-thes*). Genus of flat-bodied worms.

pleocytosis (*plē-ō-sī-tō-sis*). Increase of lymphocytes in cerebrospinal fluid.

pleomorphism (*plē-ō-mor-fism*). Occurring in more than one form as with a crystal.

plethora (*pleth'-o-ra*). Fulness; an excess of blood.

pleura (*plū'-ra*). A thin membrane which covers each lung and lines the inner surface of the thoracic cavity.

pleural rub (*plū-ral rub*). A squeaking sound produced by friction between the layers of the pleura.

pleurisy (*plū'-ri-si*). Inflammation of the pleura. There are three kinds: dry, with effusion, and empyema or purulent pleurisy.

pleurodynia (*plū-ro-din'-i-a*). Pain in the side, ordinarily in the intercostal nerves.

plexor (*plek-sor*). Small hammer used in testing deep reflexes, etc.

plexus (*pleks'-us*). A network of vessels or nerves.

plica (*pli'-ka*). A fold.

plicate (*pli'-kāt*). Folded.

plombage (*plom-barj*). Filling a cavity of a tuberculous lung with nylon or polythene substances to ensure permanent collapse.

plumbism (*plum'-bizm*). Lead-poisoning.

plumbum. See LEAD.

Plummer-Vinson syndrome (*sin-drōm'*). A functional dysphagia occurring in patients with secondary anaemia.

pneumatocele (*nū-ma-tō-sēl*). A swelling containing air or gas.

pneumaturia (*nū-mā-tū-ri-a*). Diagnostic feature of vesico-intestinal fistula. Air is passed through the urethra.

pneumococcal (*nū-mō-kok'-kal*). Pertaining to the pneumococcus.

penumococcus (*nū-mō-kok'-us*). A microbe which causes pneumonia See BACTERIA.

pneumoconiosis (*nū'-mō-kō-ni'-ō-sis*). Fibrosis of the lungs caused by working in an atmosphere full of powdered grit and stone.

pneumo-encephalography (*nū-mō-en-kef-a-log'-rafi*). X-ray examination of cerebral ventricles after they have been injected with air.

pneumogastric (*nū-mō-gas'-trik*). Pertaining to the lungs and stomach. *P. Nerve*, vagus. The tenth pair of cranial nerves which supply the lungs, heart, stomach, and intestines.

pneumomycosis (*nū-mō-mī-kō'-sis*). Fungus disease of the lungs.

pneumonectomy (*nū-mo-nek'-to-mi*). Surgical removal of a lung.

pneumonia (*nū-mō'-ni-a*). An infective disease characterized by inflammation of the lungs. Double pneumonia, both lungs are diseased. *Hypostatic p.* is caused by lack of movement in a debilitated patient. May occur after operation or in the aged. *Lobar p.*, affecting one or more lobes of the lung. *Lobular p.*, see BRONCHO-PNEUMONIA.

pneumonitis (*nū-mo-nī-tis*). Inflammation of the lung.

pneumoperitoneum (*nū-mō-pe-ri-to-nē'-um*). Air in the peritoneal cavity.

pneumoradiography. X-ray examination of a part after injection with air.

pneumothorax (*nū-mō-tho'-raks*). Air in the pleural space. *Spontaneous p.* due to rupture of one of the air passages which may lead to a rise in pressure inside the chest (*tension pneumothorax*) and difficulty in breathing. *Artificial pneumothorax.* Air is introduced into the chest through a needle or incision.

pressure indicator
lead to chest
pump
valve

APPARATUS FOR
ARTIFICIAL
PNEUMOTHORAX

pock (*pok*). A pustule or the scar left by it.

podalic version (*pod-al'-ik ver-shon*). A turning round of the fetus in utero, so that the breech presents in delivery.

poikilocytosis (*poy'-ki-lō-sī-tō-sis*). Variation in the form of the red blood corpuscles.

poison (*poy'-son*). A substance deleterious to the body if absorbed in toxic concentrations. The term is usually reserved for substances which are toxic in low concentrations, *e.g.* cyanide.

polar body. Two small cells formed after mitotic division of the primary oocyte.

polio (*pō'-li-ō*). Prefix denoting grey. Journalese abbreviation of poliomyelitis.

polioencephalitis (*pōliō-en-kef-a-li'-tis*). Inflammation of the grey matter of the brain.

poliomyelitis (*pōliō-mī-e-lī'-tis*). Acute virus-mediated infection causing degeneration of the anterior horn cells of the spinal cord and consequent paralysis of the appropriate muscles.

Politzer's bag (*po-lit'-serz*). An india-rubber bag with long tube and nozzle. Used for inflating the middle ear through the nose and Eustachian tube.

pollution (*po-lū'-shon*). The act of rendering impure.

poly- (*poli*). A prefix denoting much or many.

polyarteritis nodosa (*po-li-ar-te-rī'-tis no-dō-sa*). See PERIARTERITIS NODOSA.

polyarthritis (*po-li-ar-thrī'-tis*). Inflammation of many joints.

Polya's operation (*pol-yus ope-rā-shon*). Operation for duodenal ulcer in which the stump of the stomach is anastomosed to the side of the jejunum.

polycystic (*pol-i-sis'-tik*). Composed of many cysts.

polycythaemia (*pol'-i-sīt-hē'-mi-a*). (1) *Primary polycythaemia.* Neoplasm of erythropoietic cells. (2) *Secondary polycythaemia.* Increase in the number of red blood cells in the blood due to stimulation of the bone marrow, *e.g.* by anoxia at high altitudes or due to respiratory disease.

polydactyly (*pol-i-dak'-ti-li*). The presence of supernumerary fingers or toes.

polydipsia (*po-li-dip-si-a*). Abnormal thirst.

polyglandular (*pol-i-glan'-dū-lar*). Pertaining to several glands.

polyhedral (*pol-i-hē'-dral*). Having many surfaces.

polymorphonuclear (*pol-i-mor-fō-nū'-kle-ar*). Having nuclei of various shapes. Name given to the most numerous form of white blood corpuscle, of which there are normally about 70 per cent of total. These are the chief phagocytes, and therefore they are increased in number in the presence of pus.

polymyositis (*po-li-mī-ō-sī-tis*). Weakness and wasting of muscles due to inflammation of unknown aetiology.

polymyxin B (*po-li-mik'-sin bē*). Antibiotic used mainly for local treatment of infections with certain Gram negative organisms.

polyneuritis (*po-li-nū-rī'-tis*). Multiple neuritis.

polyopia (*pol-i-ō'-pi-a*). Seeing multiple images of the same object.

polyosteotic fibrous dysplasia (*po-li-o-stē-o-tik fī-brus dis-plā-si-a*). Albright's syndrome. A congenital disorder characterized by widespread osteitis fibrosa, segmental hyperpigmentation of the skin and, in girls, precocious sexual development.

polypeptide (*pol-i-pep'-tīd*). A complex compound of several amino-acids.

polypoid (*po-li-poyd*). Like a polypus.

polypus (*pol'-i-pus*). A small simple tumour occurring in the ear, nose, uterus or rectum. *See* below.

POLYP IN POSTERIOR NARES

polysaccharides (*pol-i-sak'-ar-īdz*). A group of carbohydrates which contain more than three molecules of simple carbohydrates combined with each other, *e.g.* starch, glycogen.

polyuria (*pol-i-ū'-ri-a*). Excessive flow of urine.

polyvalent (*po-li-vā'-lent*). As applied to sera, meaning those which are active against many different strains of the same micro-organisms.

pompholyx (*pom'-fo-liks*). A dermatitis with vesicles. A vesicular eruption occurring on the palms and soles. Probably a form of eczema.

pons Varolii (*ponz va-rō'-li-ē*). That portion of the base of the brain which connects together the medulla oblongata, cerebrum and cerebellum. *See* BRAIN.

pontine (*pon-tīn*). Pertaining to the pons.

popliteal (*pop-li-te'-al*). Pertaining to the popliteal space, the area behind the knee.

pore (*por*). A minute passage in the skin for perspiration; an opening between the molecules of a body.

porphyria (*por-fī'-ri-a*). Rare metabolic disturbance which may cause mental damage in young children. There are convulsions, delirium, polyneuritis, etc.

porphyrins (*por'-fi-rins*). Pyrrole derivatives produced in the metabolism of haemoglobin.

portal hypertension (*por-tal hi-per-ten-shon*). Hypertension, *q.v.*, in the hepatic portal system, *q.v.*, usually resulting from cirrhosis of the liver.

portal vein (*por'-tal vān*). The vein which conveys to the liver the blood circulating through the gastro-intestinal system and spleen.

position (*po-si'-shon*). Attitude or posture.

positive pressure ventilation. Air is pushed into the lungs either by manual method such as the Holger Nielsen or by a mechanical device.

posological (*pos-ol-oj-i-kal*). Pertaining to dosage.

posset (*pos'-set*). In infant feeding, regurgitation of a feed.

post (*pōst*). Behind or after.

postclimacteric (*post-klī-mak-te-rik*). After the menopause.

postdiphtheritic paralysis (*post-dif-the-ri-tik pa-ra'-li-sis*). Paralysis as a result of the diphtheria toxin acting on the central nervous system. These may be palatal, ocular, cardiac, pharyngeal, laryngeal and respiratory paralysis.

postencephalitis (*pōst-en-ke-fa-lī-tis*). Condition which may remain after encephalitis.

posterior chamber of eye (*pō-stēr'-i-or chām'-ber*). Small space lying behind iris and containing aqueous humour.

postganglionic (*pōst-gan-gli-o-nik*). Behind a ganglion.

posthumous (*pos'-tū-mus*). After death; a posthumous child is one born after the father's death.

postmature (*pōst-ma-tūr*). Occurring after the due time.

post mortem (*pōst mor'-tem*). The opening and examining of a dead body.

post-natal (*nā-tal*). Following birth.

post-operative (*pōst-o'-per-ā-tiv*). After operation.

post-partum (*par'-tum*). After labour. *Post-partum haemorrhage* is excessive vaginal bleeding occurring either immediately after the birth of the baby (primary), or within a few days (secondary).

postprandial (*pōst-pran-di-al*). After a meal.

postural (*pos'-tū-ral*). By means of posture; thus the 'knee-elbow' posture is sometimes useful in treating retroversion of the gravid uterus, prolapse of the umbilical cord during labour. *See diagram*, p. 162. *P. Drainage*, the position adopted to drain the lungs in pulmonary abscess or bronchiectasis.

post-vaccinial (*pōst-vak-si-ni-al*). Occurring after vaccination.

Potain's aspirator (*pō'-tuz as-pi-rā-tor*). Used to aspirate fluid from the chest.

potassium (*po-tas'-sē-um*). A useful alkali. Many of its salts are used as drugs, *e.g.* the *bromide* as a sedative; the *chlorate* is a mild astringent and used as a mouthwash; the *chloride* is given in potassium deficiency; the *citrate* as a diuretic and given when treating bladder infection, to make the urine alkaline and to prevent crystals forming as

a result of sulphonamide therapy; the *hydroxide* is a powerful caustic; the *iodide* a diuretic and expectorant, and the *permanganate* an antiseptic.

potential (*pō-ten'-shal*). Capable of action.

Pott's disease (*po'tz diz-ēz'*). Tuberculous disease of the spine, usually in children.

Pott's fracture (*frak'-tūr*). Fracture of the fibula close above the ankle, may also be fracture of the inner malleolus with rupture of the internal lateral ligament and displacement of the foot outwards.

pouch of Douglas (*dug'-las*). *See* DOUGLAS'S POUCH.

poultices (*pōl'-tis-es*). Soft and moist applications containing heat and applied to relieve pain. Kaolin is often used spread on lint. Formerly poultices of linseed, mustard, charcoal, bread and bran were all applied but needed to be changed frequently.

Poupart's ligament (*poo-parz'*). The ligament of the groin, stretching between the anterior superior spine of the ilium and the os pubis.

p.r. Per rectum—Examination made with one finger in the rectum, by which information can be obtained of the condition of the rectum and adjacent structures.

pre- (*prē*). Prefix meaning before.

precancerous (*prē-kan'-se-rus*). A state before a cancer has arisen but which may become cancerous.

precipitate labour (*pre-sip'-it-āt*). Labour which is concluded in a time very much shorter than the average.

precipitation (*pre-sip-i-tā-shon*). The process of separating solids from the liquids which hold them in solution, by the application of heat or cold, or the addition of chemicals.

precipitins (*pre-sip'-it-ins*). Protective substances in the blood which kill bacteria by 'precipitating' their protein content.

precordium (*pre-kor'-dium*). The area of the chest over the heart.

precursor (*pre-ker'-sor*). Forerunner.

predigestion (*pre-di-jes-chon*). Food is partially digested artificially before it is eaten as with a junket when rennet has curdled the milk.

predisposed (*pre-dis-pōsd*). Susceptible.

pre-eclampsia (*pre-e-klamp'-si-a*). State before eclampsia develops and when it can still be prevented. There are albuminuria, raised blood pressure and swelling of the ankles.

prefrontal (*pre-frun'-tal*). Lying in the anterior part of frontal lobe of the brain. *P. Leucotomy. See* LEUCOTOMY.

pregnancy (*preg'-nan-si*). The state of being with child.

Usual period 280 days. *See also* ECTOPIC GESTATION.

premature labour (*prē'-ma-tūr*). Labour resulting in birth of premature baby, i.e. one weighing 2,500 G. or less.

premedication (*prē-me-di-kā'-shon*). Drug given as a narcotic before a general anaesthetic.

premenstrual (*prē-men-stroo-al*). Before menstruation. *P. tension syndrome.* Syndrome consisting of tension, anxiety, aches, depression and often accident-proneness which occurs for a few days before menstrual period in some women. It is thought to be hormonal in origin.

premolar (*prē-mō-la*). The two biscuspid teeth in each jaw which lie between the canine and the molars. *See* TEETH.

premonitory (*prē-mon'-it-ori*). Giving warning beforehand.

prenatal (*prē-nā'-tal*). Prior to birth, during the period of pregnancy.

preparalytic (*prē-pa-ra-li-tik*). State before paralysis has occurred.

prepuce (*pre'-pūs*). Loose skin covering the glans penis: foreskin.

presbyopia (*pres-bi-ō'-pi-a*). Long-sightedness due to inability to make lens of the eye convex by contraction of the ciliary muscles, i.e. failure of adaptation of the lens.

prescription (*pre-skrip'-shon*). A formula written by the physician to the dispenser.

Consists of the heading, usually the symbol R meaning 'take', the names and quantities of the ingredients, the directions to the dispenser, the directions to the patient, the date and the signature.

presentation (*prez-en-tā'-shon*). The part of the foetus which first engages or tends to engage in the pelvis is said *to present*, and the description of this part is the presentation.

pressor (*pres'-sor*). Substance causing blood pressure to rise.

pressure areas (*pre-shor ā-rē-us*). Parts of the body where the bone is near the skin surface and where a bed sore is likely to occur if there is prolonged pressure owing to diminished blood supply to these parts.

pressure points. Points at which pressure may be applied to check haemorrhage. *See* illustration, p. 172.

presystole (*prē-sis'-to-li*). Period in the cardiac cycle before systole.

priapism (*prī-a-pism*). Persistent erection of the penis.

prickle cells (*pri-kl*). Epidermal cells furnished with radiating processes which connect with similar cells. *P. Layer*, the lowest stratum of the dermis.

prickly heat. Miliaria papillosa.

primary focus (*fō-kus*). First site of infection in tuberculosis. Healing usually takes place uneventfully.

primary lesion. Original lesion from which others may arise.

primary sore. Initial site of infection in syphilis.

primidone (*pri-mi-dōn*). Anticonvulsant drug used in epilepsy.

primigravida (*prī-mi-gra-vi-da*). A woman pregnant for the first time.

primipara (*prī-mip'-a-ra*). A woman who has borne one child.

primordial (*prī-mor'-dial*). Pertaining to the beginning.

Priscol (*pris'-kol*). Tolazoline hydrochloride. Vasodilator used in Raynaud's disease.

probe (*prōb*). A slender rod, sometimes of silver, used for exploring wounds.

procaine (*prō'-kān*). Novocain, *q.v.*

process (*prō'-ses*). A prolongation or eminence of a part.

procidentia (*pro-sid-en'-shi-ah*). Prolapse. A falling down.

proctalgia (*prok-tal'-ji-a*). Pain about the rectum.

proctectomy (*prok-tek'-to-mi*). Excision of rectum.

proctitis (*prok-tī'-tis*). Inflammation of the rectum.

proctocele (*prok'-to-sēl*). Prolapsed rectum.

proctoclysis (*prok-to-klī-sis*). Introduction into the rectum of saline solution for absorption.

proctorrhaphy (*prok-to-ra-fi*). Suturing of the rectum.

proctoscope (*prok'-tō-skōp*). An instrument for viewing the interior of the rectum. See illustration, p. 450, plate IV E.

prodromal period (*prō-drō'-mal*). The period that elapses in an infectious disease between the appearance of the first symptoms and the development of the rash, *e.g.* in smallpox, 3 days.

progeria (*prō-jē'-ri-a*). A condition in which premature senility is combined with infantilism.

progesterone (*prō-jes'-ter-ōn*). The hormone of the corpus luteum which causes secretory changes in the uterine mucous membrane in pregnancy and during the menstrual cycle.

progestogen (*prō-jes-tō-jen*). Substance having similar action to progesterone.

proglottis (*prō'-glo-tis*). Segment of tapeworm.

prognosis (*prog-nō'-sis*). The considered opinion as to the course of a disease.

progressive muscular atrophy. Loss of power and wasting of muscles. Degenerative changes are found in the motor cells of the brain and anterior horns of the spinal cord.

proguanil (*prō-gwa'-nil*). Antimalarial drug used in prophylaxis.

projection (*pro-jek'-shon*). Painful thoughts, feelings and motives are relieved by transferring them on to someone else, *e.g.* blaming one's own mistake on to another.

prolactin (*prō-lak'-tin*). Milk-producing hormone of the anterior lobe of the pituitary.

prolan (*prō'-lan*). The original name given to the secretion of the anterior lobe of the pituitary gland. *Prolan A* stimulates the Graafian follicle to ripen, and the production of oestrin. This is now called the follicle stimulating hormone or F.S.H. *Prolan B* stimulates the formation of the corpus luteum and the secretion of progesterone. This is now called luteinizing hormone or L.H.

prolapse (*prō'-laps*). Falling forwards or downwards.

prolapsed intervertebral disc (*prō-lapst in-ter-ver-te-bral disk*). Slipped disc due to prolapse of the central part of the cartilaginous intervertebral disc. See NUCLEUS PULPOSUS.

proliferation (*prō-lif-er-ā-shon*). Reproduction. Cell-genesis.

promazine (*prō-ma-zēn*). A tranquillizing drug.

promethazine hydrochloride (*prō-me-tha-zēn hi-drō-klo-rīd*). Antihistamine drug. Phenergan, *q.v.*

promontory (*prom'-on-to-ri*). A projecting part. An eminence.

pronation (*pro-nā'-shon*). Downward turning of the palm of the hand. (*See* p. 290.)

PRONATION

prone. Lying with the face downwards.

propamidine isethionate (*pro-pa-mi-dēn ī-se-thē-ō-nāt*). Used as a cream for treatment of wounds and burns.

propantheline bromide (*pro-pan-the-lēn brō-mīd*). Antispasmodic drug given in gastric and duodenal ulcer, etc.

propensity (*prŏ-pen-si-ti*). Inclination or tendency.

prophylactic (*prŏ-fi-lak'-tik*). Tending to prevent disease.

proprietary drug (*prop-rī'-et-ar-i*). A remedy with a registered trade name.

proprioceptor (*prŏ-pri-ō-sep-tor*). Sensory end organ which detects changes in position, *e.g.* of muscles or joints or fluid in the balancing apparatus of the inner ear.

proptosis oculi (*prop-tŏ'-sis ok'-ū-lē*). Protrusion of eyeballs.

prostate (*pros-tāt*). A gland associated with the male reproductive system. Its size and secretion are under the influence of androgens. Its function is not clear but it

appears to supply supportive substances to the spermatozoa in the seminal vesicle.

POSITION OF THE PROSTATE

prostatectomy (*pros-tat-ek'-to-mi*). Operation of removing the prostate gland. The operation may be suprapubic when the bladder is first incised, or retropubic (*see* MILLIN'S PROSTATECTOMY) or transurethral.

prostatic (*pros-ta'-tik*). Pertaining to the prostate.

prostatitis (*pros-ta-tī'-tis*). Inflammation of the prostate gland.

prosthesis (*pros-thē'-sis*). The replacement of an absent limb or organ by an artificial apparatus.

Prostigmin Methylsulphate (*prŏ-stig-min me'thil-sul-fāt*). Neostigmine methylsulphate. A derivative of physostigmine. Given by injection in paralytic ileus and post-operative retention of urine. Also used in the palliative treatment of myasthenia gravis.

prostration (*pros-trā'-shon*). Extreme exhaustion.

protamine sulphate (*prō'-ta-mēn sul-fāt*). Drug used to allay haemorrhage caused by overdosage of heparin.

protamine insulin (*prō-ta-mēn in-sū-lin*). See INSULIN.

protein (*prō'-tēn*). Very complex organic compound made up of a large number of amino-acids which are synthesized by living systems. There are 20 different amino-acids commonly found in proteins and these are arranged in different sequences which give the specific characteristics to the proteins.

proteinuria (*pro-ti-nū-ri-a*). Protein in the urine.

proteolysis (*pro-te-ol'-is-is*). The change of proteins into peptones.

prothrombin (*prō-throm'-bin*). The substance which when activated by thrombokinase in the presence of calcium ions becomes the fibrin-ferment thrombin.

protoplasm (*prō'-tō-plasm*). The living jelly-like substance which forms the main part of a cell. It is made up chiefly of water, proteins, and inorganic salts.

prototype (*prō'-tō-tīp*). The original form from which others are copied.

protozoa (*prō-tō-zō'-a*). A class of unicellular organisms, forming the lowest

division of the animal kingdom, *e.g.* an amoeba.

proud flesh (*prow'd*). Excessive granulation tissue in a wound.

provitamin (*prō-vi'-ta-min*). A precursor of a vitamin.

proximal (*prok'-si-mal*). Nearest to the centre.

Prunus serotina (*prū'-nus se-rot-ē-na*). Wild black cherry bark; sedative; given mostly as a linctus.

prurigo (*pru-rī'-go*). A skin disease marked by irritating papules.

pruritus (*pru-rī'-tus*). Itching.

prussic acid (*prus-sik as'-id*). Hydrocyanic acid. Violent poison found in bitter almonds and laurel leaves. For treatment in case of poisoning *see* Cyanides, p. 388.

pseudarthrosis (*sū-dar-thrō'-sis*). A false joint.

pseudo (*sū'-dō*). A prefix meaning false or spurious.

pseudo-angina (*sū-dō-an-jī-na*). A neurotic disease resembling angina pectoris.

pseudocyesis (*sū-dō-sī'-ē-sis*). Changes mimicking pregnancy but without a fetus.

pseudohermaphrodite (*sū-dō-her-ma-frō-dīt*). The external sex organs are of different sexual type to the sex glands.

pseudoplegia (*sū-dō-plē'-ji-a*). Hysterical paralysis.

pseudopodium (*sū-dō-pō'-di-um*). Temporary protrusion of cell serving as method of locomotion and phagocytosis, *q.v.*

psittacosis (*sit-a-kō′-sis*). A virus disease found in parrots and other birds which is communicable to man. It manifests itself as an atypical pneumonia, and is usually fatal.

psoas (*sō′-as*). An important muscle attached above to the lumbar vertebrae and below to the femur. It flexes the femur on the trunk. *P. Abscess. See* ABSCESS.

psoriasis (*so-rī′-a-sis*). Genetically determined abnormality of keratinization producing skin lesions consisting of raised, red, scaly areas.

psyche (*sī′-ki*). The mind.

psychiatric social worker (*sī-ki-a-trik′ sō-shal wer-ker*). One who works under a psychiatrist to rehabilitate mentally ill people.

psychiatrist (*sī-kī′-a-trist*). A doctor who specializes in psychiatry.

psychiatry (*sī-kī-at′-ri*). The study and treatment of mental disorders.

psychical (*sī′-ki-kal*). Relating to the mind.

psycho-analysis (*sī-kō-an-al′-is-is*). A method of treatment, based upon the theories of Freud, tracing nervous conditions to their antecedent causes.

psychodynamics (*sī-kō-dī-na-miks*). Science of mental processes.

psychogenic (*sī-kō-je′-nik*). Originating in the mind.

psychologist (*sī-ko′-lo-jist*). One who studies psychology but is not a doctor of medicine.

psychology (*sī-ko′-lo-ji*). The study of behaviour patterns.

psychoneurosis (*sī-kō-nū-rō′-sis*). A functional mental disease.

psychopath (*sī-ko-path*). A mentally deranged person.

psychopathology (*sī-kō-pa-tho-lo-ji*). Study of the mechanism of mental disorders.

psychosis (*sī-kō′-sis*). Any disorder of the mind. (Plu. psychoses.)

psychosomatic (*sī-kō-sō-ma′-tik*). Relating to mind and body.

psychotherapeutics, psychotherapy (*sī-kō-the-ra-pū′-tiks, sī-kō-ther′-a-pi*). Treatment of the mind. A term which includes any treatment for functional nervous disorders, *e.g.* by hypnotism, suggestion, psycho-analysis, etc.

psychotic (*sī-ko′-tik*). Relating to a psychosis.

pterygium (*te-rij′-ēum*). Mucous membrane growing on the conjunctiva and tending to grow on to the cornea.

pterygoid (*te-ri-goyd*). Wing-shaped.

pterion (*te′-rē-on*). The point of junction of the frontal, parietal, temporal and sphenoidal bones.

ptomaine (*tō-mān*). Poisonous amines from bacterial decomposition of animal or vegetable matter.

ptosis (*tō'-sis*). Drooping of the upper eyelid.

ptyalin (*tī'-a-lin*). A ferment which is present in saliva. It has the power of digesting starch. Now called salivary amylase.

ptyalism (*tī'-a-lizm*). Excessive flow of saliva.

puberty (*pū'-ber-ti*). The period of sexual development.

pubes (*pū'-bēz*). The two pubic bones. Also applied to the area above the bones.

pubiotomy (*pū-bē-ot'-o-mi*). Cutting the pubis; an operation sometimes performed to enlarge a contracted pelvis and so facilitate delivery.

pudenda (*pū-den'-da*). The external genital organs.

pudendal block (*pū-den-dal blok*). Method of anaesthesia in second stage of labour by injecting pudendal nerves transvaginally.

puerperal (*pū-er'-per-al*). Relating to the six weeks following childbirth.

puerperal fever. A continued fever following labour, and due to infection.

puerperal insanity (*pū-er'-per-al in-san'-i-ti*). Mental disorder following childbirth. A rare occurrence.

puerperium (*pū-er-pē-rē-um*). The period after a confinement until the uterus is involuted.

Pulex irritans (*pū-leks i'-ri-tans*). Common flea. *See* FLEA.

pulmonary (*pul'-mun-a-ri*). Relating to the lungs. *P. stenosis.* Narrowing of the pulmonary valve of the heart. *P. valve.* The valve at the exit of the right ventricle into the pulmonary artery.

pulp (*pulp*). The interior, fleshy part of vegetable or animal tissue.

pulsation (*pul-sā'-shon*). Beating of the heart, or of the blood in the arteries.

pulse (*puls*). Can be felt where an artery crosses a bone. It is usually taken at the wrist with three fingers on the radial artery. The pulse in health beats about 120 to the minute in infants; 80 in children; 60 to 70 in maturity, and 50 in old age. *See* DICROTIC PULSE and CORRIGAN'S PULSE.

pulsus alternans (*pul-sus orl-ter-nans*). The pulse is alternately strong and weak though regular in time.

pulvis (*pul'-vis*). A powder.

punctate (*punk'-tāt*). Dotted.

puncture (*punk'-tūr*). To make a hole with a sharp instrument.

pupa (*pū'-pa*). Second stage of insect development following the larval stage.

pupil (*pū'-pil*). The orifice in the centre of the iris.

pupillary (*pū-pil'-a-ri*). Pertaining to the pupil.

purgative (*per'-ja-tiv*). A medicine for causing evacuation of the bowels.

purine (*pū'-rin*). A protein substance from which may be derived a series of compounds including uric acid.

purine diet, low (*pū'-rin*). Prescribed for gout. *See* Appendix, p. 420.

Purkinje cells (*per-kin-ji- sels*). Nerve cells found in the cortex of the cerebellum.

purpura (*per'-pū-ra*). Red or purple spots or patches due to haemorrhages into the skin. May be a symptom in severe illnesses such as bacterial endocarditis cerebrospinal meningitis. *P. Haemorrhagica.* A severe form with diminished number of blood platelets.

purulent (*pu'-rū-lent*). Pus-like.

pus. Matter. Consists of dead leucocytes in an albuminous fluid.

pustula maligna (*pus'-tū-la mal-ig-na*). Anthrax, *q.v.*

pustulation (*pus-tū-lā-shon*). The formation of pustules.

pustule (*pus'-tūl*). A pimple containing pus.

putrefaction (*pū-tre-fak'-shon*). The rotting away of animal matter. Decomposition advanced to an offensive stage.

p.v. Abbreviation for *per vaginam.* Examination of the pelvic organs by inspection or palpation through the vagina.

pyaemia (*pī-ē-mi-a*). The circulation of septic emboli in the blood stream causing multiple abscesses.

pyarthrosis (*pī-ar-thrō'-sis*). Suppuration in a joint.

pyelitis (*pī-e-lī'-tis*). Inflammation of the pelvis of the kidney. The organism is usually the bacillus coli communis.

pyelography (*pī-el-og'-raf-i*). Investigation of the condition of the pelvis of the kidney by photographing it with X-rays after it has been rendered opaque. Methods, (1) Retrograde Pyelography, Injection of sodium iodide into the kidney through ureteric catheters, or (2) Intravenous Pyelography. Injection of iodoxyl (*q.v.*) intravenously.

pyelolithotomy (*pī-e-lō-li-tho'-tō-mi*). Operation to remove a stone from the renal pelvis.

pyelonephritis (*pī-el-ō-nef-rī'-tis*). Inflammation of the kidney and its pelvis.

pyknic (*pik-nik*). One of Kretschmer's types, *q.v.*, fat and jolly.

pylorectomy (*pī-lo-rek'-tom-i*). Removal of the pyloric end of the stomach.

pyloric stenosis (*pī-lo'-rik sten-ō'-sis*). Narrowing of the pylorus. (1) A condition found in infants, more commonly male than female. It is not apparently present at birth and is usually noted after the age of ten days. Projectile vomiting after all feeds, constipation, wasting, are the chief symptoms, while on examination visible peristalsis may be present and a hard tumour to the right of the umbilicus may be felt. Condition is supposed to be due to muscular spasm and consequent hypertrophy of muscle surrounding the pylorus, so preventing the passage of food. The stomach is always dilated. The condition can be treated in its early stages by gastric lavage, and small and frequent feeds; but once a tumour is felt, it is best to open the abdomen and divide hypertrophied muscle (Ramstedt's operation). (2) In adults when it is usually due to a gastric ulcer, or to a growth.

pyloroplasty (*pī-lo'rō-plas'-ti*). Operation for widening a contracted pylorus.

pylorus (*pī-lor'-us*). Region of the junction between the stomach and the duodenum. There is a thickening of the circular muscle at this point which acts as a sphincter allowing the passage of food out of the stomach.

pyocolpos (*pī-o-kol'-pos*). Pus retained in the vagina.

pyoderma (*pī-ō-der'-ma*). Any septic skin lesion.

pyogenic (*pī-o-jen'-ik*). Producing, forming pus.

pyometra (*pī-o-mĕ'-tra*). Pus retained in the uterus.

pyonephrosis (*pī-ō-nef-rō'-sis*). Pus in the kidney.

pyopericardium (*pī-ō-per-i-kar'-di-um*). Pus in the pericardium.

pyopneumothorax (*pī-ō-nŭ'-mō-thor'-ax*). Pus and air in the pleural cavity.

pyorrhoea (*pī-ō-rē'-a*). A flow of pus. Generally used as meaning the same as *pyorrhoea alveolaris*, a condition in which pus oozes out from the gums around the roots of the teeth. This is also known as Rigg's disease.

pyosalpinx (*pī-ō-sal-pinks*). Abscess in a Fallopian tube.

pyramid (*pi'-ra-mid*). Elevation on the medulla oblongata caused by the pyramidal tract.

pyramidal (*pi-ram'-id-al*). Shaped like a pyramid. *P. Cells.* Cells in the cerebral cortex giving out impulses to voluntary muscles. *P. System.* Tracts in the brain and spinal cord transmitting impulses from the pyramidal cells.

pyrexia (*pī-reks'-i-a*). Fever. Elevation of the body temperature. *Intermittent P.*, temperature high at night, below normal in the morning. *Remittent P.*, temperature high at night, down in the morning, but never reaching normal. *Continuous P.*, with a variation of less than two degrees F.

pyridoxin (*pi-ri-dok'-sin*). Vitamin B, or adermin, *q.v.*

pyrosis (*pī-rō'-sis*). A burning pain in the stomach with eructation; heart-burn.

pyroxylin (*pi-rok'-si-lin*). A substance prepared by the action of sulphuric and nitric acids on cotton wool. Very inflammable. Is the basis of collodion.

pyuria (*pī-ū'-ri-a*). Pus in the urine.

Q

'Q' fever. Also called Queensland fever. An acute disease resembling pneumonia and caused by Rickettsia burneti.

quack (*kwak*). One who pretends to knowledge or skill which he does not possess.

quadriceps (*kwod'-ri-seps*). Four-headed: name given to four separate muscles, covering the front of the thigh, which are all inserted into the tubercle of the tibia, and extend the knee.

quadriplegia (*kwo-dri-plē-ji-a*). Paralysis of both legs and arms. *See* TETRAPLEGIA.

quadruple vaccine (*kwo-droopl vak-sēn*). Vaccine immunizing against tetanus, diphtheria, whooping cough and poliomyelitis.

quarantine (*kwo-ron-tēn*). A period of separation of infected persons or contacts from others, necessary to prevent the spread of disease.

quartan (*kwor'-tan*). An intermittent fever rising and falling in periods of 72 hours.

quassia (*kwash'-i-a*). A bitter tonic produced from a South American and West Indian tree.

quaternary ammonium compounds (*kwa-ter-na-ri*). Bactericides such as cetrimide, benzalkonium and domiphen.

Queckenstedt's test (*kwek-enstetz*). To elicit the presence of spinal block, *e.g.* tumour. A lumbar puncture is performed. If the manometer shows no increase of intraspinal pressure when the jugular veins are pressed, there is spinal block.

quickening (*kwik'-ning*). The first perception of movement of the fetus in the womb, usually felt by the mother at the end of the fourth month.

quiescent (*kwē-es-sent*). Not active. Dormant.

quinalbarbitone (*kwi-nal-barbi-tōn*). Short-acting barbiturate.

quinidine (*kwin'-id-ēn*). An active principle of cinchona bark. It slows and regulates the atrial beat in cases of atrial fibrillation.

quinine (*kwi-nēn'*). An alkaloid of the cinchona bark. Uses: (1) as a tonic, (2) as a prophylactic and cure in malaria, (3) as an oxytocic to strengthen or initiate uterine contractions.

quinism (*kwi-nizm*). *See* CINCHONISM.

quinophan (*kwin'-ō-fan*). Cinchophen, *q.v.*

quinsy (*kwin'-zi*). A peritonsillar abscess, situated immediately outside the capsule of the tonsil. *See* TONSILLITIS.

quintan (*kwin'-tan*). Remittent fever, which recurs every fifth day.

quotidian (*kwo-tid'-ē-an*). Recurring daily. Intermittent malarial fever.

quotient (*kwō'-shent*). Result obtained by dividing one quantity by another. *See also* INTELLIGENCE QUOTIENT.

R

rabid (*ra-bid*). Having rabies.

rabies (*rā'-bēz*). A specific infective disease: affects dogs chiefly, but may be transferred to human beings, *See* HYDROPHOBIA.

racemose (*ras'-e-mōs*). Resembling a bunch of grapes. *R. Glands*, having the cells arranged in saccules with numerous ducts leading to a main duct, *e.g.* Salivary glands.

rachis (*rak'-is*). The spine.

rachitic (*rak-it'-ik*). Due to rickets. A *rachitic flat pelvis* is a deformity of the pelvis due to rickets during childhood.

rachitis (*ra-kī'-tis*). *See* RICKETS.

rad. A unit of measurement for energy absorbed by tissue exposed to X or gamma radiation.

radial (*rā'-dē-al*). Relating to the radius.

radiation (*rā-di-ā'-shon*). Emanation of energy from a source. The usual form is that of *photons* which according to their frequency of emission are known as radio waves, light, X-rays, gamma rays, etc. Subatomic particles such as *electrons*, *neutrons*, *protons*, and *positrons*, *mesons* and many sub-nuclear particles may also be radiated.

radiation sickness. Diarrhoea and vomiting resulting from radiation.

radical (*rad'-i-kal*). That which goes to the root; thus radical treatment aims at an absolute cure, not a palliation.

radioactive fall out (*rā-di-ō-ak-tiv fawl owt*). Radioactive isotopes distributed in the atmosphere as the result of atomic explosions. Constitutes a biological hazard as isotopes give off damaging radiations.

radioactive isotopes (*rā-dē-ō-ak'-tiv ī-sō-tōps'*). Varieties of chemical elements which exhibit radioactivity.

radioactivity (*rā'-di-ō-ak-tiv'-i-ti*). A radio-active substance is one which emits spontaneously some form of radiation, and which in course of time by spontaneous disintegration becomes converted into another substance. *See* RADIUM.

radiobiology (*rā-di-ō-bī-ol-o-ji*). Science studying the results of radiation on living tissue.

radiocarbon (*rā-di-ō-kar-bon*). Radioactive isotope of carbon.

radiographer (*rā-dē-og'-raf-er*). Person trained to take X-rays.

radiography (*rā-di-og'-ra-fi*). Science of examination by means of X-rays.

radiologist (*rā-di-ol'-oj-ist*). A doctor who has made a special study of radiology.

radiology (*rā-di-ol'-o-ji*). The study of diagnosis by means of radiography.

radioscopy (*rā-di-o-sko-pi*). Direct vision of X-ray picture by means of a fluorescent screen.

radiosensitive (*rā-di-ō-sen-si-tiv*). Term applied to a structure, especially a tumour, responsive to radiotherapy.

Radiostoleum (*rā-di-ō-stōl'-e-um*). Brand of vitamin A and D solution. An anti-rachitic preparation.

radiotherapy (*rā-di-ō-the'-ra-pi*). The treatment of disease by radium, X-rays or other radioactive substances.

radium (*rā-di-um*). A disintegration product of uranium. It belongs to the group of radioactive elements; when isolated it is a white metal, but for medical purposes it is used as a compound, *i.e.* radium bromide for the production of radon, and radium sulphate for use in needles, plaques, etc. Radium disintegrates slowly, reaching half-strength in 1690 years. Radium is a valuable therapeutic agent, and is used chiefly to destroy malignant growths.

radium rays (*rā'-di-um rāz*). The rays emitted by radium are of three types, *i.e.* alpha, beta, and gamma rays.

radius (*rā'-di-us*). The outer bone of the forearm, from the elbow to the wrist. *See* SKELETON.

radon (*rā-don*). Radioactive gas derived from radium. *R. seeds.* Sealed containers of radon.

râle (*rahl*). Slight rattling sound heard in the air passages upon auscultation.

Ramstedt's operation (*ram'-stet*). *See* PYLORIC STENOSIS.

ramus (*rā'-mus*), (plu. rami). A branch; thus *ramus abdominalis*, branch from lumbar artery to abdominal walls. The term is also applied to branches of nerves.

ranula (*ran'-ū-la*). Cyst of mucous gland.

raphe (*rā'-fē*). Fibrous junction between muscles.

rapport (*ra-paw*). A good relationship between two people.

rarefaction (*rā-re-fak'-shon*). The process of becoming less dense.

rash. Skin eruption.

raspatory (*ras'-pa-tor-i*). A blunt instrument for dissecting tissues.

RASPATORY

rat-bite fever (*rat'-bīt*). Disease which occurs in China and Japan. It is conveyed by the bite of an infected rat. The organism is known as the spirillum minus.

rationalization (*ra-shon-al-ī-zā'-shon*). A justification to oneself of one's action or behaviour. The explanation is based on unconscious or instinctive motives.

raucous (*raw'-kus*). Hoarse.

rauwolfia (*row-wol-fē-a*). Alkaloid derived from an Indian shrub and used for the reduction of high blood pressure.

ray fungus. The organism which causes actinomycosis.

Raynaud's disease (*rā-nō'*). Recurring vascular spasm of the extremities. The fingers become cold and white. Occasionally dry gangrene occurs.

reaction (*rē-ak'-shon*). Response to stimulus.

reagent (*rē-ā'-jent*). An agent taking part in a reaction.

recalcitrant (*rē-kal-si-trant*). Resistant, esp. of a disease to its treatment.

recall (*re-kawl*). Bringing back a memory.

receptaculum chyli (*re-sep-tak'-ū-lum kil'-ē*). The lower expanded portion of the thoracic duct.

receptor (*re-sep'-ter*). Sensory nerve ending.

recessive (*re-ses'-siv*). Tending to disappear.

recipient (*re-si-pē-ent*). The person receiving blood by a transfusion.

Recklinghausen's disease (*rek'-ling-how-sen*). See VON RECKLINGHAUSEN'S DISEASE.

recrudescence (*re-krū-des'-sens*). Return of symptoms.

rectal. Relating to the rectum.

rectified spirit. See ALCOHOL.

rectocele (*rek'-tō-sēl*). Prolapse of posterior vaginal wall. Strictly the term applies to any herniation of the rectum.

rectopexy (*rek-tō-pek'-si*). Surgical procedure to fix a prolapsed rectum.

rectoscope (*rek'-to-skōp*). Proctoscope *q.v.*

rectosigmoidectomy (*rek-tō-sig-moy-dek'-to-mi*). Operation to excise the rectum and the sigmoid colon.

rectovesical (*rek-tō-ve-sī'-kal*). Of the rectum and bladder.

rectum (*rek'-tum*). The lower part of the large intestine from the colon to the anal canal. See BOWEL.

rectus (*rek'-tus*). Straight; applied to certain muscles. *R. Abdominis.* Two external abdominal muscles one each side of mid-line running from pubic bone to ensiform cartilage and the fifth, sixth and seventh ribs. It is enclosed in a strong sheath. There are also four short muscles of the eye, external, internal, superior and inferior rectus. *R. Femoris*, muscle on the front of the thigh, one of the four forming the Quadriceps Extensor.

recumbent (*re-kum'-bent*). Lying down.

recuperate (*re-kū'-pe-rāt*). To get better.

recurrent (*re-ku'-rent*). Returning again after an interval. *R. Laryngeal Nerve*, supplying vocal cords. If cut or compressed by a tumour loss of voice results.

red blood cell or corpuscle. These are the blood cells which contain haemoglobin (*erythrocytes*). There are about 5,000,000 in each ml of blood and they carry nearly all the oxygen required by the body cells. Red blood cells are formed in the bone marrow, normally at a rate of about one million a second, and are notable for the absence of a nucleus in the mature state. They do not divide and have a lifetime of about 120 days when they are destroyed in the spleen.

red lotion (*red lō'-shon*). Astringent, contains sulphate of zinc.

reduction (*re-duk'-shon*). (1) Replacing to a normal position, *e.g.* after fracture, dislocation or hernia. (2) In chemistry, the addition of electrons to the reduced substance.

reef knot (*rēf not*). It does not slip; the ends lie parallel. (*See illustration*).

referred pain (*re-ferd'*). Pain felt at a point quite different from the position of the affected part.

reflex (*rē-fleks*). Simplest form of nervous behaviour whereby a stimulus produces an almost instantaneous response due to an inborn nerve pathway, the *reflex arc*.

reflux (*rē-fluks*). Flowing back, *e.g.* oesophageal reflux is the flow of stomach acid into the oesophagus.

refraction (*rē-frak'-shon*). The bending of light rays as they pass from one medium to another. This bending is an essential part of the process by which the image of an object is focused on the retina of the eye. Errors of refraction are caused when the eyeball is too short or too long from before backwards which prevents the rays of light from converging on the retina. Spectacles will correct the error.

REEF KNOT

refractory (*rē-frak'-to-ri*) Stubborn; not amenable to treatment.

refrigeration (*re-fri-je-rā'-shon*). The cooling of part of the body to reduce its metabolic requirements or to anaesthetize a part.

regeneration (*rē-je-ne-rā'-shon*). Renewal of damaged tissue such as regenerating nerve fibres.

regimen (*rej'-i-men*). A rule of diet or of hygiene, or of life.

regional ileitis (*rē-jo-nal ī-lē-ī-tis*). See CROHN'S DISEASE.

regression (*rē-gre'-shon*). Reverting to a more primitive stage. In psychology, reverting to childlike behaviour as is often seen in illness.

regurgitation (*re-ger-ji-tā'-shon*). A backward flow of blood through defective valves. Also used when fluid taken by the mouth regurgitates through the nose. This occurs with paralysis of the pharynx or soft palate, and may be one of the complications of diphtheria. See MITRAL VALVE.

rehabilitation (*rē-ha-bi-li-tā-shon*). Fitting a patient to take his place in the world again, *e.g.* rehabilitation of an amputee.

Reiter protein complement fixation test (*rī-ter*). One of the three screening tests for syphilis. The other two tests are the W.R. and the Kahn test.

Reiter's syndrome (*rī-ters sin-drōm*). Urethritis combined with arthritis and conjunctivitis.

relapse (*re-laps'*). A return of disease after convalescence has once begun.

relapsing fever (*re-lap'-sing*). Famine fever. A tropical disease caused by spirochaetes of the genus Borrelia.

relaxant (*re-lak-sant*). Applied to drug used to relax muscle tone.

relaxation (*rē-lak-sā-shon*). Reduction of muscle tone.

relaxin (*re-lak-sin*). Ovarian product which softens the cervix and ligaments at childbirth.

remission (*re-mi'-shon*). Period when a disease subsides and shows no symptoms.

remittent (*re-mit'-tent*). Returning at regular intervals; applied to certain fevers. *R. Pyrexia.* See PYREXIA.

renal (*rē'-nal*). Relating to the kidney, *R. calculus.* Stone in the kidney.

R. threshold *see* THRESHOLD.

renin (*re-nin*). Enzyme produced by the kidneys which may cause hypertension when there is a poor blood supply to the kidneys.

rennin (*ren'-nin*). A milk-curdling ferment present in the gastric juice.

repression (*rē-pre-shon*). Psychiatric term when the individual keeps painful memories away from consciousness thus distorting reality for him.

resection (*re-sek'-shon*). A complete removal.

resectoscope (*rē-sek-to-skōp*). Instrument to view and remove pieces of tissue in transurethral prostatectomy.

reserpine (*re-ser'-pin*). An alkaloid from rauwolfia. The drug is a sedative which lowers blood pressure and slows the heart.

residual air (*re-zi'-dū-al*). That remaining in the lungs after forced expiration. *R. Urine*, that left in the bladder after the organ has apparently been emptied naturally, measured by catheterization.

resistance (*re-zis'-tans*). The degree of opposition to an action.

resolution (*rez-ol-ū'-shon*). 1. A resolve. 2. Absorption—as for instance when an inflammatory tumour or exudate disappears without suppurating. This term is also applied to the process whereby the lung returns to normal after an attack of pneumonia.

resonance (*rez'-o-nanz*). Increase of sound by reverberation, applied to voice sounds in auscultation.

resorcinol (*re-sor'-si-nol*). Antiseptic and anti-pruritic drug for skin infections. May be dangerous if applied over large areas.

resorption (*re-sorp-shon*). Absorption of secreted matter.

respiration (*re-spi-rā'-shon*). Breathing. Rate should be in infants 50 to the minute, in children 36, in adults 16. *Inverted R.* The pause is after inspiration instead of after expiration; noticed in babies with broncho-pneumonia.

respirator (*res'-pi-rā-tor*). (1) Appliance worn over the mouth and nose to prevent the inhalation of poisonous gas. (2) Apparatus used to assist the muscles of respiration when paralysed, *e.g.* in poliomyelitis. There is a variety of types of these respirators.

respiratory distress syndrome. *See* HYALINE MEMBRANE.

restitution (*res-ti-tū'-shon*). In obstetric practice this term means the rotation of the foetal head towards the right or left side immediately after it has completely passed the vulva; the occiput is thus turned (in a vertex presentation) towards the same side of the mother as that on which it originally entered the pelvis.

resuscitation (*re-sus-si-tā'-shon*). Reviving those who are apparently dead.

retardation (*re-tar-dā'-shon*). A slowing down of activity; backwardness.

retching (*retsh'-ing*). Ineffectual efforts to vomit.

retention (*rē-ten'-shon*). A holding back. Inability to void urine.

reticular (*ret-ik'-ū-lah*). Resembling a network. Applied to tissue.

reticulocyte (*re-ti'-kū-lō-sīt*). Immature erythrocyte found in blood regeneration.

reticulocytosis (*re-ti-kū-lō-sī-tō'-sis*). Excessive reticulocytes found in the blood stream.

reticulo-endothelial system (*re-ti-kū-lō- en-dō-thē'-lē-al sistem*). Special endothelial cells which are phagocytic and are found in spleen, lymph glands, liver and bone marrow. These cells aid in the destruction of red cells and form bilirubin from haemoglobin.

reticuloses (*re-ti-kū-lō-sis*). A group of neoplasms arising from lymphoid tissue, *e.g.* Hodgkin's disease, lymphosarcoma.

retina (*ret'-i-na*). The delicate inner coat of the eye between choroid and vitreous humour. It is the termination of the optic nerve upon which objects are focused. *See* EYE.

retinal (*ret'-i-nal*). Pertaining to the retina.

retinitis (*ret-in-ī-tis*). Inflammation of the retina.

retinoblastoma (*re-ti-nō-bla-stō'-ma*). Tumour arising from germ cells in the retina.

retinopathy (*re-ti-no-pa-thi*). Pathological lesion affecting the retina, *e.g.* diabetic retinopathy, hypertensive retinopathy.

retractile (*re-trak-tīl*). That which can be drawn back.

retraction (*re-trak'-shon*). Shortening, drawing backward. The process whereby the muscular fibres of the uterus remain permanently shortened to a slight degree after each contraction or labour pain; by this process the uterus when empty does not require to continue in a state of active contraction in order to maintain its lessened bulk and for the prevention

Thick upper segment

Retraction ring

Thin lower segment

Bony pelvis

RETRACTION RING

of haemorrhage. The *retraction* ring, or *Bandl's* ring, is a ridge, which can sometimes be felt on the uterus above the pubes in cases of prolonged or obstructed labour. Its appearance is an indication for immediate completion of labour by artificial means.

retractor (*re-trak'-ter*). Instrument used to withdraw structures obscuring the field of operation.

ABDOMINAL RETRACTOR

retro- (*re-trō*). Prefix denoting backwards.

retrobulbar (*re-trō-bul'-ba*). Behind the globe of the eye.

retrocaecal (*re-trō-sē'-kal*). Behind the caecum.

retroflexion (*re-trō-flek'-shon*). A bending back, as of the body of the uterus on the cervix.

retrograde pyelography (*ret'-rō-grād pī-el-og'-ra-fi*). See PYELOGRAPHY.

retrogression (*rē-trō-gre-shon*). Moving backwards.

retrolental fibroplasia (*re-trō-len'-tal fi-brō-plā-sē-a*). The posterior part of the capsule of the lens of the eye becomes fibrosed and blindness may result. Found in premature babies who have been given too much oxygen.

retro-ocular (*re-trō-o-kū-la*). Posterior to the eye.

retroperitoneal (*re-trō-pe-rit-on-ē-al*). Behind the posterior layer of the peritoneum.

retropharyngeal (*re'-trō-far-in-jē'-al*). Behind the pharynx. *R. Abscess*, a collection of pus behind the wall of the pharynx and anterior to the cervical vertebrae. An acute abscess may develop from inflammation of two glands near mid-line, a chronic one from cervical caries.

retropubic (*re-trō-pū-bik*). Behind the pubis. *R. Prostatectomy.* See MILLIN'S PROSTATECTOMY.

retrospection (*re-trō-spek'-shon*). Looking back into the past.

retrosternal (*re-trō-ster'-nal*). Behind the sternum.

retroversion (*re-trō-ver'-shon*). A turning backwards. The uterus is normally turned considerably forwards, that is, the cervix is directed towards the lower end of the sacrum and the fundus towards the suprapubic region. Any deviation from this in the backward direction is termed retroversion. *Retroversion of the gravid uterus* may prevent the enlarging uterus from rising out of the pelvis.

retroverted gravid uterus (*retrō-ver'-ted gra-vid ū'-te-rus*). See RETROVERSION.

Reverdin's needle (*rev-er-dinz nē'-dl*). A long handle with a curved needle at right angles. Used for deep work in pelvis. Needle is inserted beneath tissue required to be tied, threaded, then withdrawn, leaving ligature *in situ.* It can thus be tied.

rhagades (*rag'-ad-ēz*). A crack or fissure of skin causing pain; a term especially used of radiating scars at angle of mouth due to congenital syphilis.

Rhesus (Rh) factor (*rē'-sus*). See BLOOD GROUPING.

rheum (*re'-um*). Rhubarb: a purge. An ingredient of Gregory's powder.

rheumatic (*rū-ma'-tik*). Pertaining to rheumatism. *R. fever.* Acute rheumatic fever is a disorder affecting connective tissue, particularly that of the heart and the joints. The cause is considered to be an allergic reaction to toxins from haemolytic streptococcus

(Lancefield group A). *R. heart disease.* Chronic rheumatic heart disease is the result of severe damage and deformation of the heart due to rheumatic fever.

rheumatism (*ru-ma-tizm*). General term covering diverse conditions which have in common rather ill-defined pains of the muscles and joints.

rheumatoid (*rū-ma-toyd'*). Similar to rheumatism.

rheumatoid arthritis (*rū-matoyd arth-rī'-tis*). A subacute or chronic form of arthritis. Gross changes occur in the joints leading to deformity and ankylosis.

rheumatologist (*ru-ma-to'-lojist*). One who studies rheumatic disease.

rhinitis (*rī-nī'-tis*). Inflammation of the nose.

rhinoplasty (*rī-nō-plas'-ti*). Making a false nose.

rhinorrhoea (*rī-no-re'-a*). Discharge from the nose.

rhinoscope (*rī'-no-skōp*). Nasal speculum.

rhizodontropy (*rī-zō-don-tropi*). Dental term for crowning the root of a tooth.

rhizotomy (*rī-zo'-to-mi*). Division of spinal nerve roots.

rhodopsin (*rō-dop'-sin*). Visual purple contained in the retina.

rhonchus (*rong'-kus*). A rattling bronchial sound heard on auscultation.

rhubarb (*rū'-barb*). *See* RHEUM.

rhythm (*ri'-thum*). Movement following a definite pattern.

The *Alpha R.* is the normal pattern recorded by electro-encephalogram of changes in electrical potential. The *Beta R.* is the rhythm recorded occasionally from the front of the brain.

riboflavin (*ri-bō-flā'-vin*). Part of vitamin B complex.

ribonuclease (*rī-bō-nū-klē-ās*). Enzyme which degrades R.N.A.

ribonucleic acid (*rī-bō-nū-klā-ik a-sid*). Chemical substance in animal cells. It is concerned in synthesis of protein.

ribs. Long lateral bones enclosing the chest. The upper seven ribs on each side join the sternum by separate cartilages, and are called true ribs, the lower five ribs being termed false ribs. Of the latter, the upper three pairs are attached to the sternum by a common cartilage on each side; while the lower two ribs on each side are not attached to the sternum at all, and are therefore called floating ribs.

rice-water stools (*rīs-waw-ter stoolz*). Stools of cholera which look like water in which rice has been boiled.

Richter's hernia (*rik-ters her'-nē-a*). Hernia which involves only a portion of the lumen of the intestine.

ricinoleic acid (*rī'-sin-ō-le-ik*). The fatty acid of castor oil.

rickets (*ri'-ketz*). Disease of childhood due to a diet lacking in vitamin D and lack of fresh air and sunshine. The child is fat but flabby, irritable: delay in walking and teething, profuse sweats, head large, anterior fontanelle open at 2 years, bossing of frontal bones, pigeon breast, beading of ribs, enlargement of epiphyses, deformities of long bones, enlarged abdomen, tendency to bronchitis and gastro-enteritis. *See* VITAMINS.

Rickettsia (*ri-ket-sē-a*). Minute organisms responsible for typhus and similar infections.

Riggs's disease (*rigz*). *See* PYORRHOEA.

rigor (*rī'-gor*). Sudden feeling of cold accompanied by shivering which raises the body temperature above normal. Due to disorder of thermoregulatory centre of the brain caused by toxins, etc.

rigor mortis (*rī'-gor mor'-tis*). The stiffening of the body after death.

rima (*rī'-ma*). A fissure; thus *rima glottidis*, slit between vocal cords.

Ringer's solution (*rin-gers so-lā'-shon*). Physiological saline, *q.v.*, which includes, in addition to sodium, potassium, calcium, magnesium and some other ions normally present in extracellular fluid.

ring pessaries (*ring pes'-a-riz*). *See* PESSARY.

ringworm (*ring'-werm*). Also called tinea, fungus infection or dermatophytosis. Infec-

tion of the skin, hair or nails by various kinds of fungi. Some forms of ringworm as *microsporon audouini* only affect man; *tinea verrucosum* affects cattle but may be passed on to man, affecting the scalp. *Microsporon felinum* affects dogs and cats and man secondarily. In body ringworm, *tinea circinata*, there are spreading rings with blistery or scaling edges; in *tinea pedis* or athlete's foot, the skin between and behind the toes is specially affected; *onychomycosis* is ringworm of the nails usually caused by trychophyton rubrum. Ringworm of the scalp may be caused by *microsporon audouini* or infection from cattle, dogs or cats. There are circular patches of dull colour, The hairs in the infected areas break off just above the scalp. Diagnosis is made with Wood's light and also microscope. Modern treatment is a course of griseofulvin by mouth for at least six weeks.

Rinne's test (*rin-ners*). A vibrating tuning-fork is placed on the mastoid process until no longer heard, then quickly put in front of the meatus; normally the vibration is still heard. The test is negative when obstruction exists in the external or middle ear.

Ripple mattress. Apparatus designed to reduce the incidence of bed sores by rhythmically shifting weight of the patient from one side to the other by means of pumping air into linear compartments causing the mattress to 'ripple'.

risus sardonicus (*rē-sus sar-do'-ni-kus*). A convulsive grin, symptomatic of tetanus.

R.N.A. *See* RIBONUCLEIC ACID.

rodent ulcer (*rō'-dent ul'-ser*). Basal cell carcinoma of skin.

rods. Retinal organs giving night vision.

Romberg's sign (*rom'-bergz sīn*). Inability to stand erect when the eyes are closed and the feet placed together; seen in tabes dorsalis.

Röntgen rays (*rern-shen*). X-rays. *See* RADIATION.

Röntgen unit. Unit of radiation defined as the quantity of radiation necessary to produce 1 electrostatic unit of charge (1 e.s.u.) in 1 ml. of dry air under standard pressure and temperature conditions. This is not a satisfactory unit for estimating the biological effects of radiation and a number of alternative units have been introduced.

rosacea (*rō-zā'-se-a*). Vasculomotor disturbance affecting the face with associated hyperplasia of the sebaceous glands.

roseola (*rō-zē-ō'-la*). A rose-coloured rash.

rotation (*rō-tā'-shon*). Twisting. Applied to the twisting of the head upon the shoulders of the foetus as it passes

down the birth canal and follows its curves.

rotators (*rō-tā'-tors*). Muscles which cause circular movement.

Rothera's test. *See* URINE TESTING, p. 383.

roughage (*ru'-fij*). Cellulose part of food which gives bulk and aids peristalsis.

round ligaments (*row'nd lig-a-ments*). Two thin cords passing from the uterus through the broad ligaments, and terminating in the canals of Nuck in the inguinal regions. When these are shortened for retroverted uterus, this is called Mackendrodt's operation.

Round ligament
Ext. iliac vessels
Uterus
Inguinal canal
Broad ligt.
Labium majus

ROUND LIGAMENT

roundworm. *See* ASCARIS LUMBRICOIDES.

Rovsing's sign (*rōv-sings sīn*). In appendicitis, pressure in the left iliac fossa will cause pain in the right iliac fossa.

R.P.C.F.T. Reiter protein complement fixation test, *q.v.*

rubefacients (*ru-be-fā'-sē-ents*). Mild irritants which cause redness of the skin.

rubella (*roo-bel'-la*). Also called German measles. A

mild infectious disease caused by a virus. Incubation period 14–20 days, infectivity less than measles. There may be slight catarrh and fever and swelling of suboccipital glands. The rash begins on the face and spreads to the body and fades quickly. Complications are few but if a woman has the disease during the first four months of pregnancy, she may have a deformed child.

rugae (*roo-jē*). Wrinkles or creases.

rugine (*rū-jēn*). Instrument for elevating the periosteum.

RUGINE

rugose (*rū'-jōs*). Wrinkled.

rumination (*roo'-min-a'-shon*). Act analogous to chewing the cud. Infant brings up some of feed and plays with it in mouth. Considered to have a psychological basis.

rupia (*roo'-pi-a*). A skin disease with crusts due to tertiary syphilis.

rupture (*rup'-tūr*). A bursting. In popular language a rupture means a hernia, *q.v.* In obstetric practice *rupture of the perineum* is not uncommon as a result of labour, especially in primiparae; *rupture of the uterus* is a rare event due to unrelieved obstructed labour, or more rarely still to unskilful attempts at delivery by the use of instruments; *rupture of the membranes* is the normal sequence of full dilatation of the cervix in labour, and marks the commencement of the second stage. *Rupture of a tubular extra-uterine pregnancy* may result in severe internal haemorrhage and would require immediate operation.

Russell traction (*ru'-sel trak-shon*). Method to reduce a fractured femur. There is an upward pull to a Balkan beam from a sling beneath the knee and from the lower part of the leg a longitudinal pull towards the foot of the bed. The resultant direction of the pull helps to straighten the femur.

Ryle's tube (*rīls-tūb*). Narrow bore rubber tube, slightly weighted, used for giving a test meal or aspirating the stomach.

S

Sabin's vaccine (*sā-bins vak-sēn*). One of the poliomyelitis vaccines. It is taken orally.

sac. A small pouch, such as a hernial sac.

saccharin (*sak'-ka-rin*). A glucoside. A substitute for sugar. It has no food value.

Saccharomyces (*sak-a-rō-mī'-sez*). A group of fungi including yeasts. One is the cause of thrush, *q.v.*

sacculated (*sak'-ū-la-ted*). Bagged, or pursed out.

sacral (*sā-kral*). Pertaining to the sacrum. *S. analgesia, see* CAUDAL ANALGESIA. *S. canal.* This passes through the sacrum and contains the cauda equina.

sacro-iliac synchondrosis or **joint** (*sak-ro-i-li-ak sin-kon-drō-sis*). The articulation between the sacrum and the hip-bone. Normally there is no movement at this joint. During pregnancy the joint becomes more movable and this, to a slight extent, facilitates the birth of the child.

sacro-anterior, sacrolateral and **sacroposterior.** These terms indicate positions of breech presentations.

sacrococcygeal joint (*sā-krō-kok-si-jē-al joynt*). The joint between the sacrum and coccyx. When the baby is delivered there is a backward movement of the coccyx.

sacrum (*sā'-krum*). A wedge-shaped bone consisting of five fused vertebrae. They form the posterior wall of the pelvic cavity.

saddle-nose (*sa-dle-nōs*). A flattened bridge of the nose.

sadism (*sā-dism*). A sexual perversion in which pleasure is derived from inflicting cruelty upon another.

sagittal (*saj-it-tal*). In the median plane. *S. section.* Section made by cutting through a specimen from top to bottom so that there are equal right and left halves. *S. suture,* the suture between the parietal bones.

St. Vitus' dance (*vī'-tus*). Chorea, *q.v.*

sal. A salt.

salicylate (*sa-li-si-lāt*). A salt of salicylic acid, *e.g.* *sodium salicylate* used in rheumatism. It relieves pain and reduces the temperature. *Methyl salicylate* (chief constituent of oil of wintergreen) is applied to painful joints.

salicylic acid (*sal-i-sil'-ik as'id*). An antiseptic used on the skin. See SALICYLATE. Acetyl-salicylic acid is aspirin.

saline (*sā'-lin*). Containing salt. *Normal saline solution* is 0·91 per cent, *i.e.* 80 gr. (large teaspoonful) of common salt in a pint of water. This is isotonic with the blood. Sterile saline is given intravenously or subcutaneously.

saline aperient (*sā'-lin ap-ē'-ri-ent*). Sod. sulph. = Glauber's salts; mag. sulph. = Epsom salts.

saliva (*sa-lī'-va*). The secretion of the salivary glands.

salivary glands (*sal-ī'-va-ri*). Three pairs of glands. The sublingual and submaxillary situated in the floor of the mouth; the parotid above the angle of the lower jaw. See PAROTID.

salivation (*sal-i-vā'-shon*). The act of secretion of saliva.

Salk vaccine (*salk vak-sēn*). One of the vaccines given to protect against poliomyelitis. It contains dead virus.

Salmonella (*sal-mon-el'-la*). Group of bacilli; common cause of food poisoning in England.

salpingectomy (*sal-pin-jek'-tō-mi*). Removal of one or both Fallopian tubes.

salpingitis (*sal-pin-jī'-tis*). Inflammation of a tube, usually applied to the Fallopian tubes.

salpingocyesis (*sal-ping-gō-sī-ē'-sis*). Tubal pregnancy.

salpingography (*sal-pin-gō-gra-fi*). Examination of the Fallopian tubes by X-rays.

salpingo-oophorectomy (*sal-pin'-go-oo-for-ek'-to-mi*). Removal of Fallopian tubes and ovaries.

salpingostomy (*sal-pin-gos'-to-mi*). Opening artificially a Fallopian tube whose aperture has been closed by inflammation.

salpinx (*sal'-pinks*). A tube, either Eustachian or Fallopian.

salt (*sor'lt*). Any union of a base with an acid, *e.g.* sodium chloride (common salt) is formed by the union of sodium and hydrochloric acid.

saltpetre (*sawlt-pē'-tr*). Nitrate of potassium.

Saluric (*sa-lū'-rik*). See CHLOROTHIAZIDE.

salvarsan. Formerly a remedy for syphilis. Also known as '606'. Has been superseded by less toxic arsenical compounds, such as neoarsphenamine and antibiotic drugs.

salve (*salv*). An ointment.

sal volatile (*sal vo-lat-'il-ē*). Stimulant, antacid and expectorant.

sanatorium (*san-at-or'-ium*). Any institution for convalescent patients can technically be called a sanatorium; but usually indicates an institution for the open-air treatment of tuberculosis.

sandfly fever (*sand-flī fē'ver*). Tropical disease due to infection by organism transmitted by sandfly bites.

sanguine (*san-gwin*). (1) Full-blooded. (2) Hopeful.

sanguineous (*san-gwin'-e-us*). Bloodstained. Containing blood.

sanitary (*sa-ni-ta-ri*). Pertaining to health.

sanitation (*san-i-tā'-shon*). The use of methods conducive to the public health.

sanity (*sa-ni-ti*). Being of sound mind.

Sanocrysin (*san-o-krī'-sin*). A salt of gold. GOLD THERAPY, *q.v.*

saphena varix (*sa-fē-na vā-riks*). Saccular enlargement of the termination of the long saphenous vein often without obvious varicose veins.

saphenous nerve. Large branch of the femoral nerve.

saphenous opening (*saf-ē'-nus*). Just below groin near inner side of thigh where superficial saphenous vein passes deep to enter femoral vein.

saphenous veins (*sa-fē-nus vāns*). Superficial leg veins. *Long s.v.* begins on the foot and extends to the groin. *Short s.v.* joins the popliteal vein at the knee.

sapo. Soap. *S. Mollis.* Soft soap.

saponify (*sa-po'-ni-fī*). To make into a soap.

saprophytes (*sap'-rō-fīts*). Organisms that exist only in dead matter.

Sarcina (*sar'-sin-a*). A genus of Schizomycetes which form rectangular bundles as they divide; usually non-pathogenic.

sarcoid (*sar'-koyd*). Resembling flesh.

sarcoidosis (*sar-koy-dō'-sis*). A disease with cutaneous nodules, pulmonary changes and rarefication of the phalanges.

sarcolemma (*sar-kō-lem'-ma*). The membrane which covers each fibril of muscle.

sarcology (*sar-kol'-o-ji*). Anatomy of the soft tissues as distinguished from osteology.

sarcoma (*sar-kō'-ma*). A malignant tumour composed of embryonic connective tissue. Spread is by way of the blood-stream, and metastases are found in lungs, brain, and other organs.

Sarcoptes scabiei (*sar-kop'-tēz skā-bē-ā-ē*). The itch mite or insect causing scabies. It burrows into the skin where it lays its eggs which hatch out. The 'burrows' often terminate in a papule on the skin. The disease is treated with benzyl benzoate.

sartorius (*sar-tor'-ē-us*). The long ribbon-shaped muscle of the front of the thigh.

sassafras oil (*sas'-sa-fras*). An aromatic oil formerly used in cleansing heads infected with pediculi capitis.

saturation (*sat-ū-rā'-shon*). The condition of holding in solution the full amount of a solid capable of being dissolved.

scab. An incrustation formed over a wound.

scabies (*skā'-bēz*). A contagious skin disease due to a parasitic insect, the acarus scabiei or Sarcoptes scabiei, *q.v.*

scald (*skawld*). Burn caused by hot fluids.

scalenus anterior syndrome (*ska-lē-nus an-tā-ri-or sin-drōm*). Characterized by pain in the arm and tingling of the fingers with loss of power and muscle wasting due to compression of the lower fibres of the brachial plexus by the scalenus anterior muscle.

scale (*skāl*). The horny epidermis the skin sheds.

scalp (*skal'-p*). The skin covering the cranium.

scalpel (*skal'-pel*). A straight knife with convex edge, used in dissecting and surgery.

scanning speech. *See* STACCATO or SCANNING SPEECH.

scaphoid (*skāf'-oyd*). Boat-shaped. The name of a bone

of the carpus and of the tarsus.

scapula (*skap'-ū-la*). The shoulder blade. (*See illustration.*)

acromion process
coracoid process
glenoid fossa

SCAPULA

scar (*skar*). The connective fibrous tissue found after any wound has healed.

scarification (*skar-i-fi-kā'-shon*). Shallow incisions just penetrating the epidermis. A technique used in vaccination.

scarlatina (*skar-la-tē'-na*). Scarlet fever; an infectious fever. There is a widespread erythematous rash produced by a toxin released by haemolytic streptococci.

scarlet red (*skar'-let red*). A derivative of naphthol. Used as ointment 2–8 per cent, to promote granulation in clean but slow-healing ulcers.

Scarpa's triangle (*skar'-pas tri-angle*). The femoral tri-

angle bounded by Poupart's ligament, the adductor longus and sartorius.

S.C.A.T. Sheep cell agglutination test. A serum test for rheumatoid arthritis.

Schäfer's method of artificial respiration (*shā'fers*). *See* Appendix, p. 433.

Scheuermann's disease (*shoy'-er-mans*). Vertebral osteochondritis found in adolescents. It affects the two rings of cartilage and bone around the margin of both superior and inferior surfaces of the vertebral body. The condition does not cause general ill-health.

Schick test (*shik*). A test for antibody in the patient's blood to the Klebs-Loeffler bacillus which causes diphtheria. A minute amount of diphtheria toxin (and protein) is injected into the patient's left forearm. If there is antitoxin in the patient's blood the toxin will be neutralized and there will be no reaction. If the patient's blood has little or no antitoxin, there will be an area of redness on the skin 1 cm in diameter, within 24 hours, reaching its height in four days. This patient is susceptible to diphtheria. A control solution containing protein and inactive toxin is injected into the right arm. If there is a protein reaction or false reaction, this reaches its height in 24 hours and then fades.

schistosomiasis (*skis-tō-so-mī-a-sis*). See BILHARZIA.

schizoid temperament (*skit-zoyd*). One that is reticent and aloof.

Schizomycetes (*skiz-o-mī-sē'tēz*). The fission fungi which are micro-organisms of vegetable composition such as yeast.

schizophrenia (*skit-zō-frē-ni-a*). Term used for a group of mental disorders characterized by a progressive loss of emotional stability, judgement and contact with reality.

Schlatter's disease (*shla'-ters*). Osteochondritis of the anterior tubercle of the tibia. Also called Osgood-Schlatter's disease.

Schlemm's canal (*shlem*). Lymphatic channel leading to a venous plexus at the root of the ciliary body of the eye. It allows the intra-ocular fluid (aqueous humour) to drain. Failure to do so results in raised hydrostatic pressure in the anterior chamber of the eye (glaucoma).

Schultz-Charlton reaction (*shootz-charl'-ton*). Test to confirm scarlet fever. Antitoxin is injected into the skin where the rash is bright red. If the disease is present, there is a blanching ring round the injection site in about 18 hours.

Schwann substance (*shwon substans*). White sheath of nerve fibre.

sciatica (*sī-at'-ik-a*). Neuralgia of the sciatic nerve—the large nerve of the thigh. It may be caused by pressure on the nerves in the spinal canal or the pelvis.

scilla (*sil'-la*). Plant from which white squill is obtained. See SQUILL.

scirrhous (*ski'-rus*). Hard and fibrous.

scissor-leg deformity (*si-zer-leg di-for'-mi-ti*). Deformity due to exaggerated tone in the adductor muscles usually resulting from cerebral damage.

sclera (*sklē-ra*). The opaque outer coat of the eyeball, forming five-sixths of the globe of the eye, the remaining one-sixth being formed by the cornea. See EYE.

scleritis (*skle-rī'-tis*). An inflamed sclera.

scleroderma (*sklēr-ō-der'-ma*). A chronic disease of the skin, causing hardness.

sclerosis (*skler-ō'-sis*). Hardening. See also DISSEMINATED SCLEROSIS.

sclerosis-tuberose (*skle-rō-sis-tū-be-rōs*). Epiloia. Dominantly inherited defect characterized by sebaceous adenomas in a butterfly distribution on the face, multiple gliomas of the brain, and tumours of the heart, kidney and retina.

sclerotic (*skle-rot'-ik*). Pertaining to the sclera.

sclerotomy (*skler-ot'-to-mi*). An operation on the sclerotic coat of the eye, for the relief of glaucoma.

scolex (*skŏ'-leks*). Head of a tapeworm.

scoliosis (*skŏ-li-ŏ'-sis*). Lateral curvature of the spine.

SCOLIOSIS SHOWING THE SPINAL VERTEBRAE MARKED

scopolamine (*sko-po'-lam-ēn*). Hyoscine, *q.v.*

scorbutus (*skor-bū-tus*). Scurvy, *q.v.*

scotoma (*sko-tō'-ma*). A blind spot in the field of vision.

Scott's dressing. Compound mercurial ointment; applied to chronically inflamed joints.

'screening' (*skrēn'-ing*). Radiological examination by means of a fluorescent screen.

scrofuloderma (*skro-fū-lō-der'-ma*). Tuberculous condition of the skin.

scrotocele (*skrŏ'-tō-sēl*). Hernia in the scrotum.

scrotum (*skrŏ'-tum*). The bag which holds the testicles.

scruple (*skrū'-pl*). A weight equal to 20 gr. apothecaries' weight, or 1·296 grams.

scurf (*skerf*). Dandruff. Scales from the epidermis of the scalp.

scurvy (*sker'-vi*). A deficiency disease, due to absence of the vitamin C. *See* VITAMINS. Characterized by swelling of the gums, haemorrhages into skin and subcutaneous tissues, and from mucous membranes, and by anaemia. *Infantile S.* A type of the above occurring in infancy, characterized by subperiosteal haemorrhages and anaemia. Due to same cause.

scybala (*sib'-a-la*). Faeces passed as hard dry masses.

sebaceous (*se-bā'-shus*). Fatty, secreting oily matter, *S. Glands*, of skin, secrete fatty material called sebum. *S. Cysts*, dilatation of one of these glands, due to blocking of its opening on to the skin. Cyst is filled with sebum.

seborrhoea (*seb-o-rē'-a*). Excessive secretion of the sebaceous glands.

sebum (*sē'-bum*). The fat of the skin, secreted by the sebaceous glands.

Seconal Sodium (*se'-ko-nal sō-dē-um*). Quinalbarbitone sodium. A barbiturate hypnotic.

secondary areola (*a-rē-o-la*). A peculiar pigmentation of the skin often seen on the breast around the nipple during pregnancy. *See* AREOLA.

secondary disease. A disease consequent on another disease already active.

secondary haemorrhage (*hem-o-rāj*). *See* HAEMORRHAGE.

secondary uterine inertia (*sek-on-da-ri ū'-te-rin in-er'-sha*). *See* INERTIA OF UTERUS.

second intention (*in-ten-shon*). The healing of a wound by means of granulation, and the growing of new skin.

second stage (of labour) (*stāj*). From complete dilatation of the cervix, usually associated with rupture of the membranes, to the complete expulsion of the child. During this stage, which lasts normally two to four hours in primigravidae, and up to one hour in multiparae, the pains are very severe, and the uterine contractions are assisted by those of the abdominal muscles. This is the stage for which anaesthetics are often given. *See also* LABOUR.

secretin (*se-krē'-tin*). A hormone formed in the mucous membrane of the duodenum. It is carried by the blood to the pancreas, exciting it to activity. It also stimulates the secretion of bile.

secretion (*se-krē'-shon*). The active production, filtering or extrusion of material from cells. Gland cells have specialized secretory activity.

section (*sek-shon*). Usually applied to thin slices of tissue cut for microscopical examination.

sedative (*sed'-a-tiv*). Allaying excitement or pain, *e.g.* morphia and barbiturates.

sedimentation rate (*se-di-men-tā-shon rāt*). *See* E.S.R.

segment (*seg'-ment*). A small piece; section; a subdivision.

segregation (*se-gre-gā'-shon*). A setting apart. Isolation.

Seidlitz powder (*sed'-lits*). A saline aperient in the form of two powders. Sodium potassium tartrate and sodium bicarbonate is in the powder found in the blue paper. They are dissolved in a tumbler of water and then the contents of the white paper, tartaric acid, is added to it and the liquid effervesces.

sella turcica (*ter'-si-ka*). Pituitary fossa of the sphenoid bone.

semen (*sā'-men*). The secretion of the testicles mixed with that of the seminal vesicles and prostate.

semi (*se'-mi*). Half.

semicircular canals (*sem-i-ser'-kū-la can-als'*). Three canals of the internal ear, the sense organs of equilibrium or balance. *See* EAR.

semilunar cartilages (*sem-i-lū-na kar'-til-āj-es*). Two crescentic cartilages, an internal and an external, lying in the knee joint between the femur and tibia. These may be torn and displaced, giving rise to pain and deformity and fluid in the knee joint. Usually removed by operation.

seminal (*sem'-in-al*). Relating to the semen. *S. Vesicles.* Two small structures in the male genito-urinary system which secrete part of the seminal fluid.

senega (*sen'-e-ger*). A vegetable drug chiefly used as an expectorant.

senescence (*se-nes-sens*). Growing old.

Sengstaken tube (*seng-sta-ken tūb*). Oesophageal tube used to compress bleeding varices.

senility (*se-nil'-i-ti*). Degenerative changes due to advanced age.

senna (*sen'-na*). An aperient. The syrrup of senna is best disguised if given in coffee.

sensible (*sen'-si-bl*). That which the senses perceive.

sensitive (*sen'-si-tiv*). Able to react to a stimulus.

sensitization (*sen-si-ti-zā-shon*). Act of producing an immunological state in which there is a disproportionate reaction to a substance which normally acts as an antigen.

sensory nerves (*sen'-sor-i*). Afferent nerves carrying sensory information to the central nervous system. *Cf.* motor nerves.

sepsis (*sep'-sis*). The condition of being infected by pyogenic bacteria.

septic (*sep'-tik*). Pertaining to sepsis.

septicaemia (*sep-ti-sēm-i-a*). The circulation and multiplication of micro-organisms in the blood; a very serious condition.

septum (*sep'-tum*). The division between two cavities; such as *septum ventriculorum*, which separates the right ventricle of the heart from the left.

sequelae (*se-kwe'-lē*). Morbid conditions remaining after, and consequent on, some former illness.

sequestrectomy (*se-kwes-trek'-to-mi*). Operation to remove sequestrum.

sequestrum (*se-kwes'-trum*). A fragment of dead bone.

serosa (*se-rō'-sa*). A serous membrane. Serous membranes line the large lymph spaces, *e.g.* pleural, pericardial, peritoneal cavities.

serositis (*se-rō-sī'-tis*). An inflamed serous membrane.

serotonin (*se-rō-tō-nin*). Amine found in blood platelets, the intestines and brain substance. Mono-amine oxidase inactivates it.

Serpasil (*ser-pa-zil*). Reserpine, *q.v.*

serpiginous (*ser-pij'-in-us*). Serpent-like in shape.

serrated (*se-rā-ted*). With a saw-like edge.

serum (*sār'-um*). (1) The fluid part of the blood, after clot and corpuscles have been removed. (2) Fluid used for providing passive immunity, *q.v.* against infection. The serum is taken from an animal which has been rendered immune against a certain pathogenic germ, and which therefore must contain a large quantity of antibodies, *q.v.* to that germ. The best known are the antidiphtheritic and the antitetanic sera. The antibodies contained in the injected serum combine chemically with the disease toxins, rendering the latter harmless. *S. Sickness.* Late reaction to serum injections, arising eight to ten days after. *Symptoms*: Oedema, urticarial rash, joint pains, slight temperature.

sesamoid bones (*ses-a-moyd*). Small foci of bone formation in the tendons of muscles. The patella is the largest.

sessile (*ses'-īl*). Having no stem (applied to tumours).

sex (*seks*). State of being male or female. *S.-linked.* Characteristics not inherited equally by both sexes.

Sheehan's syndrome (*shē-hans sin-drom*). Panhypopituitarism resulting from thrombosis of the pituitary blood supply occurring in association with post-partum haemorrhage.

Shiga's bacillus (*shē-gus ba-si-lus*). The Shigella dysenteriae. A cause of dysentery, especially in the Far East.

shin-bone. The tibia. *See* SKELETON, p. 320.

shingles. *See* HERPES.

shock. General depression of the vital functions. Most common after haemorrhage, severe injuries, or operations or in toxaemic states. The essential factor in shock is a deficiency in the volume of blood in active circulation. Primary or neurogenic shock is seen where the injury is severe and the patient under the influence of pain. Secondary shock is due to the absorption of toxic substances, including histamine, which damage the walls of the capillaries. The capillaries dilate and a good deal of blood stagnates there, and the blood pressure is lowered. *Symptoms*: Pulse, short, quick and rising in rate; respiration, shallow, quick, irregular; face, blanched; nose, pinched and cold; skin, pale, cold and clammy; temperature, subnormal. *Treatment*: Warmth, gradually applied; posture, raise end of bed so that blood may flow to brain. *Stimulants*: Coramine, noradrenaline. If there is pain, morphia is ordered. Administration of fluid is most essential to give the heart something further to work on and to stimulate the circulation. Blood, plasma or saline are given by the appropriate route.

short circuit (*shawt ser-kit*). Anastomosis between gut or blood vessels which allows the contents to by-pass a section of the normal pathway.

short-sighted (*shawt-sī-ted*). Myopic.

shoulder presentation (*shōl'-der*). A form of transverse lie which must be converted into breech or vertex before delivery is possible.

show (*shō*). Popular term for the discharge of slightly blood-stained mucus common at the beginning of labour.

sialectasis (*si-a-lek-ta-sis*). Dilatation of salivary gland due to obstruction to the flow of saliva.

sialogogue (*si-al'-o-gog*). A medicine causing increased salivation, *e.g.*, pilocarpine, mercury.

sialolith (*sī-al-ō-lith*). A salivary calculus.

sibilus (*sib'-il-us*). A hissing sound heard on auscultation of the chest during respiration in bronchitis, etc.

sibling (*sib'-ling*). One of two or more children of the same parents.

sickle-cell anaemia (*sikl-sel a-nē-mi-a*). Hereditary anaemia found sometimes in negroes. The red blood cells become sickle-shaped or crescentic.

siderosis (*si-de-rō-sis*). (1) Inhalation of iron particles causing pneumoconiosis. (2) Excess of iron in the blood.

sight (*sīt*). The power of seeing.

Sigmamycin (*sig-ma-mī-sin*). Oleandomycin and tetracycline hydrochloride.

sigmoid (*sig'-moyd*). Like the Greek letter *s*, applied especially to a bend in the pelvic colon just before it becomes the rectum.

sigmoidoscope (*sig-moyd'-os-cōp*). An instrument for viewing the interior of the rectum and sigmoid flexure of the colon.

sigmoidostomy (*sig-moy-dos-to-mi*). Operation made into the sigmoid colon.

sign (*sīn*). An indication of the presence of disease.

signatura (*sig-na-tū'-ra*). A label.

silicones (*si-li-kōns*). Water-repellent organic compounds.

silicosis (*sil-i-kō'-sis*). Lung disease due to the inhalation of very fine particles of silica which irritate the lungs causing fibrotic changes.

silkworm gut (*silk'-werm gut*). A suture material much used by surgeons for sewing up abdominal wounds. It is very strong, not absorbed, and can be sterilized by boiling.

silver nitrate (*sil'-ver nī'-trāt*). When solid this substance constitutes *lunar caustic*: used to destroy excess granulation tissue; it burns the skin and stains it dark brown or black. In weak solution it is used as an antiseptic.

Silvester's method of artificial respiration. Rarely used now. Patient lies on his back.

Simmonds' disease (*sim-mons di-sēz*). See PANHYPOPITUITARISM.

simple fracture. See FRACTURE.

Sims' position. The patient lies in the semi-prone position, across the bed. The buttocks are brought to the edge of the bed. The right knee is flexed more than the left. Used for vaginal examination.

SIMS' POSITION

Sims' speculum (*spek-ū-lum*). See under SPECULUM.

sinapism (*sin'-a-pizm*). A mustard plaster.

sinciput (*sin'-si-put*). The upper fore part of the head.

sinew (*sin'-nū*). A tendon uniting a muscle to a bone.

sinistral (*sin-is'-tral*). Pertaining to the left side.

sino-atrial node (*sī-nō-ā'-tri-al nōd*). Cells found in the heart at the junction of the superior vena cava and the right atrium. The node is the pacemaker of the heart.

sinus (*sī'-nus*). (1) A passage leading from an abscess, or some inner part, to an external opening. (2) A dilated channel for venous blood, *e.g. Lateral s.*, a large venous channel on inner side of the skull. It passes near the mastoid antrum and empties itself into the jugular vein. (3) Air sinuses, hollow cavities in the skull bones which communicate with the nose. They are the frontal, maxillary, ethmoidal and sphenoidal sinuses.

sinus arrhythmia (*sī-nus a-rith-mi-a*). Irregular cardiac rhythm due to the controlling effect of the vagus on the sino-atrial node. The heart rate increases on inspiration and slows during expiration.

sinusitis (*sī-nu-sī-tis*). Inflammation of a sinus, especially one of the air sinuses of the bones of the skull.

sinusoid (*sī-nu-soyd*). Like a sinus. Channels for small blood vessels as found in the liver, suprarenal glands, etc.

siphonage (*sī-fo-nij*). The method of drawing fluid from one vessel to another by means of a bent tube and the use of atmospheric pressure.

Sjögren's syndrome (*shergrens sin-drōm*). Kerato conjunctivitis and dry mouth usually in postmenopausal women.

skatol (*skā-tol*). A nitrogenous compound found in the faeces.

skeleton (*skel'-e-ton*). The bony framework of the body. (*See illustration, p. 320.*)

Skene's glands (*skēns*). These open into posterior wall of the female urethra, just within the orifice; almost always infected in acute gonorrhoea.

skiagram (*skē'-a-gram*). A photograph taken by means of X-rays.

SKELETON

skin. The outer covering of the body consisting of epidermis and its appendages (hair, sweat glands) supported by specialized dermal connective tissue.

SECTION OF SKIN
1. Epidermis.
2. Dermis.
3. Subcutaneous fatty tissue.

skull. The bony framework of the head.

sleeping sickness. (1) Tropical disease due to a trypanosome. The tsetse fly carries the organisms which are transferred to healthy individuals by the bite of the fly. (2) *See* ENCEPHALITIS LETHARGICA.

slough (*sluf*). Dead matter thrown off by gangrene or ulcers.

smallpox (*smawl-poks*). A highly infectious disease caused by a virus. Incubation period 12–14 days. There is high temperature, headache, backache and cough, Rash appears on the fourth day and the temperature falls, but rises again and pustula-

tion occurs and the patient becomes very ill. *The main differences between smallpox and chickenpox* are that in smallpox the prodromal illness is much more severe. The smallpox rash is centrifugal (fleeing from the centre), whereas the chickenpox rash is centripetal (seeking the centre). The pustules in smallpox take 6–8 days to mature, whereas in chickenpox from a few hours to a day or two. The smallpox

A = Sphenoid   C = Lacrymal
B = Zygomatic   D = Ethmoid

TWO VIEWS OF THE SKULL

rash lies deep in the skin compared to the superficial one of chickenpox. Recent vaccination usually protects against smallpox which is also known as variola.

smear (*smare*). Material for examination or culture which is spread on a slide or culture medium.

smegma (*smeg'-ma*). Thick white secretion forming under the prepuce.

Smith-Petersen nail (*smith-pē-ter-sen nāl*). Inserted to fix the two fragments of bone in a fracture of the neck of the femur.

SMITH-PETERSEN NAIL

Snellen's test types (*snel'-lens*). A chart showing letters of different size and used for testing vision. The patient sits at a distance of six metres from it. If only the large top letter can be seen the patient's vision is termed 6/60, *i.e.* he can see at 6 metres what the normal eye can see at a distance of 60 metres.

snow (*snō*). See CARBON DIOXIDE.

snow blindness (*blī'-nd-ness*). Ophthalmia with photophobia caused by the glare from snow.

snuffles (*snufls*). Occurs in babies with congenital syphilis, due to changes in the mucous membrane of the nose.

sodium (*sō'-di-um*). An alkaline metal. It forms an important part of animal tissue.

sodium acid phosphate (*sō-di-um a-sid fos'-fāt*). Drug given to make the urine acid.

Sodium Amytal (*sō'-di-um am'-i-tal*). See AMYTAL.

sodium aurothiomalate (*so'-di-um aw-ro-thī-ō-ma'-lāt*). A gold salt, given by intramuscular injection for rheumatoid arthritis. See GOLD THERAPY.

sodium bicarbonate (*sō'-di-um bī-kar-bo-nāt*). An antacid.

sodium chloride (*sō'-di-um klaw'-rīd*). Common salt. It is found in the body and maintains the osmotic tension of the blood. Given in infusions with dextrose for fluid replacement in dehydration. Given in Addison's disease to maintain electrolyte balance.

sodium citrate (*sō'-di-um si-trāt*). Same uses as potassium citrate. Also prevents clotting of blood and formation of large curds in milk.

sodium morrhuate (*sō-di-um mo'-roo-āt*). Used in the treatment of varicose veins by injection.

sodium propionate (*sō'-di-um pro-pī-o-nāt*). An antimycotic drug used in fungus infections.

sodium sulphate (*sō'-di-um sul-fāt*). A purgative.

soft sore (*so-ft sor'*). A venereal sore not due to syphilis. Also known as *chancroid*, and *non-infecting sore*. The infecting organism is Ducrey's bacillus.

solar plexus (*sō-la plek'-sus*). A plexus of nerves and ganglia in the upper region of the abdomen.

soleus (*so'-le-us*). A muscle in the calf of the leg.

solution (*so-loo'-shon*). A liquid containing a solid which has been dissolved in it.

solvent (*sol'-vent*). A liquid able to dissolve another substance.

somatic (*so-ma'-tik*). Pertaining to the body.

somnambulism (*som-nam'-bū-lizm*). Walking and carrying out other activities whilst asleep. There is dissociation which may be hysterical.

Soneryl (*son'-e-ril*). Butobarbitone, *q.v.*

Sonne dysentery (*son-ni dis'-en-te-ri*). A type of bacillary dysentery, common in Britain. There is abdominal pain, diarrhoea and vomiting.

The disease is usually slight except in infants and debilitated persons. The fluid intake must be adequate to prevent dehydration. Sulphonamides and antibiotics may be used.

soporific (*so-po-rif'-ik*). An agent which induces sleep, *e.g.* chloral.

sordes (*sor-dēz*). Brown crusts about the lips and teeth of a feverish patient. They should be carefully washed away with soft linen dipped in a weak solution of Condy's fluid, or glycerin and borax.

souffle (*soofl*). A soft blowing sound. During late pregnancy the *funic souffle* can sometimes be heard by auscultation of the maternal abdomen, a sound synchronous with the fetal heart and supposed to be produced in the umbilical cord. The *uterine souffle* is a blowing murmur heard over the uterus due to pulsations in the maternal arteries.

sound (*sownd*). A probe-like instrument used for exploring cavities such as the uterus, bladder, etc. *See illustration.*

BLADDER SOUND

graduated in inches

UTERINE SOUND

Southey's tubes (*sow-thēz*). Small perforated metal tubes, used to drain oedematous tissue.

Soxhlet bottle. An upright bottle used in infant feeding.

Spalding's sign (*sporl-dings sīn*). Sign of foetal death. There is overlapping of the skull bones on X-ray.

Spanish fly (*span-ish flī*). The dried beetle from which cantharides is extracted. It is used as a counter-irritant. Very poisonous. *See* CAN-THARIDES.

spasm (*spazm*). (1) Sudden convulsive involuntary movement. (2) Sudden contraction of a muscle or muscles, especially of the unstriped muscle coats of arteries, intestines, heart, bronchi, etc. The effect of such spasm depends on the part affected: thus asthma is believed to be due to spasm of the muscular coats of the smaller bronchi; and renal colic is due to spasm of the muscle coat of the ureter.

spasmolytic (*spaz-mo-li'-tik*). Substance which relieves spasm.

spasmus nutans (*spaz-mus nū-tanz*). A condition known as nodding spasm in babies, in which the head is continually nodding or turning from side to side.

spastic (*spas'-tik*). (1) In a state of spasm. (2) Popular term for cerebral palsy, *q.v.* In patients with this disease the muscles are often spastic,

i.e. hypertonic, and there is excessive neuromuscular excitability.

spasticity (*spas-tis'-i-ti*). The condition of being spastic. Occurs in an upper motor neurone lesion.

spatula (*spat'-ū-la*). (1) A flat, flexible, blunt knife, used for spreading ointments and poultices. (2) A tongue depressor.

species (*spē-sēz*). A group of organisms having many of the same characteristics. In natural history various species form a genus or class of animals.

specific (*spe-sif'-ik*). Applied to a medicine or treatment, it means the particular remedy for a certain disease; applied to a disease, it means due to a distinct specific microorganism which causes that disease alone.

specific gravity (*spe-sif-ik gra'-vi-ti*). By this is meant the ratio between the weight of a substance and the weight of an equal volume of water, the latter being taken, as a matter of convenience, to be 1·000, formerly written as 1000. The specific gravity of a liquid depends on the amount of solid in solution. *See* URINE TESTING in Appendix, p. 380.

spectroscope (*spek'-tro-skōp*). An instrument for the production and examination of spectra in luminous bodies.

spectrum (*spek'-trum*). The band of colours formed when rays of white light are passed through a prism.

speculum (*spek'-ū-lum*). A polished instrument for examining the interior cavities of the body, especially the vagina, the rectum, the ear, and the nose. *See following illustrations.*

a. AUVARD'S VAGINAL SPECULUM

b. FERGUSSON'S VAGINAL SPECULUM

c. SIMS' VAGINAL SPECULUM

speech (*spē-tch*). The power of speaking; conveying a meaning by vocal sounds.

speech centre. The parts of the brain controlling speech.

speech therapist (*spē-tch the'-ru-pist*). One trained to treat

defects and disorders of language, voice and speech.

Spencer-Wells forceps. The usual forceps for haemostasis during operations. *See* FORCEPS.

sperm (*sper'm*). Semen, *q.v.*

spermatic cord (*sper-mat'-ik*). Composed of arteries, veins, lymphatics and nerves, and the vas deferens (the duct of the testicle); it suspends the testicle from the abdomen.

spermatocele (*sper-ma-tō-sēl*). A retention cyst from some part of the epididymis.

spermatozoa (*sper-ma-tō-zō'-a*). The male generative cells; minute animated cells found in the semen, which are possessed of the power of self-propulsion by means of a flagellum, and which can fertilize the ovum, or female germ cell.

spermicide (*sper-mi-sīd*). Substance destroying spermatozoa.

sphenoid (*sfē-'noyd*). Wedge-shaped. The name of one of the bones forming the base of the skull.

sphenoidal (*sfen-oy'-dal*). Pertaining to the sphenoid bone.

sphincter (*sfink'-tur*). A circular muscle which contracts the orifice of an organ.

sphincterotomy (*sfink-te-ro'-to-mi*). Division of sphincter muscles.

sphygmocardiograph (*sfig-mō-kar'-dē-ō-graf*). Apparatus recording both pulse and heart beats.

sphygmograph (*sfig'-mō-graf*). An instrument affixed to the wrist, which moves with the beat of the pulse and registers the rate and character of the beats.

sphygmomanometer (*sfig-mō-ma-no'-mē-ter*). An instrument for measuring the arterial tension (or blood pressure) of the circulation.

SPICA FOR SHOULDER

SPHYGMOMANOMETER

spica (*spī'-ka*). A spiral bandage done with a roller in a series of figure eights. Most used for the shoulder, groin, thumb, and great toe.

spicule (*spi-kūl*). Fragment of bone.

spigot (*spi'-got*). Wooden peg closing a tube.

spina bifida (*spī-na bi-fid-er*). A congenital malformation of the spine due to the neural arch of one or more vertebrae failing to fuse in the midline. The vertebral canal is exposed at this site and may herniate through the opening. *See* MENINGOCELE. The defect most commonly occurs in the lumbo-sacral region.

SPINA BIFIDA WITH MENINGOCELE

spinal column (*spī'-nal ko'-lum*). The backbone. It is composed of seven cervical, twelve thoracic and five lumbar vertebrae and the sacrum with its five fused vertebrae and the coccyx or tailbone.

SPICA FOR GROIN

spinal cord (*spī'-nal kord*). The portion of the central nervous system within the spine. It contains many nerve cells and bundles of nerve fibres connecting the various levels of the spinal cord with the brain. Thirty-one pairs of nerves form the connections with the peripheral nervous system of the trunk and limbs. *See also* NERVE ROOT.

spinal curvature (*spī-nal ker'-va-tūr*). The *normal* curvature of the spine is divided into primary curvature (giving an ape-like stooping posture) and secondary curvatures (cervical and lumbar). For abnormal spinal curvature *see* SCOLIOSIS, KYPHOSIS, LORDOSIS.

spine (*spīn*). The backbone or spinal column, *q.v.*

spirillum (*spi-ril'-lum*). Cork-screw-shaped bacteria.

spirochaete (*spī-ro-kēt*). Elongated spiral bacteria which move by flexions of the body. Parasitic spirochaetes cause syphilis and Weil's disease.

spirochaetaemia (*spī-rō-kē-tē-mi-a*). The presence of spirochaetes in the blood.

spirograph (*spī'-rō-grarf*). Instrument for recording respirations.

spirometer (*spi-rom'-e-ter*). An instrument for measuring the capacity of the lungs.

splanchnic (*splank'-nik*). Pertaining to the viscera. *S. nerves*. Group of sympathetic nerve fibres which supply the viscera.

splanchnicectomy (*splank-ni-sek'-to-mi*). Surgical removal of the splanchnic ganglia and transection of the splanchnic nerves.

splanchnology (*splank-no'-lo-ji*). The study of the viscera.

splanchnoptosis (*splank-nop-tō'-sis*). Prolapse of the viscera, *e.g.* of the stomach, intestines or kidney.

splay foot (*splā*). Flatfoot. Pes planus.

spleen (*splēn*). A mass of lymphoid tissue situated in the mesentery of the abdomen. Unlike the lymph nodes, the spleen acts as a filtration organ for blood. The spleen forms an important part of the reticulo-endothelial system, *q.v.*, and is the generative centre for the formation of many lymphocytes. The spleen is largely responsible for the removal of red blood corpuscles at the end of their lifespan.

splenectomy (*splen-ek'-to-mi*). Removal of the spleen.

splenic anaemia (*a-nē'-mi-a*). Banti's syndrome. It is characterized by anaemia and splenomegaly associated with portal hypertension due to hepatic cirrhosis.

splenic flexure (*splen'-ik flek'-cher*). Bend of the colon on the left side, near the spleen.

spleniculus (*sple-ni'-kū-lus*). A second little spleen.

splenitis (*splen-i'-tis*). Inflammation of the spleen.

splenomegaly (*sple-nō-me'-ga-li*). An enlarged spleen.

'splinter' haemorrhages (*splinter he-mo-rā-jes*). Bleeding from the longitudinal capillaries in the nail bed giving the appearance of splinters under the nail. Characteristically occur in subacute bacterial endocarditis.

splints (*splin'-tz*). Used to immobilize a limb in the case of fracture, disease or deformity. They are now made chiefly of plaster of Paris, metal, rarely of wood, and the limb is slung on pieces of material attached to sides of splints. The aim of modern splints is to leave joints free for movement and massage, and to facilitate the correct application of methods of extension. For illustrations of special splints, *see* under own name.

spondyle (*spon'-dīl*). A vertebra.

spondylitis (*spon-di-lī'-tis*). Inflammation of a vertebra or vertebrae. *Ankylosing s.* Condition of unknown origin occurring characteristically in young men. There is ossification of spinal ligaments with ankylosis, *q.v.*, of the cervical and sacro-iliac joints.

spondylolisthesis (*spon-di-lō-lis-thē'-sis*). The vertebral arch of the fifth lumbar vertebra gives way so that the body of the affected vertebra becomes displaced.

spondylosis (*spon-di-lō'-sis*). Degenerative changes in the intervertebral discs with peripheral ossification. Known as 'osteo-arthritis' of spine'.

sponging (*spun'-jing*). A method of bringing down high temperature. It is also useful for calming restlessness and inducing sleep. It can be done with hot, tepid, cold, or iced water, and the whole body and limbs of the patient are sponged down, part only of the patient being exposed at a time. During the treatment the patient must be watched carefully for signs of collapse.

spontaneous fracture (*spon-tā'-ne-us frak'-tūr*). Fracture due to disease affecting the bone, either from abnormal development or rarefaction of the bone from other causes.

spontaneous version (*spon-tā'-nē-us ver'-shon*). The unaided conversion of a transverse lie into a cephalic or podalic one.

sporadic (*spo-rad'-ik*). A disease which is not epidemic, but occurs in one or two isolated cases in a district.

spore (*spaw*). Reproductive body which gives rise to a new individual organism. Produced by protozoa, fungi and bacteria, spores increase rapidly and can survive in unfavourable conditions. Important spore-forming bacteria are Clostridium Welchii and Clostridium botulinum.

sporotrichosis (*spo-rō-tri-kō'-sis*). Disease due to a fungoid organism causing subcutaneous abscesses.

spotted fever (*spo'-ted*). Cerebrospinal meningitis.

sprain (*sprān*). Severe strain of a joint without fracture or dislocation, but with swelling and often with effusion into joint.

Sprengel's deformity (*spreng'-els de-for'-mi-ti*). Congenital upward displacement of the scapula.

sprue (*sproo*). A disease of tropical climates which causes inflammation of the mucous membrane of the alimentary canal, characterized by soreness of tongue and mouth, chronic diarrhoea, wasting and anaemia.

spurious pains (*spū'-rē-us*). False labour pains, leading to no result, and sometimes occurring several days before confinement.

sputum (*spū'-tum*). Expectorated matter. Different types are; *Mucoid*, occurs in the early stage of irritation. *Muco-purulent* develops at a later stage, pus is mixed with mucus. *Rusty*, tenacious sputum occurs in lobar penumonia. Copious foul smelling sputum occurs in bronchiectasis. *Foaming sputum* occurs in oedema of the lung. Separate pellets or nummular sputum occurs in pulmonary tuberculosis. It may be streaked with blood.

squamous (*skwā'-mus*). Scaly.

squill (*skwil*). Drug used as an expectorant.

squint (*skwi'nt*). *See* STRABISMUS.

stable (*stā'-bl*). Not moving, fixed. *Stable current*. Steady application of an electrode to a part.

staccato or scanning speech (*stak-ar'-tō*). Hesitation between syllables, and when the sound comes it comes explosively. It is a type of inco-ordination, and occurs in cerebellar lesions and disseminated sclerosis.

Stacke's operation (*staks*). Operation used in chronic infection to join the middle ear cavity with that of the mastoid cells.

stages of labour. *See* LABOUR.

stain (*stān*). Dye used to colour tissues before microscopical examination, or to produce certain reactions.

stamina (*sta'-min-a*). Vigour. Staying power.

stapedius (*sta-pē'-di-us*). A muscle of the middle ear.

stapes (*stā'-pēz*). One of the three ossicles of the middle ear; stirrup-shaped. *See* EAR.

Staphylococcus (*staf-i-lō-kok'-us*). Genus of Gram-positive bacteria which grow in clusters when cultured. Many staphylococci are commensals on the skin. Some are serious pathogens and several strains have evolved which are insensitive to penicillin and other antibiotics.

staphyloma (*staf-i-lō'-ma*). Any protrusion of the sclerotic or corneal coats of the eyeball due to inflammation.

staphylorrhaphy (*sta-fi-lor'-ra-fi*). Operation to suture cleft soft palate.

starch (*star'-ch*). Carbohydrate. It can be obtained from maize, rice, wheat and potato. *S. bandage*. Muslin bandage impregnated with starch powder as plaster bandages. *S. poultice*. Used to remove scabs, especially in impetigo. Two tablespoonfuls of starch powder and one teaspoonful of boric acid powder are mixed with one pint of water brought to the boil whilst stirring. The mixture is spread on old linen. *S. powder*. Widely used dusting-powder for the skin.

Starr valve. Artificial heart valve.

stasis (*stā'-sis*). Standing still. Most commonly used for arrest of the circulation of either blood or lymph, but also for intestinal stasis, a holding up of the contents of the bowel.

status asthmaticus (*stā-tus asthma'-ti-kus*). Severe attack of asthma.

status epilepticus (*stāt'-us epil-ep'-ti-kus*). A condition in which a series of epileptic fits occur in rapid succession.

status lymphaticus (*stāt'-us lim-fat'-i-kus*). A rare condition in which the patient is believed to be liable to sudden death for very slight (or no apparent) reason.

steapsin (*stē-ap'-sin*). Lipase, *q.v.*

steatoma (*stē-at-ō'-ma*). A fatty encysted tumour. A sebaceous cyst.

steatorrhoea (*ste-at-or-ē'-ah*). The passage of excessive fat in the stools. Thought to be due to pancreatic deficiency, or deficiency of bile, or inability on the part of the lacteals to absorb fat. Sometimes produced by allergy to protein in wheat flour. A diet without fat and wheat gluten is given.

steatosis (*stē-at-ō'-sis*). Fatty degeneration.

Stegomyia (*steg'-ō-mi'-ē-a*). A variety of mosquito which acts as the carrier of the parasite of yellow fever from a patient to a healthy individual.

Stein-Leventhal syndrome (*stīn-le-ven-thal sin-drōm*). Sterility, uterine hypoplasia, masculinization and polycystic ovaries.

Steinmann's pin (*stīn'-marn*). A fixation pin inserted through a bone in order to apply extension in the case of fractures. *See* EXTENSION.

stellate ganglion (*stel-lāt gan'-glē-on*). Star-shaped sympathetic ganglion situated in the neck.

stenosis (*ste-nō'-sis*). Contraction of a canal or an orifice.

Stensen's duct (*sten'-sens dukt*). The duct of the parotid salivary gland. Its opening is opposite the upper first molar tooth.

stercobilin (*ster-kō-bī'-lin*). The colouring matter of the faeces. It is derived from bile pigment.

stercolith (*ster'-kō-lith*). Small hard mass of faeces. Faecolith.

stereognosis (*ste-rē-og-nō'-sis*). Recognition of the form of bodies by handling them.

sterile (*ste'-rīl*). Barren; unable to have children. In *surgical practice*, sterile means entirely free from germs of all kinds, a result brought about by heat or by the use of antiseptic chemicals.

sterility (*ste-ril'-it-i*). The condition of being sterile.

sterilization (*ster-il-ī-zā'-shon*). (1) Made incapable of progeny, e.g. by removal of ovaries, tying the Fallopian tubes, hysterectomy or, in the male, castration, tying the vas deferens. (2) Rendering germ-free.

sternal puncture (*ster-nal pungk'-cher*). Technique employed to obtain sample of red bone marrow for investigation. A needle is inserted into the sternum under local anaesthesia and a small amount of marrow aspirated.

sterno-mastoid muscle (*sternō-mas'-toyd mus-l*). Muscle of neck, running from the inner end of clavicle and upper border of sternum to behind the ear. *See* TORTICOLLIS.

sternum (*ster'-num*). The breastbone.

steroids (*ste'-royds*). Group of compounds resembling cholesterol. They include sex hormones, bile acids, sterols and some hydrocarbons.

sterols (*ste'-rols*). Steroids with an alcohol (—OH) side group, e.g. Cortisol (=hydrocortisone).

stertor (*ster'-tor*). Snoring type of respiration.

stethoscope (*steth'-o-skōp*). Instrument for listening to sounds, e.g. heart sounds, respiratory sounds. The *binaural* stethoscope has two flexible ends, to apply to the ears of the listener.

STETHOSCOPE

Stevens-Johnson syndrome (*stē-vens-jon-son sin-drōm*). Severe form of erythema multiforme in which mucous membranes may be extensively involved.

sthenic (*sthen'ik*). Strong, active.

stibophen (*sti'-bo-fen*). An antimony compound used to treat schistosomiasis.

stigma (*stig'-ma*) (plu. **stigmata**). Mark on the skin. Also any permanent condition indicative of some constitutional peculiarity.

stilboestrol (*stil-bēs'-trol*). A synthetic compound possessing a high degree of oestrogenic activity. Used to control menopausal symptoms, suppress lactation and, in the male, for prostate carcinoma.

stilette (*sti-let'*). A probe.

stillborn (*stil'-born*). Dead when born.

Still's disease. A form of rheumatoid arthritis occurring in children. The syndrome is characterized by polyarthritis, lymphadenopathy, splenomegaly, calcification of the cornea and formation of cataract.

stimulant (*stim'-ū-lant*). That which causes temporary increase in the output of the vital energy.

stimulus (*sti'-mū-lus*). An agent provoking activity.

stitch (*stich*). (1) Suture, *q.v.* (2) Pain in the side due to spasm of the diaphragm.

Stokes-Adams' syndrome (*sin-drōm'*). Syncope due to cerebral hypoxia resulting from heart block.

stoma (*stō'-ma*). The mouth.

stomach (*stum'-ak*). The dilated portion of the intestinal canal into which the food passes from the oesophagus, and where it undergoes partial digestion.

stomach pump (*stum'-ak pum'p*). A thick rubber tube, at least 18 inches long, attached to a glass receptacle which has a rubber bulb inserted into its neck by means of which a vacuum is created in the glass flask.

SECTION OF STOMACH

STOMACH PUMP

Used to aspirate the contents of the stomach.

stomatitis (*stom-a-tī'-tis*). Inflammation of the mouth.

stone (*stōn*). (1) A measure of weight, 14 pounds. (2) A concretion.

stools (*stū'ls*). Discharge of faeces from the bowels. *See* MOTIONS.

strabismus (*stra-biz'-mus*). Squint; *divergent* when the eye turns out; *convergent* when it turns in.

strabotomy (*stra-bot'-o-mi*). Operation to remedy squinting.

strain (*strān*). (1) To filter. (2) Condition resulting from unsuitable use of a part.

stramonium (*stra-mo'-nē-um*). A drug similar to belladonna used as a sedative and antispasmodic. Overdose poisons. Prescribed in asthma.

strangulated (*strang'-gū-lā-ted*). Constricted, so that the blood-supply is cut off. *See* HERNIA.

strangury (*stran'-gu-ri*). Painful passage of urine. Usually the result of disease of the bladder, urethra, broad ligament, etc., but occasionally occurs after labour.

strapping (*strap'-ping*). Material used to bind up injuries.

stratified (*strat'-if-īd*). In layers.

stratum (*stra'-tum*). A layer.

streptococcus (*strep-to-ko-kus*). Germs of Gram-positive bacteria which grow in chains. Pathogenic cocci produce toxins responsible for scarlet fever, rheumatic fever and acute glomerulo-nephritis.

streptomycin (*strep-to-mī'-sin*). An antibacterial agent produced by the organism Streptomyces griseus. It has a bacteriostatic effect chiefly on Gram-negative organisms. Used in the treatment of tuberculosis. It is injected intramuscularly. Also given orally for pre-operative cleansing of the intestinal tract.

Streptothrix (*strep'-to-thriks*). Filamentous bacteria.

stress incontinence. Incontinence of urine or faeces when the intra-abdominal pressure is raised as in coughing or sneezing.

striae (*stri-ē*). Scars on the abdomen and thighs due to stretching of the dermis during rapid expansion of the abdomen. Frequently seen in association with pregnancy.

striae gravidarum (*strī'-ē gravid-ar'-um*). The numerous marks which develop on the skin of the abdomen in the later months of pregnancy. They never quite disappear. Striae are due to the stretching of the skin, and are seen also in any condition of *rapid* enlargement of the abdomen, and also sometimes on the thighs of boys who are growing very rapidly. They are thought to be associated with increased activity of the suprarenal cortex. Syn. LINEAE ALBICANTES.

striated muscle (*strī-ā-ted musel*). Striped voluntary muscle, cf. *smooth muscle.*

stricture (*strikt'-ūr*). Contraction. Usually applied to the urethra, with consequent inability to pass urine.

stridor (*strī'-dor*). A harsh sound during breathing, cau-

sed by obstruction to the passage of air.

stroke (*strōk*). Cerebrovascular accident, *q.v.* See also HEATSTROKE.

stroma (*strō'-ma*). The connective tissue.

strophanthin (*strō-fan'-thin*). The active principle of strophanthus.

strophanthus (*strō-fan'-thus*). A poison, used in small doses as a heart stimulant. Diuretic.

strychnine (*strik'nēn*). An alkaloid of Nux Vomica. Poison; used as a nerve and spinal stimulant. It stimulates the vital centres in the medulla. *Antidotes:* an emetic, strong tea, and *see* p. 390.

stupe (*stūp*). A fomentation sprinkled with a counter-irritant, *e.g.* turpentine. See FOMENTATIONS.

stupor (*stū'-por*). State of unconsciousness.

Sturge-Weber syndrome (*sterj-we-ber sin-drōm*). Syndrome characterized by capillary naevus on the face in the distribution of the fifth cranial nerve. Associated with angiomas of the cerebral cortex which may cause focal epilepsy, hemiparesis and mental deficiency.

stye (*stī*). Suppuration around an eyelash follicle.

stylet (*sti-let'*). See STILETTE.

styptic (*stip'-tik*). Agent applied to arrest bleeding; astringent, *e.g.* adrenaline.

Stypven (*stīp'-ven*). Local haemostatic containing Russell's viper venom.

styrax (*stī'raks*). Storax: a constituent of Tinct. Benzoin Co.

sub. A prefix denoting beneath or under.

subacute (*sub-a-kūt*). Fairly severe.

subacute bacterial endocarditis (*sub-a-kūt bak-tā-ri-al en-dō-kar-dī-tis*). Bacterial colonization of defective heart valves with consequent bacteraemia and distribution of septic emboli throughout the body.

subacute combined degeneration of the cord. Degeneration of the posterior and lateral columns of the spinal cord due to vitamin B_{12} deficiency.

subarachnoid haemorrhage (*sub-a-rak-noyd he-mo-rāg*). Haemorrhage into the subarachnoid space.

subarachnoid space (*sub-ar-ak-noyd'*). The space between the arachnoid membrane and the pia mater. It contains cerebrospinal fluid.

subclavian (*sub-klā'-vē-an*). Under the clavicle: thus the subclavian artery and vein are vessels passing under the clavicle.

subclinical (*sub-kli'-ni-kal*). Without any obvious signs of the disease.

subconscious (*sub-kon'-shus*). The part of the mind outside an individual's awareness, but able to affect the way of acting or thinking.

subcutaneous (*sub-kŭ-tā'-ne-us*). Under the skin.

subinvolution (*sub-in-vō-lŭ'-shon*). Failure of the lately pregnant uterus to regain the normal unimpregnated size within the usual time (six weeks) of delivery.

subjacent (*sub-jā'-sent*). Lying below.

subjective (*sub-jek'-tiv*). Internal: pertaining to one's self.

sublimation (*sub-li-mā'-shon*). (1) The process of vaporizing and condensing a solid substance without melting it; (2) 'shunting off' the energy from an impulse or urge from the subconscious by changing its character and aiming at something more attainable.

subliminal (*sub-li'-mi-nal*). Beneath the threshold of consciousness.

sublingual (*sub-ling'-gwal*). Under the tongue.

subluxation (*sub-luks-ā'-shon*). Sprain and partial dislocation.

submaxillary (*sub'-mak-sil'-ari*). Under the lower jaw. *S. glands.* One of the three pairs of salivary glands.

submucous (*sub-mū'-kus*). Under a mucous membrane; a uterine fibroid is submucous when it projects into the cavity of the uterus.

subnormal (*sub-nor'-mal*). Below normal.

subphrenic (*sub-fren'-ik*). Under the diaphragm. *S.*

abscess, a collection of pus beneath the diaphragm.

substrate (*sub-strāt*). Compound on which an enzyme acts.

subtotal hysterectomy (*sub-tō'-tal his-to-rek'-to-mi*). The removal of the uterus, excluding the cervix.

succenturiate placenta (*suk-sen-tūr'-i-āt pla-sen'-ta*). An accessory placenta.

succus entericus (*suk'-us en-te'-rik-us*). The digestive juice secreted by the glands in the small intestine.

succussion (*suk-kush'-on*). Sound made on shaking a patient if fluid is present in a hollow cavity.

sudamina (*su-dam'-ēn-a*). Sweat rash.

Sudol (*sū-dol*). A phenol preparation having the same wide range of bactericidal power as Lysol, but with reduced necrotic action on the skin.

sudorific (*sū-do-rif'-ik*). An agent causing perspiration.

suffused (*su-fūz'-d*). Congested.

suggestibility (*su-jes'-ti-bi-li-ti*). A state when the patient readily accepts other people's ideas and influences.

suicide (*soo-'i-sīd*). (1) The person who kills himself by intent. (2) Self slaughter.

sulcus (*sul'-kus*). A furrow.

Sulfasuxidine (*sul-fu-suk'-si-dēn*). Succinylsulphathiazole.

sulphacetamide (*sul-fu-se'-ta-mīd*). Sulphonamide drug

used in eye infections, and as an ointment for burns and wounds. Syn. Albucid.

sulphadiazine (*sul-fu-dī'-a-zēn*). A sulphonamide drug given in meningitis, etc.

sulphadimidine (*sul-fu-di'-mi-dēn*). Sulphonamide drug especially suitable for children as there is small risk of crystals being formed in the urinary tract.

sulphafurazole (*sul-fu-fūr'-a-zol*). Sulphonamide drug used especially in urinary tract infections.

sulphamerazine (*sul-fu-me'-ru-zēn*). A long-acting sulphonamide.

sulphate (*sul'-fāt*). A salt of sulphuric acid, *e.g.* atropine sulphate.

sulphonamide drugs (*sul-fon'-am-īd*). A group of drugs used as internal germicides (chemotherapeutic agents), particularly in strepto-, pneumo-, meningo-, and gonococcal infections and in those due to the colon bacillus. Soluble sodium salts are caustic with the exception of sulphacetamide. They can be given intravenously but should never be injected intramuscularly or under the skin. The standard pharmaceutical unit is a half-gram tablet. Children and infants require relatively larger doses than adults. A four-hourly plan of administration is accepted to sustain a steady concentration of the drug in the blood and tissues. Toxic effects, sometimes of a serious nature, tend to occur if treatment is continued for longer than a week. Possible complications are granulocytopenia, drug rash, anuria. Some degree of cyanosis is common but rarely necessitates withdrawal of the drug. Saline aperient sulphates are harmless.

sulphones (*sul-fōns*). Group of synthetic drugs used in the treatment of leprosy.

sulphuric acid (*sul-fūr'-ik*). Vitriol. A poison; some of the antidotes are limewater, potash water, oil and milk.

sunstroke (*sun'-strōk*). See HEATSTROKE.

superciliary (*su-per-sil'-ya-ri*). Having to do with the eyebrows.

supercilium (*su-per-sil'-i-um*). The eyebrow,

superego (*soo'-per-e-go*). Term used in psychology for the part of the subconscious, founded on early experiences, which acts as a sort of conscience and sets forth standards and ideals. The superego can cause feelings of guilt and anxiety.

superfecundation (*su-per-fe-kun-dā'-shon*). The fertilization of two ova discharged at the same ovulation by two distinct acts of insemination effected at a short interval.

superior (*soo-pār'-i-or*). Above. The upper of two organs.

supination (*su-pi-nā'-shon*). Turning the palm of the hand upwards.

supine (*sū'-pīn*). Lying face upwards; in the case of the forearm, having the palm uppermost.

supplemental air (*sup-lē-ment'-al ā-er*). That part of the residual air of the lung which after the tidal air has been expelled may be driven out by forced respiration.

suppository (*sup-pŏz'-i-to-ri*). Rectally administered cones containing a medicament in a base which is soluble at body temperature.

suppression (*sup-presh'-on*). Failure to secrete or when some activity is prevented. In psychology, the voluntary dismissal from the mind of painful or unsuitable urges.

suppuration (*sup-pū-rā'-shon*). The formation of pus.

supra-orbital (*sū-pra-or'-bi-tal*). Above the orbit.

suprapubic (*sū-pra-pū'-bik*). Above the pubes.

suprarenal (*sū-pra-rē'-nal*). Above the kidney. *S. glands*, two small ductless glands situated above the kidney and secreting adrenaline. They are also concerned with the development of the secondary sexual characteristics. Disease of suprarenals is called Addison's disease, *q.v.* The suprarenals may be the seat of growths, especially of hypernephromata. *See* ADRENALINE and HYPERNEPHROMA.

sural (*sū'-ral*). Relating to the calf of the leg.

surface (*ser'-fes*). The outer part. *S. markings*. Lines drawn on the skin to show the position of structures beneath it.

surgery (*ser'-je-ri*). (1) The part of medicine concerned with diseases needing treatment by operation. (2) A physician or surgeon's consulting room.

surgical (*ser'-ji-kal*). Pertaining to surgery. *S. kidney*. Pyelitis or diffuse suppuration in the kidney. *S. neck*. Narrow part of the humerus, below the tuberosities.

susceptible (*su-sep'-tibl*). Liable to, *e.g.* infection.

suspension (*sus-pen-shon*). (1) Hanging. (2) Particles in water which are not dissolved by it. *See* VENTROSUSPENSION.

suspensory bandage (*sus-pen'-so-ri ban-dāj*). A bandage to support the testicles.

sutures (*soo'-tūrs*). (1) Silk, thread, catgut, nylon, etc., used to sew a wound. (2) The union of flat bones by their margins, *e.g.* bones of the skull.

swabs (*swobz*). Small pieces of wool, gauze over wool, or gauze only, used for cleaning wounds and for removing blood at operations.

sweat (*swet*). Perspiration. The fluid secreted on to the skin by the sweat glands.

sycosis (*sī-kō'-sis*). Inflammation of the hair follicles, especially of the beard and whiskers.

symbiosis (*sim-bī-ō'-sis*). The living together of two organisms, whose mutual association is necessary to each, although neither is parasitic on the other.

symblepharon (*sim-blef'-a-ron*). Adhesion of the eyelids to the eyeball.

Syme's amputation (*sīmz*). Amputation at the ankle joint.

sympathectomy (*sim-path-ek'-to-mi'*). Surgical transection of sympathetic nerves usually with excision of part of the sympathetic chain.

sympathetic system (*sim-pa-thet'-ik*). A nerve system consisting of a chain of ganglia beside the spine supplying nerves to the heart, blood-vessels and other internal viscera.

symphysiotomy (*sim'-fiz-ē-ot'-o-mi*). The operation of dividing the symphysis pubis (of the mother) so as to facilitate delivery in certain cases of contracted pelvis.

symphysis (*sim'-fi-sis*). Growing of bones together. The *symphysis pubis* is the bony mass bounding the front of the pelvis, at the lower end of the abdomen. *See* PELVIS.

symptom (*simp'-tum*). A noticeable change in the body and its functions, evidence of disease. Usually meaning the change complained of by the patient.

symptomatology (*simp'-tō-ma-to'-lo-ji*). A study of the symptoms of disease.

synapse (*sī-naps*). Region where nerve cells communicate. There is no continuity between the neurons and impulses are transmitted from one nerve cell to another by the passage of chemical messengers which stimulate the post-synaptic nerve cell.

synarthrosis (*sin-ar-thrō-sis*). Immovable union of bones, *e.g.* the cranial bones.

synchondrosis (*sin-kon-drō'-sis*). A joint whose surfaces are united by cartilage.

synchysis (*sin'-ki-sis*). Softening of the vitreous humour of the eye. *S. scintillans*. Bright particles found in the vitreous humour.

synclitism (*sin'-klit-ism*). Descent of the fetal head through the pelvis with its planes parallel to those of the pelvis.

syncope (*sin'-kō-pē*). Fainting.

syndactyly (*sin-dak'-ti-li*). Webbed fingers or toes.

syndesmitis (*sin-des-mī'-tis*). Inflammation of ligaments.

syndrome (*sin'-drōm*). Collection of symptoms and signs which form a recognizable pattern of disease.

synechia (*sin-ek'-i-a*). Adhesion of the iris to the cornea, or to the crystalline lens.

synergy (*si'-ner-ji*). The working together of two or more agents.

Synkavit (*sin'-ka-vit*). A vitamin K analogue.

synonyms (*sin'-ō-nims*). Different words having the same meaning.

synostosis (*sīn-os-tō'-sis*). Abnormal osseous union of bones.

synovectomy (*sī-nō-vek'-tō-mi*). Operation to remove synovial membrane.

synovial fluid (*sī-nō-vi-al flū-id*). The liquid which lubricates the joints.

synovial membrane (*sī-nō'-vial mem'-brān*). That lining a joint cavity but not covering the articular surfaces.

synovitis (*sī-nō-vī'-tis*). Inflammation of the synovial membrane of a joint.

synthesis (*sin'-the-sis*). The building up of complex substances by the union and interaction of simpler materials.

synthetic (*sin-thet'-ik*). Pertaining to synthesis. Artificial.

syphilide (*sif'-il-īd*). Lesion of the skin due to syphilis. May be papular, macular, squamous, etc.

syphilis (*sif'-i-lis*). A venereal disease. Caused by a specific spirochaete, the Treponema pallidum. S. may be congenital or acquired. *Congenital* may be inherited from the mother. The chief symptoms in young babies: wasting, snuffles, rashes, enlargement of liver and spleen. If child survives, he may later show pallor, malnutrition, depressed bridge of nose, rhagades, square skull, thickening of tibiae, corneal opacities, Hutchinson's teeth (*see* RHAGADES, HUTCHINSON'S TEETH). *Acquired* is divided into three stages. (1) First stage or primary S. with local symptoms, two–three weeks after infection. Hard chancre on penis, vulva, or cervix. Inflamed glands in groin. Lesions infective (*see* CHANCRE). (2) Second stage or secondary S., one to two months after infection, with rashes, sore throat, mucous patches, condylomata, general enlargement of glands, anaemia, and fever. Infective (*see* CONDYLOMA). (2) Third stage or tertiary S., two to ten years or even longer after infection. Non-infective, giving, among other manifestations, gummata, tabes, G.P.I., *see* GENERAL PARALYSIS.

syringe (*si-rinj*). An instrument for injecting fluids, or for exploring and aspirating cavities.

syringomyelia (*se-rin'-go-mī-ēl'-i-a*). Progressive degenerative disease affecting the brain stem and spinal cord in which the tracts of the fibres subserving pain and temperature are mainly affected.

syringomyelocele (*si-rin-gō-mī-el'-ō-sēl*). A type of spina bifida. There is a communication between the projecting mass and the central canal of the spinal cord.

syringotomy (*sir-ing-got'-o-mi*). Cutting open a fistula.

system (*sis'-tem*). An organized scheme. A series of parts concerned in a basic function such as nutrition by the alimentary system.

systemic (*sis-te-mik*). Affecting the whole body.

systole (*sis'-tō-lē*). The period when the heart contracts. See DIASTOLE.

systolic blood-pressure (*sis-to-lik blud-pre-shor*). The force with which the left ventricle contracts and which is measured in the peripheral arteries.

systolic murmur (*sis-to-lik mer'-mer*). Murmur heard during systole. It may be due to aortic or tricuspid obstruction.

T

T.A.B. Triple vaccine to prevent typhoid, paratyphoid A and paratyphoid B.

T bandage. A special bandage used for keeping dressings on the perineum.

SHOWING T BANDAGE IN POSITION

T BANDAGE WITH SPLIT ENDS

tabes (*tā-bēz*). Wasting. *T. dorsalis*, a disorder of the spinal cord, due to tertiary syphilis, also called locomotor ataxia, and characterized by loss of power over muscles. See SYPHILIS. *T. mesenterica*, tuberculosis of the mesenteric glands. Seen in children.

tachycardia (*tak-ē-kar'-di-a*). Abnormally rapid action of the heart, as in atrial fibrillation.

tactile (*tak'-tīl*). Relating to the touch. *T. corpuscles*. Cutaneous end organs of the tactile nerves.

taenia (*tē-ni-a*). A flat strip.

Taenia (*tē'-ni-a*). The tapeworm. The adult worm consists of a head and numerous segments. It has the appearance of jointed tape and may be several feet long. The *Taenia solium* is a common variety which gains entrance to the body through underdone infected pork. The head attaches itself to the mucous membrane of the intestines and the worm continues to grow. The treatment is (1) little food for several hours, (2) purge, (3) ext. filix mas, (4) purge.

T.A.F. Toxoid-antitoxin floccules. Used to immunize against diphtheria.

talc. French chalk. Used as dusting powder.

talipes (*tal'-i-pēz*). Clubfoot. *Talipes valgus*, the foot turned outwards; *varus*, the foot turned inwards; *equinus*, the heel lifted from the ground; *calcaneus*, heel projected downwards.

TALIPES EQUINO-VARUS

TALIPES VALGUS, FLATFOOT

TALIPES CALCANEUS, WITH SOME CAVUS DEFORMITY

TALIPES EQUINUS

talus (*tāl'-us*). The ankle.

tampon (*tam'-pon*). A plug of wool or gauze introduced into the vagina.

tamponade (*tam-pō-nād*). Compression (usually *cardiac T.*) in which the action of the heart is impeded by the presence of fluid in the pericardium.

Tannafax (*tan'-a-faks*). Tannic acid in jelly form.

tannin (*ta'-nin*). Tannic acid. An astringent vegetable principle, used as a styptic. A constituent of many astringent drugs given internally for haemorrhage, dysentery, etc., formerly used in the treatment of burns.

tantalum (*tan'-ta-lum*). A resistant metal sometimes used in bone surgery for plates or wire.

tapeworm (*tāp'-werm*). See TAENIA.

tapping. See ASPIRATION.

tar (*tah*). Dark liquid obtained from pine-wood. It has antipyretic and antiseptic properties. *Coal-t.* Black liquid distilled from coal. It contains benzene, phenol, cresols, naphthalene, etc.

tarsal (*tar-sal*). Bones of the ankle, *cf.* carpal bones. There are seven in man, forming a group which articulate with the tibia and fibula and the metatarsal bones.

tarsalgia (*ta-sal'-ji-a*). Pain in the foot.

tarsectomy (*ta-sek-to-mi*). Excision of part of the tarsal group of bones.

tarsoplasty (*ta-sō-plas'-ti*). Plastic surgery of the eyelid.

tarsorrhaphy (*ta-so'-ra-fi*). Stitching the eyelids together.

tarsus (*tar'-sus*). (1) The seven small bones of the foot. (2) The cartilaginous framework of the eyelid.

tartar (*tar'-ta*). Deposit on the teeth of calcium salts derived from saliva.

tartar emetic (*tar'-tar em-et'-ik*). Antimony tartrate, *q.v.*

tartaric acid (*tah-ta'-rik a'-sid*). Used in making effervescent preparations. It should be taken well-diluted if not neutralized.

tartrate (*tar'-trāt*). A salt of tartaric acid.

taste bud. Specialized sensory end organ which is sensitive to taste.

taurocholic acid (*taw-rō-kō-lik a'-sid*). One of the bile acids.

taxis (*tak'-sis*). Hand-manipulation for restoring a part to its natural position, such as reducing a hernia.

Tay-Sach's disease (*tā-saks*). Amaurotic family idiocy.

tears (*tārs*). Secretion of the lacrimal gland.

tease (*tēz*). To divide a tissue into shreds.

teat (*tēt*). Nipple.

technique (*tek-nē'k*). The essential details of any process.

teeth, eruption of. The milk teeth, or first dentition of the infant, begin to erupt between the sixth and twelfth months. Occasionally they start to appear even earlier than the sixth month. The lower central incisors usually appear first, followed by the upper central incisors. As a rule there will be from eight to twelve teeth cut at a year old, and the twenty teeth which constitute the first dentition should be present at two years of age. The permanent teeth begin to erupt about the fifth or sixth year with the appearance of the first permanent molars;

SECTION OF A
MOLAR TOOTH

then about the seventh year there is shedding of the incisors. The numbers in the *top illustration* indicate the child's age in months when the teeth erupt.

TEMPORARY TEETH

PERMANENT TEETH

Teflon (*tef'-lon*). Proprietary material used in heart surgery.

tegument (*teg'-ū-ment*). The skin.

tela (*tā'-la*). Tissue formed like a web.

telangiectasis, telangioma (*te-lan-ji-ek'-ta-sis, te-lan-ji-ō'-ma*). Lesion consisting of a number of tortuous dilated capillaries which have a web-like appearance.

teleradium (*te-lē-rā-di-um*). Used in radium beam therapy.

temper tantrums (*tem'-per tan'-trums*). Outburst of temper. An infantile way of demanding that a need be satisfied.

temperament (*tem'-pe-ra-ment*). A person's mental outlook.

temperature (*tem'-per-a-tūr*). A measurement of the degree of heat. The average normal temperature of the human body is 98·4° F (37° C). The average temperature of a sick-room should be 60° to 65° F (16 to 18° C).

temples (*tem'-plz*). The part of the forehead between the outer corner of the eye and the hair.

temporal (*tem'-por-al*). Relating to the temple. Thus T. artery, T. bone, T. lobe of the brain.

temporal arteritis. *Giant cell arteritis.* A disease of unknown aetiology characterized by general malaise, aches and muscle pains and acute inflammation of the arteries, particularly those of the scalp.

tenaculum (*te-nak'-ū-lum*). An instrument like a vulsellum, but having only one pair of teeth for fixing the cervix uteri.

tendinitis (*ten-di-nī'-tis*). Inflammation of a tendon.

tendo Achillis (*ten-dō ak'-il-is*). The stout tendon of the calf muscles at the back of the heel.

tendon (*ten'-don*). A sinew, a cord of fibrous white tissue by which a muscle is attached to a bone or other structure.

tendovaginitis, stenosing (*ten-dō-va-gi-nī-tis stē'-nō-zing*). Stenosing tenosynovitis, de Quervain's disease. Fibrous thickening of tendon sheath most commonly affecting the tendons of the abductor muscles of the thumb.

tenesmus (*te-nes'-mus*). Painful straining to empty the bowel.

tennis elbow (*ten'-nis el'-bō*). Severe pain is felt over the outer aspect of the elbow and arises from excessive or unaccustomed lifting, gripping or twisting movements of the hand. There is resultant weakness and extension of elbow is painful. Treatment is rest, injection of local anaesthetic and, in obstinate cases, operation may be necessary.

tenoplasty (*te-nō-plas'-ti*). Plastic surgery to a tendon.

tenorrhaphy (*te-no'-ra-fi*). Operation to suture a tendon.

tenosynovitis (*ten'-ō-sī-nō-vī'-tis*). Inflammation in the sheath of a tendon.

tenotomy (*te-not'-o-mi*). Cutting a tendon.

tension (*ten'-shon*). Stretching.

tensor (*ten'-sor*). A muscle which stretches.

tent (*ten't*). A cylindrical rod constructed of some material such as compressed seaweed which in the presence of moisture swells to a much larger size. Used for dilating the cervix uteri so as to allow the introduction of instruments or dilating bags. One or more are introduced into the cervix overnight, and the vagina lightly plugged to prevent its escape. Rarely used at present time. Steam T., erected around a bed to provide a moist atmosphere. Screens and an old sheet or blanket are used. Steam is directed inside from a bronchitis kettle. Temperature of tent, 70° F (21°C.)

tentorium cerebelli (*ten-tor'-i-um se-ri-bel-li*). A septum of the dura mater which lies between the cerebrum and cerebellum. This may be torn in a breech delivery and may prove fatal to the child.

tepid (*te'-pid*). Just warm.

teratogen (*te-ra-tō-jen*). Any agent able to produce a fetal monster.

teratoma (*te-ra-tō'-ma*). *See* EMBRYOMA.

terebene (*ter'-e-bēn*). A preparation of oil of turpentine.

terebinthina (*ter-e-bin'-thi-na*). Turpentine. Turpentine enema. *See* ENEMA and FOMENTATIONS.

teres (*te'-rās*). Round and smooth. *Ligamentum T.* Ligament of the head of the femur.

terminology (*ter-mi-no'-lo-ji*). Nomenclature. The science of the proper use of terms, as in medicine.

Terramycin (*te-ra-mi-sin*). Oxytetracycline. Antibiotic produced by growth of streptomyces rimosus. Has wide range of action and is active orally.

tertian (*ter'-shan*). A form of malaria with attacks every third day.

tertiary (*ter-she-ri*). Third.

tertiary syphilis. *See* SYPHILIS.

test. (1) Trial. (2) A reaction distinguishing one substance from another.

test meal. *See* FRACTIONAL TEST MEAL.

testicles (*tes'-ti-kls*). The two glands of the scrotum, which secrete the semen.

testis (*tes'-tis*). A testicle.

testosterone (*tes-tos'-te-rōn*). Endocrine secretion of the testis. Promotes growth and secondary sexual development.

tetanus (*tet'-a-nus*). Lock-jaw. Disease caused by *clostridium tetani* characterized by rigidity and spasm of the muscles. The causative organism is anaerobic and thrives in wounds contaminated by soil or road dust containing the spores. A powerful toxin is produced by the clostridium which reaches the spinal cord by retrograde spread up the motor nerves, and is responsible for the clinical features.

tetany (*tet'-an-i*). A condition marked by spasms of the extremities, particularly of hands and feet (carpopedal spasm) due to faulty calcium metabolism. It may be due to dysfunction of the parathyroid glands, alkalosis, rickets.

tetrachloroethylene (*te'-tra-klo-rō-e'-thi-lēn*). Anthelmintic effective against hookworm.

tetracyclines. Group of chemically related antibiotics which include Aureomycin (chlortetracycline), Terramycin (oxytetracycline) and Achromycin (tetracycline hydrochloride).

tetraethylthiuram disulphide (*te'-tra-e-thil-thi-ū-ram di'-sul-fĭd*). Substance used for the treatment of alcoholic addiction by inducing aversion to alcohol.

tetralogy of Fallot (*te'-tra'-lo-ji*). A congenital heart disease. The aorta is displaced to the right so that it receives blood from the right ventricle, which is hypertrophied, as well as from the left ventricle. The interventricular septum is patent and there is narrowing of the pulmonary artery.

tetraplegia (*te-tra-plē'-ji-a*). Paralysis of all four limbs. Syn. quadriplegia.

thalami (*thal-a-mi*). (Sing. thalamus.) Two areas of grey matter at the base of the brain; concerned with the appreciation of crude sensations.

thalassaemia (*tha-la-sē-mi-a*). Anaemia found in the Mediterranean area. The red cells contain some abnormal haemoglobin of the type usually found in the fetus. It is detected by the alkali resistance test.

theca (*thē'-ka*). A sheath. Examples are the meninges of the spinal cord, and the synovial sheaths of the flexor tendons of the fingers.

theine (*thē'-in*). The alkaloid of tea, same as caffeine.

thenar (*thē'-nar*). Relating to the palm of the hand at the base of the thumb.

Theobroma (*thē-o-brō'-ma*). A genus of trees. The seeds of *T. cacao* furnish cocoa and cocoa butter.

theobromine (*thē-ō-brō'-min*). Drug with similar action to caffeine but with less effect on the central nervous system and greater effect on the heart and kidneys. Used chiefly as a diuretic.

theophylline (*thē-ō-fi'-lin*). A diuretic. Its derivative, aminophylline, is often administered.

theory (*thē-o-ri*). (1) General principles of a subject. (2) A supposition.

therapeutics (*ther-a-pū'-tiks*). The branch of medicine which deals with treatment.

therm (*therm*). A unit of heat. The amount of heat required to raise one gram of water through one degree centigrade.

thermolabile (*ther-mō-lā-bil*). Substance which undergoes change with temperature.

thermometer (*ther-mom'-e-ter*). An instrument used to record variations of temperature. *Clinical thermometer*, a small thermometer used for taking the temperature of the body. It is graduated from 95° F to 110° F. It is made so that the mercury does not fall when the thermometer is taken from the patient. After the temperature has been recorded the mercury is shaken down. *See* ZERO, TEMPERATURE, and p. 20.

thermophilic (*ther-mō-fi-lik*). Applied to organism which flourishes at high temperatures.

thermostat (*ther'-mō-stat*). Apparatus which is made to regulate heat automatically.

thermotherapy (*ther-mō-the'-ra-pi*). Treatment by applying heat.

thesis (*thē-sis*). The essay of a candidate for a degree.

thialbarbitone sodium (*thī-al-bar'-bi-tōn sō'-di-um*). Short-acting anaesthetic given intravenously.

thiamine (*thī-a-min*). Synthetic vitamin B₁. Also called aneurine. *See* VITAMINS.

Thiersch (*tersh*). Type of skin graft in which the epidermis and upper part of the dermis is employed. *See* GRAFT.

thigh (*thī*). The portion of the lower limb above the knee.

Thiomerin Sodium (*thī-ō-me′-rin sŏ′-di-um*). Mercaptomerin sodium. Mercurial diuretic. Unlike mersalyl can be given by subcutaneous injection.

thiomersal (*thī-ō-mer-sal*). A preparation of mercury which is antiseptic. Thiomersal ointment is used to treat fungus infections of the skin.

thiopentone sodium (*thī-ō-pen-tōn sŏ-di-um*). A barbiturate drug. Proprietary names, Intraval Sodium and Pentothal. Given intravenously to induce anaesthesia. Often used with curare to give good muscle relaxation.

Thomas's splint. (1) Knee splint for immobilizing a fractured femur or tibia and fibula. It consists of two sidepieces of metal with a crosspiece at foot, and an oblique ring for fixation in groin. Leg is kept

THOMAS'S KNEE SPLINT

THOMAS'S ARM SPLINT

in position by pieces of material slung between sidepieces and adjusted to the fracture. (2) Arm splint.

thoracic (*thor-as′-sik*). Pertaining to the thorax.

thoracic duct. The largest lymphatic vessel. It receives the fat absorbed from the intestine and the lymph from the greater part of the body. It ascends from the abdomen through the thorax to the left side of the neck, where it empties itself into the angle of union between the left internal jugular vein and the subclavian vein.

thoracocentesis (*tho′-ra-kō-sen-tē′-sis*). Puncture of the thorax, *e.g.* aspiration of pleural effusion.

thoracolysis (*thor-a-kō-li′-sis*). The severing of adhesions between the two layers of the pleura.

thoracoplasty (*thor′-a-kō-plas′-ti*). Operation in which part of the chest wall is resected in order to collapse the lung.

thoracoscopy (*tho-ra-kos′-ko-pi*). The pleural cavity is inspected by an endoscope.

thoracotomy (*tho-ra-ko′-to-mi*). Operation of opening the thorax.

thorax (*tho′-raks*). The chest; the cavity which holds the heart and lungs. (*See* p. 348.)

Thorium X (*thaw′-ri-um eks*). Radioactive isotope, *q.v.*, of radium (224 R) which is primarily an emitter of α particles which penetrate about 1 mm. in tissues.

THORAX

threadworm (*thred'-werm*). Oxyuris vermicularis, *q.v.* Small parasitic worm in the rectum; common in children.

threonine (*thrē-ō-nin*). An amino-acid essential for protein metabolism.

threshold (*thresh'-hōld*). (1) The smallest stimulus which can yet produce a reaction. (2) The lowest level of concentration of a substance, such as sugar, in the blood. Above the level it is excreted in urine and this is called the renal threshold.

thrill (*thril*). A vibratory impulse perceived by palpation.

thrombectomy (*throm-bek'-to-mi*). Removal of a blood clot.

thrombin (*throm'-bin*). Enzyme necessary for the clotting of shed blood. It causes fibrinogen to become fibrin.

thromboangiitis (*throm-bō-an-ji-i'-tis*). Inflamed blood vessel with formation of a blood clot. *T. Obliterans.* Inflammatory, obliterative disease of the blood vessels, especially in the limbs.

thrombo-arteritis (*throm-bō-ar-ter-i'-tis*). Arteritis with thrombosis.

thrombocytes (*throm'-bō-sīts*). Blood platelets.

thrombocytopenia (*throm-bō-sī-tō-pē-ni-ah*). Deficiency of platelets in the blood.

thromboendarterectomy (*throm-bō-en-dar-te-rek'-to-mi*). Operation to remove a clot from a blood vessel.

thrombokinase (*throm-bō-ki'-nāz*). The active principle of a substance liberated when the blood platelets are disintegrated. It is necessary for the clotting of blood.

thrombolytic (*throm-bō-li-tik*). Causing a clot to disintegrate.

thrombophlebitis (*throm-bō-fle-bi'-tis*). Inflammation of a vein with thrombosis.

thromboplastin (*throm-bō-plas-tin*). Syn. thrombokinase.

thrombosis (*throm-bō'-sis*). Coagulation of blood in the vessels. The clot thus formed is termed a *thrombus*.

thrombus (*throm'-bus*). (Plu. **thrombi**.) A clot of blood found in the heart or in a blood vessel.

thrush (*thru'-sh*). Growth of white patches of fungus (*oidium albicans*) in the mouth.

thymectomy (*thī-mek'-to-mi*). Operation to remove the thymus gland. Sometimes performed for myasthenia gravis.

thymol (*thī'-mol*). An antiseptic often used for mouthwashes and gargles.

thymoma (*thi-mō-ma*). Malignant neoplasm of the thymus.

thymus (*thī'-mus*). A gland at the root of the neck. It is largest in children and then gradually atrophies. The function of the thymus is not clear. It appears to be concerned with the immunological mechanisms of the body. It has been suggested that it acts as a 'priming station' for lymphocytes where they are selected for release into the general circulation. It is not yet possible to be certain of its function. The gland, which is situated in the anterior mediastinum, reaches its maximum size at puberty and thereafter atrophies slowly.

thyroglossal cyst (*thī'-rō-glos-al*). A type of dermoid cyst which appears in the midline of neck between hyoid bone and sternum.

thyroid cartilage (*thī'-royd*). The largest cartilage of the larynx. It forms an angle in front, more prominent in the male.

thyroid crisis. Acute severe thyrotoxicosis which may follow subtotal thyroidectomy in the absence of preoperative antithyroid treatment.

thyroid extract (*thī'-royd eks'-trakt*). This is prepared from the glands of sheep, oxen or pigs. The active principle is thyroxine. Used in thyroid deficiency.

thyroidectomy (*thī-roy-dek'-to-mi*). Operative removal of the thyroid gland.

thyroid gland (*thī-'royd gland*). A bi-lobed ductless gland lying in front of the trachea. Its secretion, thyroxine, controls metabolism, growth and development. Congenital lack causes cretinism. Under-secretion in later life causes myxoedema. Excessive secretion causes thyrotoxicosis.

THYROID GLAND

thyroidism (*thī'-royd-izm*). The symptoms caused by too rapid an absorption into the system of the secretion of the thyroid gland or by the administration by mouth of too large doses of thyroid extract. *Symptoms:* rapid pulse, sweating, diarrhoea, weight loss in spite of increased appetite, prominence of the eyeballs, fine tremor of the fingers and anxiety.

thyrotoxicosis (*thī-rō-tok-si-kō'-sis*). A condition produced by over-activity of the thyroid gland, *See* THYROIDISM.

thyrotrophic (*thī-rō-trō-fik*). Stimulating the thyroid. *T. hormone* is produced by the pituitary.

thyroxine (*thī-roks'-in*). The active principle of the secretion of the thyroid gland. A substance rich in iodine.

tibia (*tib'-i-a*). The shin bone; the larger bone of the leg below the knee, *See* SKELETON.

tic. Spasmodic twitching of muscles; usually of face and neck.

tic douloureux (*tik-doo-loo-rer*). Trigeminal neuralgia, *q.v.*

tick (*tik*). A blood-sucking parasite. *T. fever.* (1) Relapsing fever. (2) Rocky Mountain fever, a rickettsial fever.

tidal air (*tī-dal ā-r*). That which is inspired and expired during normal breathing.

tincture (*tink-tūr*). An alcoholic solution of a drug.

tinea (*tin'-e-a*). Disease of the skin due to a vegetable parasite. *See* RINGWORM.

tinnitus aurium (*tin-ni'-tus aw'-re-um*). A ringing in the ears.

tissue (*tish'-ū*). The arrangement of cells constituting the structure of an organ.

tissue culture. Method by which cells and tissues are grown under artificial conditions after their removal from the parent organism.

titration (*ti-trā'-shon*). Quantitative analysis by volume by means of standard solutions.

titre (*tē'-ter*). A standard of purity or strength.

T.N.T. Abbreviation for Trinitrotoluene (*q.v.*).

tobacco amblyopia (*to-bak'-ō am-blē-ō'-pia*). Dimness of vision from excessive smoking.

tobacco heart. Heart condition from too much smoking.

tocography (*to-ko'-gra-fi*). Method of recording alterations in the intra-uterine pressure.

tocopheryl (*to-ko'-fe-ril*). Vitamin E. Its precise function is unknown but it is widely used as an antioxidant in medical preparations.

tolazoline (*to-la-zo'-lēn*). Proprietary name, Priscol. Dilates the peripheral blood-vessels and increases the flow of blood in the peripheries. Used in Raynaud's disease and arteriosclerotic conditions, etc.

tolbutamide (*tol-bū'-ta-mīd*). Not a sulphonamide derivative but resembles carbutamide in its hypoglycaemic effect. It can be given orally and reduces the fasting blood sugar level but does not alter glucose tolerance. Should not be given to patients with ketosis.

tolerance (*tol'-er-ans*). Capacity to take a certain drug in unusually large dosage. Sugar tolerance test for diabetic patients ascertains the degree of metabolism of sugar as shown by the blood-sugar curve and the amount of sugar in the urine.

tomography (*tom-og'-raf-i*). A process of radiography which focuses an organ or plane, eliminating confusing shadows.

tone (*tōn*). (1) State of tension as found in muscles. (2) Quality of sound.

tongue (*tung*). The muscular organ which lies in the floor of the mouth, and whose chief functions are to assist in the mastication and tasting of food and in vocalization.

tongue tie (*tung'-ti*). When a fold of mucous membrane attaches the under surface of tongue to floor of mouth. It is very rare.

tonic (*to'-nik*). (1) A medicine which braces up the general health chiefly by increasing the appetite. (2) Term applied to continuous spasms, in opposition to clonic.

TONGUE

tonometer (*to-no'-me-ter*). Instrument for measuring tension such as that used to measure intra-ocular tension.

tonsillectomy (*ton-sil-ek'-to-mi*). The operation for total removal of the tonsils.

tonsillitis (*ton-sil-ī'-tis*). Inflammation of tonsils.

tonsillotome (*ton-sil'-o-tōm*). An instrument for cutting off a tonsil. (*See illustration, p. 453*.)

tonsils (*ton'-sils*). Two oval bodies of lymphoid tissue on either side of the throat at the opening of the pharynx.

toothed (*tootht*). Dentate, Possessing teeth.

topectomy (*to-pek-to-mi*). Operation to remove a convoluted portion of cerebral cortex.

tophus (*tō-fus*). (1) A gritty concretion due to gout, found most commonly on the edge of the auricle of the ear or in the joints. (2) A salivary calculus.

topical (*top'-ik-al*). Pertaining to a particular locality. Local.

topography (*to-po'-gra-fi*). A study of the various areas of the body.

torpor (*tor'-per*). Lethargy.

torsion (*tor'-shon*). Twisting.

torso (*tor'-sō*). The trunk.

torticollis (*tor-tē-kol'-lis*). Wry neck. The head is flexed and drawn to one side, due to damage to one of the sternomastoid muscles at birth.

tourniquet (*tor'-nē-kā*). An instrument used to exert pressure on an artery and so arrest bleeding.

SCREW TOURNIQUET

TOURNIQUET

tow (*tō*). Flax fibres, used to pad splints, etc.

toxaemia (*tok-sē'-mi-a*). Circulation of toxins in the blood. *Toxaemia of pregnancy.* The chief signs and symptoms are — oedema, rise in blood pressure, albuminuria, headache and vomiting. If not treated, eclampsia may result.

toxic (*tok'-sik*). Poisonous.

toxicology (*toks-i-kol'-o-ji*). Science of poisons.

toxicosis (*tok-si-kō'-sis*). Any disease due to poisoning.

toxin (*tok'-sin*). A poison, usually of bacterial origin, *i.e.* manufactured by the germs themselves.

toxoid (*tok'-soyd*). A non-poisonous modification of a toxin. Sometimes used to immunize against disease. *See* SCHICK TEST.

toxoid-antitoxin (*tok'-soyd-an-ti-tok'-sin*). A mixture of toxoid and its antitoxin.

toxoplasmosis (*tok-sō-plas-mō'-sis*). Infection caused by a parasite, the Toxoplasma, which can infect man as well as animals. If the foetus or young infant is infected encephalitis may occur. Other results of infection include nephritis, pneumonia, rashes and lymphadenopathy.

trabecula (*tra-bek'-ū-la*). A septum extending into an organ from its capsule or wall.

trace elements (*trās e'-le-menz*). Mineral substances whose presence in minute amounts in the diet is necessary for the maintenance of health, *e.g.* cobalt, copper, manganese, etc.

tracer (*trā-ser*). Radioactive isotope or substance containing a radioactive isotope which enables the substance to be traced in metabolic systems.

trachea (*tra'-kē-a*). The windpipe; the air passage from the larynx to the bronchi. *See* BRONCHI.

tracheitis (*tra-kē-i'-tis*). Inflammation of the trachea.

trachelorrhaphy (*trak-e-lor'-a-fi*). The operation of suturing a torn cervix uteri.

tracheobronchitis (*tra-ki-ō-bron-ki'-tis*). Inflammation of trachea and bronchi.

tracheostomy (*tra-kē-os'-to-mi*). The operation of making an opening into the windpipe, and inserting a tube. This is performed in cases such as laryngeal diphtheria. where the membrane is blocking the larynx, or scalded throat, where the swelling is closing the larynx.

tracheotomy (*tra-ki-o'-to-mi*). Surgical opening of the trachea.

trachoma (*trak-ō'-ma*). A contagious disease of the conjunctiva in which eyelids become red, rough and granular and the cornea becomes opaque.

traction (*trak'-shon*). The act of pulling or dragging. *Skeletal T.* Traction on a long bone to keep it in position after a fracture and to prevent muscle spasm.

tragacanth (*trag'-ak-anth*). A gummy exudate. It is used as a demulcent and to suspend insoluble bodies, *e.g.* resins.

tragus (*trā'-gus*). The small eminence just inside the ear.

trait (*trā*). A special characteristic of the individual.

trance (*trahn'-s*). State of unnatural sleep; catalepsy.

tranquillizer (*tran'-qwil-lī-zer*). Drug with sedative and tranquilizing action, such as chlorpromazine. Used to relieve anxiety, tension and agitation in psychotherapy. Whilst the patient is taking this drug, the action of a hypnotic or analgesic is made more powerful.

TRACHEOSTOMY TUBES
1. Bassett's cuffed tube (plastic).
2. Negus' valved tube (silver).
3. Parker's T. tube: *a.* outer; *b.* end of inner; *c.* catch to keep inner in position.

trans. Prefix meaning across, through.

transaminase (*tran-sa'-mi'-nāz*). Enzyme which transfers amino (—NH₂) groups from one substance to another.

Enzymes of this type are liberated into the bloodstream from damaged cells, particularly muscle cells, and the estimation of the serum transaminases (glutamic-oxaloacetic transaminase, or G.O.T., and glutamic-pyruvic transaminase or G.P.T.) is sometimes helpful in the diagnosis of conditions in which there is muscle damage, *e.g.* myocardial infarction, dermatomyositis, etc.

transference (*trans'-fe-renz*). A psychoanalytical term. The patient transfers his own emotions on to the analyst, *e.g.* he may develop an intense love or hatred of him. Also used if the patient transfers his own emotions on to someone else as when he blames someone else for what he has done himself.

transfusion (*trans-fū'-zhon*). *See* BLOOD TRANSFUSION.

transillumination (*tranz-il-ū-min-ā'-shon*). The method whereby suppuration in the maxillary or frontal sinus is detected. The patient is placed in a completely darkened room, and a bright light placed in the mouth. The affected side is not so highly illuminated as the sound side.

transmigration (*tranz'-mī-grā'-shon*). The passage of cells through a membrane.

transperitoneal (*tranz-pe-rit-o-ne'-al*). Through the peritoneum.

transplantation (*tranz-plan-tā'-shon*). Operation to re-move a portion of tissue from one part of the body to another.

transposition of vessels. Defect of development in which the pulmonary artery arises from the left ventricle and the aorta from the right ventricle.

transudation (*tran-sū-dā'-shon*). Oozing of fluid through a membrane or from a tissue.

transurethral (*tranz-ū-rēth'-ral*). Via the urethra.

transverse (*trans'-vers*). Across. A transverse incision is from side to side. T. process. Lateral projection of the neural arch of a vertebra with which the head of a rib articulates.

transvestism (*trans'-ves-tizm*). Psychiatric condition in which there exists an anomaly of instinct. The patient wears clothes characteristic of the opposite sex. Transvestites may identify themselves completely with the opposite sex and develop delusional convictions of this kind.

trapezium (*tra-pē'-zi-um*). First bone in second row of carpal bones.

trapezius (*tra-pē'-zi-us*). A large muscle, running from the nape of the neck and the upper part of the spine, to the clavicle and scapula.

trapezoid (*tra-pē'-zoid*). Second bone in second row of carpal bones.

trauma (*traw'-ma*). A wound or injury. Thus *traumatic*

gangrene is gangrene arising from an injury.

treatment (*trēt'-ment*). A way of curing a disease. *Conservative T.* Treatment by rest and drugs rather than by surgery. In dentistry, treatment of a tooth without extracting it. *Palliative T.* An attempt to alleviate pain, etc., but not a cure for the disease. *Prophylactic T.* A means of preventing the disease such as by immunization against it.

Trematoda (*trem-a-tō'-da*). Parasites which infect man, causing bilharzia, *q.v.*

tremor (*trem'-or*). Involuntary trembling.

Trendelenburg's operation (*tren-del'-en-bergs o-per-ā'-shon*). Used to treat varicose veins. The long saphenous vein is ligated in the groin.

Trendelenburg position (*tren-del'-en-berg poz-i'-shon*). A position often adopted for patients undergoing gynaecological operations, in which the head is at a lower level than the pelvis, and the latter is lower than the knees.

TRENDELENBURG POSITION

Trendelenburg's sign (*sīn*). Used to diagnose congenital dislocation of hip, etc. If the abductor muscles are not working properly, when the patient stands only on the affected leg the pelvis tilts downwards on the opposite side.

trephine (*tre-fīn*). An instrument for removing a disc of bone. Elliott's T. for removing a minute disc from the eyeball to relieve glaucoma, *q.v.*

TREPHINE

ELLIOTT'S TREPHINE

trephining (*tre-fīn'-ing*). Removing a circular piece of tissue to gain access to an enclosed structure, *e.g.* trephining the bone of the skull.

Treponema pallidum (*trep-ō-nē'-ma pal'-i-dum*). The infecting agent of syphilis.

tretamine (*tre'-ta-mēn*). A cytotoxic drug used in Hodgkin's disease, lymphocytic anaemia, etc.

trial of labour. Attempt to achieve spontaneous delivery in case of disproportion.

triamcinolone (*trī-am-si-nō-lōn*). Synthetic glucocorticoid steroid drug. It does not cause sodium retention.

triamterene (*trī-am-te-rēn*). A diuretic acting on distal renal tubules. Causes increased excretion of sodium and chloride and lessens excretion of potassium.

triangular bandage (*trī-an'-gū-la*). Made by cutting a 36-inch square of linen diagonally across. It is very useful in emergencies and for minor casualties.

triceps (*trī'-seps*). Certain muscles with three heads, especially the one at the back of the arm which extends the elbow.

trichiasis (*tri-kī-a-sis*). Inversion of the eyelashes towards the eye.

trichiniasis (*tri-ki-nī-a-sis*), **trichinosis** (*tri-ki-nō-sis*). Infection with a parasitic worm named *Trichina*. Trichina spiralis is parasitic in pigs and sometimes in man.

trichloroacetic acid (*trī-klo-rō-a-sē'-tik a'-sid*). An astringent and caustic used to remove warts.

trichloroethylene (*trī-klo-rō-eth'-i-lēn*). Drug used to produce analgesia by inhalation.

Trichocephalus dispar (*trik-ō-kef'-a-lus*). The whipworm. A parasite of the human large intestine.

trichomonas vaginalis (*trik-ō-mōn-as' vag-ē-nā'-lis*). A protozoon, motile by means of flagellae. It is a common cause of non-venereal vaginitis.

trichonosis, trichopathy (*trik-on-ō'-sis, trik-op'-a-thi*). Any disease of the hair.

trichophytosis (*trī-kō-fī-tō'-sis*). Fungus infection of the hair.

trichuris (*tri-kū-ris*). Kind of whipworm.

tricuspid valve (*trī-kus'-pid*). Valve with three cusps, particularly the valve of the heart between the right atrium and right ventricle.

Tridione (*trī-dē-ōn*). Troxidone. Anti-convulsant used in petit mal.

trigeminal (*trī-jem'-in-al*). Triple.

trigeminal nerves (*trī-jem'-in-al*). Fifth pair of cranial nerves. They are motor and sensory and each has three branches supplying the skin and structures of the face, tongue and teeth.

trigeminal neuralgia (*trī-jem'-in-al nū-ral'-jia*). Pain in the face of unknown cause. The distribution is confined to branches of the trigeminal nerve. The pain is paroxysmal and precipitated by mild stimuli such as washing the face or eating. Syn. tic douloureux.

trigger finger (*trig'-ger fin'-ger*). A thickening of the tendon sheath at the metacarpophalangeal joint often of the first finger of the right hand. The finger can be bent but not straightened without help.

trigone (*trī'-gōn*). A triangle. *T. Vesicae*. Triangular space in the bladder, immediately behind the opening to the urethra.

Trilene (*trī'-lēn*). Official name, Trichloroaethylenum. An analgesic gas, used in midwifery.

trimester (*tri-mes'-ter*). A three-month period.

trinitrin (*trī'-nī'-trin*). A name for nitro-glycerin, given in angina pectoris; it reduces blood pressure.

trinitrotoluene (*trī-nī-tro-tol'-ū-ēn*). T.N.T. A high explosive; harmful to workers with it.

triplegia (*trī-plē-ji-a*). Paralysis of three limbs.

triplets (*trip'-letz*). Three children resulting from a single pregnancy. This occurs about once in 7,800 labours.

trismus (*tris'-mus*). Lockjaw. Occurs as a reflex in dental caries. Is also a symptom of tetanus.

trisomy (*tri-so-mi*). Division of chromosome 21 into three as in mongolism.

trocar (*trō'-kar*). The perforating instrument used with

a cannula to draw off fluids from the body.

TROCAR AND CANNULA USED FOR PARACENTESIS ABDOMINIS

trochanter (*tro-kan'-ter*). Two processes at the juncture of the neck and shaft of femur.

trochlear (*trok'-lē-ar*). (1) Relating to a pulley. (2) Relating to the trochlear nerve.

trochlear nerves (*trok'-lē-ar*). The fourth pair of cranial nerves. Motor nerves to the eyes.

trophic (*trŏf'-ik*). Relating to nutrition. Trophic ulcers occur where nutrition is poor, particularly if there is paralysis.

trophoblast (*trŏ'-fŏ-blarst*). The outer ectodermal layer of the embedding ovum.

Trousseau's sign (*troo'-sōs sīn*). A spasm of the muscles, occurring in tetany, if pressure is applied over large arteries or nerves.

troxidone (*trok'-si-dōn*). An anticonvulsant drug given in petit mal. Proprietary name, Tridione.

trunk. The torso.

truss (*trus*). An apparatus for retaining a hernia in place.

Trypanosoma (*trip'-an-o-sō-ma*). A genus of microscopic parasites which cause sleeping sickness and other diseases.

trypanosomiasis (*trip'-an-ō-so-mī'-a-sis*). Infection with trypanosomes.

trypsin (*trip'-sin*). The digestive ferment of the pancreatic juice; acts on proteins.

trypsinogen (*trip-sin'-ō-jen*). A precursor of trypsin.

tryptophane (*trip'-to-fān*). *See* AMINO-ACIDS.

tsetse (*tet'-sē*). *See* SLEEPING SICKNESS.

tubal (*tū'-bal*). Relating to a tube, and especially to an oviduct. *T. gestation* or *T. pregnancy*, pregnancy in a Fallopian tube. *See* EXTRA-UTERINE GESTATION.

Tubegauz (*tūb'-gawz*). Proprietary bandage of fine tubular cotton gauze made in many sizes from finger to body width. It is cool and light and does not ruck up.

tubercle (*tū'-ber-kl*). (1) A small eminence. (2) The small greyish nodule which is the specific lesion of the tubercle bacillus.

tuberculide (*tū-ber'-kū-līd*). Any skin rash due to tuberculous infection.

tuberculin (*tū-ber'-kū-lin*). A preparation from cultures of the tubercle bacillus used in the diagnosis of tuberculosis. Many different tuberculins have been prepared in many different ways, but few are in common use. Old tuberculin is used for the intradermal Mantoux test,

and for tuberculin patch tests. Tuberculin P.P.D. is also used for intradermal test. B.C.G. vaccine is used for prophylaxis as an immunizing agent.

tuberculoma (*tū-ber-kū-lō'-ma*). Walled-off region of caseating tuberculosis.

tuberculosis (*tū-ber-kū-lō'-sis*). Infection with the Mycobacterium tuberculosis or tubercle bacillus. The human and bovine types attack man. Most infections enter by the respiratory tract and attack the lungs. Bovine bacilli, usually from infected milk, enter through the gastro-intestinal tract, causing lesions in the tonsils, glands of neck, lining of the intestinal tract and mesenteric glands. The tubercle bacillus acts slowly and a tiny nodule or tubercle forms in the affected area, which eventually calcifies. In most people, with good defences, no illness results from the primary infection and it probably serves to protect the patient against further attack. The person is termed *tuberculin positive* and this is ascertained by the Mantoux test. B.C.G. vaccination immunizes against tuberculosis by making a *tuberculin negative* person tuberculin positive. In a person who has contracted tuberculosis, the treatment is rest, good food and drug therapy, and the disease is curable, if diagnosed early, usually by X-ray.

tuberculous (*tū-ber'-kū-lus*). Connected with tuberculosis.

tuberose sclerosis (*tū'-be-rōs skle-rō'-sis*). See EPILOIA.

tuberosity (*tu-ber-os'-i-ti*). Bony eminence.

tubocurarine (*tū-bō-ku-rah'-rēn*). Drug paralysing striped muscle by blocking the nerve impulse to it. Used to give muscular relaxation during surgery and to control muscle spasms in tetany.

tubo-ovarian (*tū'-bo-ō-vā'-ri-an*). Connected with both the Fallopian tube and the ovary (abscess, cyst).

tubule (*tū-būl*). Small tube.

tularaemia (*tu-lar-ē'-mē-a*). A disease transmitted to man from rabbits by a blood-sucking insect infected with *B. tularense*.

Tulle Gras dressing (*tool'-gra dre'-sing*). Paraffin gauze dressing. Gauze impregnated with yellow soft paraffin, containing balsam of Peru. Used for burns and wounds.

tumefaction (*tū-me-fak-shon*). Becoming swollen.

tumour (*tū'-mur*). A swelling; an abnormal enlargement. Tumours may be *simple* or *malignant*; in the first case, they are not dangerous in themselves; in the second case, they are cancerous and produce secondary deposits in distant organs. Also they may be *solid* or *cystic*.

tunica (*tū'-nik-a*) A term applied to several membranes,

e.g. T. Vaginalis, the serous coat of the testicle.

tuning fork (*tū'-ning fork*). An instrument used for testing hearing. Each tuning fork bears a figure giving number of vibrations per second when it is struck, and a letter indicating the musical pitch (*see* RINNE'S TEST). It is also applied to the skin of other parts of the body to test the sense of vibration.

TUNING FORK

turbinate bones (*ter'-bin-āt bōnz*). Three thin convoluted bones situated on the lateral wall of each nasal fossa.

turbinectomy (*ter-bi-nek-to-mi*.) Operation to excise a turbinate bone.

turgid (*ter'-jid*). Swollen, distended.

Turner's syndrome (*ter-ners sin-drōm*). Ovarian agenesis. The patient is short in stature with webbed neck.

turpentine (*ter'-pen-tīn*). An oleoresin from pine. Styptic and antiseptic. Relieves flatulence and expels worms. *See* TEREBENE, ENEMA and FOMENTATIONS.

tussis (*tus'-sis*). A cough.

twilight sleep (*twī'-līt slēp*). See HYOSCINE.

twin (*twi'n*). One of two individuals born at one birth.

tylosis (*tī-lō'-sis*). Thickening of the skin of the soles and palms.

tympanites (*tim-pan-i'-tēz*). A distended state of the abdomen caused by gas in the intestines.

tympanitis (*tim-pa-nī-tis*). Otitis media.

tympanoplasty (*tim-pa-nō-plas-ti*). Operation to reconstruct sound-conducting mechanism in middle ear.

tympanum (*tim'-pan-um*). Also called tympanic cavity. A part of the middle ear, and comprises a cavity in the temporal bone deep to the tympanic membrane. *T. membrane.* The membrane separating the middle from the external ear, commonly called the eardrum.

typhlitis (*tif-lī'-tis*). Inflammation of the mucous surface of the caecum.

typhoid fever (*tī'-foyd fē-ver*). An acute infectious disease which flourishes where the standard of hygiene is poor. Caused by ingestion of the *Salmonella typhi* from contaminated food or water supplies. The germs reach the intestines and through the lymph channels produce a bacteraemia. After the first week the germs settle in the spleen, liver and intestines, especially the ileum. Here the lymph follicles known as **Peyer's** patches are attacked.

They become inflamed, raised, and eventually the tissue of the follicle sloughs off. It is at this stage that intestinal haemorrhage or perforation may occur. Incubation period for the disease is 12–14 days and the patient remains infectious until bacteriological tests are negative. The onset is gradual. For 4 or 5 days the temperature is of the step-ladder type. If untreated, the patient becomes very ill during the second week with high temperature and slow pulse and the stools are often pea-soup in character. Rose-coloured spots, in crops, appear on the abdomen, chest and between the shoulder blades. By the third week, if untreated, the patient is delirious. The treatment is chloramphenicol, usually with dramatic improvement. *See also* ENTERIC FEVER.

typhus fever (*tī'-fus fē-ver*). A highly infectious fever characterized by a petechial rash, high temperature and great prostration. It is caused by Rickettsia bodies from infected lice or rat fleas.

tyrosine (*tī'-rō-sin*). *See* AMINO-ACIDS.

tyrothricin (*tī-rō-thrī'-sin*). A drug consisting of gramicidin and tyrocidine. Used for skin infections and those of the mouth and throat. Should only be applied locally and should not be given parenterally.

ulcer (*ul'-ser*). Suppuration upon a surface. Ulcers can occur on skin or mucous membrane, and may be acute or chronic.

ulcerative (*ul'-se-ra-tiv*). Pertaining to ulceration. *U. Colitis.* A disease with inflammation and ulceration of the colon. There is diarrhoea, and mucus and blood are passed in the stools. The patient is anaemic. The disease may be mild or severe and no pathogenic organisms can be found to cause it, though emotional stress seems to precipitate it.

ulna (*ul'-na*). The inner bone of the forearm. *See* SKELETON.

ulnar. The name of an artery, a vein and a nerve running beside the ulna.

ultramicroscopic (*ul-tra-mī-krŏ-sko'-pik*). Too small to be seen with a microscope.

ultrasonic (*ul-tru-so'-nik*). Of too high a frequency to be heard by the human ear.

ultra-violet rays Beyond the visible (seven colour) spectrum into which white light is resolved by a prism, there are non-visible rays at each end, both below the red rays and above the violet rays.

umbilical cord (*um-bil-ī'-kal kord*). The funis; the cord connecting the fetus with the placenta.

umbilicated (*um-bil'-ik-ā'-ted*). Having a navel-like depression, *e.g.* the papules in smallpox.

umbilicus (*um-bi-lī'-kus*). Region of attachment of the placenta. A small depressed scar on the anterior abdominal wall.

unciform (*un'-si-form*). The hook-shaped bone of the wrist.

uncinariasis (*un'-sin-a-rī'-a-sis*). Infection with hookworm.

unconsciousness (*un-kon'-shus-nes*). A state of being insensible as when anaesthetized.

undine (*un'-dēn*). A thin glass flask with two spouts. Used for irrigation of eye.

UNDINE

undulant (*un'-dū-lant*). Wavelike. *U. Fever, Malta Fever.* A specific febrile disease. It is transmitted through cow's or goat's milk and runs a prolonged course.

unguentum (*un-goo-en'-tum*). An ointment; abbreviation, *ung.*

unguis (*ung'-gwis*). A fingernail.

unicellular (*ū-ni-sel'-lū-la*). With one cell.

unilateral (*ū-ni-la'-te-ral*). Found only on one side.

uniocular (*ū-ni-ok'-ū-la*). Relating to one eye.

union (*ū'-nē-on*). Healing. The joining up of a bone after a fracture.

uniovular (*ū-ni-ov'-ū-la*). With one ovum. Identical twins come from the same ovum.

uniparous (*ū-nip'-a-rus*). Having borne only one child.

unit (*ū'-nit*). An individual thing or group forming a complete whole. A standard of measurement.

Unna's paste (*un'-az pāst*). Useful treatment for ulcers of leg. It consists of zinc oxide, gelatin, glycerin and water. It is liquefied in a pot of hot water, and painted over a layer of gauze wrapped round the limb; if necessary a second coat may be applied and then the limb is surrounded by a thin bandage soaked in the mixture. When dry, it gives a thin plaster-like covering which keeps the part at rest.

urachus (*ū'-rā-kus*). A fibrous cord in the foetus from the bladder to the umbilicus. It becomes the median umbilical ligament.

uraemia (*ū-rē'-m-ia*). Accumulation of unknown toxic substances in the blood together with an increase in the blood urea. It is frequently the termination of nephritis and other diseases of the kidney. It may be due to a greatly diminished fluid intake.

uraemic fit (*ū-rēm'-ik*). Bears some resemblance to an epileptic seizure, but the breath has an odour of urine.

uraniscorrhaphy (*ū-ra-nis-ko'-ra-fi*). Suture of a cleft palate.

uranium (*ū-rān'-ium*). A heavy white metallic element found in pitch-blende. Radium is extracted from it.

urate (*ū-rāt*). Salt of uric acid.

urea (*ū-rē-a*). One of the end-products of protein metabolism; the chief solid constituent of urine. It is a diuretic.

urea concentration test (*ū'-rē-a kon-sen-trā'-shon test*). The normal amount of urea in urine is 2 per cent. If a definite quantity of urea, 15 grams in 100 ml. water, be given fasting—the amount of urea eliminated by the kidneys can be estimated by specimens taken 1, 2, and 3 hours after. The proper excretion of urea shows an adequately functioning kidney. The percentage should rise to 3 or 4. This test is used to estimate renal efficiency.

uresis (*ū-rē-sis*). Urination.

ureter (*ū-rē'-ter*). The canal between the kidney and the bladder, down which the urine passes. *See illustration*, p. 206.

ureteral (*ū-rē'-ter-al*). Pertaining to the ureter.

ureterectomy (*ū-rē-te-rek'-to-mi*). Excision of a ureter.

ureteric (ū-rē-te'-rik). Pertaining to a ureter.

ureteritis (ū-rē-te-rī-tis). Inflammation of a ureter.

ureterocele (ū-rē-te-rō-sēl). The result of congenital atresia of a ureteric orifice which causes a cystic enlargement of the portion of the ureter situated in the bladder wall.

ureterolith (ū-rē'-te-rō-lith'). Stone in a ureter.

ureterolithotomy (u-rē-te-rō-li-tho-to-mi). Operation for the removal of a stone impacted in the ureter.

ureterosigmoidostomy (ū-rē'-te-rō-sig-moy-dos'-to-mi). Implantation of a ureter into the sigmoid colon.

ureterovaginal (ū-rē-te-rō-va-jī'-nal). Pertaining to a ureter and the vagina.

ureterovesical (ū-rē-te-rō-ve-sī'-kal). Pertaining to a ureter and the bladder.

urethane (ū-rē-thān). Cytotoxic drug used in treatment of some of the leukaemias. See ETHYL CARBAMATE.

urethra (ū-rē'-thra). The canal between the bladder and the exterior through which the urine is discharged.

urethral (ū-rē'-thral). Pertaining to the urethra.

urethritis (ū-rē-thrī'-tis). Inflammation of the urethra.

urethrocele (ū-rē'-thrō-sēl.) Urethral diverticulum. A small pouch in the wall of the urethra more common in women than in men; the origin is probably the result of a developmental defect.

urethrography (ū-rē-thro'-gra-fi). X-ray examination of the urethra by means of retrograde injection of a radio-opaque dye.

urethroplasty (ū-rē-thrō-plas'-ti). Plastic repair to the urethra.

urethroscope (ū-rē-thros-kōp). An instrument for viewing the interior of the urethra.

urethrotomy (ū-rē-throt'-o-mi). Incision of the urethra to remedy stricture; the instrument used being a urethrotome.

uric acid (ū'-rik as'-id). Lithic acid; its presence in urine is discovered by its resemblance in colour to cayenne pepper. Frequently present in gout. Liquor potassae dissolves this red deposit.

uricosuric (ū-ri-kō-sū-rik). Drug used in gout to promote excretion of uric acid in the urine.

urinalysis (ū-ri-nal'-i-sis). Analysis of urine.

urinary (ū'-rin-a-ri). Pertaining to the urine. *U. Organs.* These include the kidneys, ureters, bladder and urethra.

urination (ū-ri-nā'-shon). Micturition. The act of discharging urine.

urine (ū'-rin). The fluid secreted by the kidneys. The normal amount secreted in the twenty-four hours varies from 1 to 1½ litres in an adult,

300 to 400 ml in a child, 250 to 300 ml in an infant. The normal constituents are water salts, urea, acid bodies. *See* URINE TESTING in Appendix, p. 380.

uriniferous tubules (*ū-rin-if'-er-us*). Numerous minute tubules in the kidney which secrete urine.

urinometer (*ū-rin-om'-e-ter*). A small glass instrument with a graduated stem, used for measuring the specific gravity of urine.

urobilin (*ū-rō-bil'-in*). One of the pigments of the urine, derived from bile pigments.

urobilinogen (*ū-rō-bi'-li'-no-jen*). Derivative of bilirubin which is made in the intestine by the gut bacteria. Some of it is absorbed and, in circumstances in which there is impaired liver function, may be excreted in the urine.

urochrome (*ū-rō-krōm*). Pigment colouring urine.

urogenital (*ū-rō-je-ni-tal*). Relating to the urinary and genital organs.

urography (*ū-ro'-gra-fi*). X-ray of the urinary tract.

urokinase (*u-ro-kī-nāz*). Enzyme found in the urine. In disease states it can cause bleeding from the kidney.

urolith (*ū-rō-lith'*). A stone found in the urine.

urologist (*ū-ro'-lo-jist*). A specialist in urology, *q.v.*

urology (*ū-ro'-lo-ji*). The study of diseases of the urinary tract.

uroscopy (*ū-ros'-ko-pi*). Examination of the urine.

Uroselectan-B (*ū-rō-sel-ek'-tan*). Synonym, Iodoxyl. *See* PYELOGRAPHY.

urticaria (*er-ti-kā'-ri-a*). Nettle-rash; hives. Allergic reaction affecting the permeability of small blood vessels. Characterized by erythema and wheals.

uterine (*ū'-ter-īn*). Relating to the uterus.

uterogestation (*ū'-te-rō-jes-tā'-shon*). The period of pregnancy.

uterosalpingography (*ū-te-rō-sal-pin'-gō-gra-fi*). X-ray of the uterus and tubes.

uterovesical (*ū-te-rō-ve-sī-kal*). Relating to the uterus and the bladder.

uterus (*ū'-ter-us*). Womb. Muscular hollow pelvic organ. In the resting state it measures about 7·5 × 5 cm and is triangular in shape with a cervix about 2·5 cm which projects into the

Fallopian tubes

Fundus

Body

Ovary

cut edge of peritoneum

Cervix

Vagina (opened.)

THE UTERUS FROM BEHIND

vagina. It is connected bilaterally to the oviducts (Fallopian tubes). The uterus has a glandular epithelium lining it and the whole structure is under the control of sex hormones, in particular oestrogens and progesterone. *See* MENSTRUATION. The uterus is the normal site of implantation of the tropho-blast, *q.v.* During pregnancy the uterus grows out of the pelvis to occupy much of the abdominal cavity.

utricle (*ū'-trikl*). (1) The larger sac of membrane in the vesti-bule of the internal ear. (2) The prostatic vesicle.

uvea (*ū-vē-a*), uveal tract. The middle coat of the eyeball. The choroid, ciliary body and iris as a whole.

uveitis (*ū-vi-ī'-tis*). Inflamma-tion of the uvea.

uvula (*ū'-vū-la*). A small fleshy body hanging down at the back of the soft palate.

uvulectomy (*ū-vū-lek'-to-mi*). Excision of uvula.

uvulitis (*ū-vū-lī'-tis*). Inflam-mation of the uvula.

V

vaccination (*vak-sin-ā'-shon*). (1) Inoculation of cow-pox lymph into the arm as a pro-tection from smallpox. (2) Protective inoculation with any vaccine.

vaccine (*vak'-sēn*). An extract or suspension of attenuated or killed organisms. The antigenic properties of the organism are retained and the vaccine is used to im-munize the recipient.

vaccinia (*vak-sin'-ia*). Cow-pox. In man, it gives immu-nity to smallpox and is there-fore used in vaccination against that disease.

vacuole (*vak'-ū-ōl*). Specialized region within a cell surroun-ded by plasma membrane.

vacuum extractor (ventouse). An alternative method to for-ceps in delivering a child. A cap is fixed to the fetal head by creating a vacuum and traction is applied to a chain attached to the cap.

vagal (*vā'-gal*). Pertaining to the vagus nerve.

vagina (*va-jī'-na*). The passage leading from the cervix uteri to the vulva. The lower limit of this canal is the hymen.

vaginal (*va-jī'-nal*). Pertaining to the vagina.

vaginismus (*vaj-in-iz'-mus*). Spasmodic contraction of vagina whenever the vulva or vagina is touched.

vaginitis (*va-jin-ī'-tis*). Inflam-mation of the vagina.

vagotomy (*vā-go'-to-mi*). Sur-gical division of the vagus nerve sometimes performed on patients with peptic or duodenal ulcers.

vagus (*vā'-gus*). The pneumo-gastric nerve, *q.v.*

valgus (*val'-gus*). *See* TALIPES.

valine (*vā'-lēn*). One of the essential amino-acids.

valve (*va'-lv*). A fold across a channel allowing flow in one direction only.

valvotomy (*val-vo'-to-mi*). Incision into a valve, especially heart valve. The purpose of the operation is to widen the orifice of a stenosed valve.

valvulae conniventes (*val-vū-lē kon-i-ven-tāz*). Transverse folds of mucous membrane in the upper part of the small intestine.

valvulitis (*val-vū-lī'-tis*). Inflammation of a valve.

valvulotomy (*val-vū-lo'-to-mi*). *See* VALVOTOMY.

van den Bergh's test (*van' den bergs*). Performed to discover the presence of bile pigment in the blood. It also differentiates between the pigment retained in the blood from obstruction of the bile passages, and that due to haemolysis.

Vaquez's disease (*vak-kāz' di-sēz*). *See* POLYCYTHAEMIA.

varicella (*var-i-sel'-la*). Chicken-pox, *q.v.*

varices (*va'-ri-sēz*). Dilated, twisted veins. Sing., varix.

varicocele (*var'-ē-kō-sēl*). A varicose condition of the veins of the spermatic cord.

varicose ulcer. Ulceration of the lower legs due to re-duction in the blood supply resulting from increased venous pressure.

varicose veins (*var'-i-kōs vānz*). Dilated veins in which the valves have become incom-petent. As a result the blood flow may become reversed or static. Most common in the legs where the blood pools by gravitation. Other examples are piles, *q.v.*, and oesophageal varices, *q.v.*

varicotomy (*va-ri-ko-to-mi*). Excision of varicose vein.

variola (*va-ri'-ō-la*). *See* SMALL-POX. *V. minor*. Much less severe disease than that of smallpox which it resembles.

varioloid (*va-ri-ō'-loyd*). A mild form of smallpox, sometimes seen in persons who have been previously vaccinated.

varix (*vā'-riks*). An enlarged and tortuous vein.

varus (*vā'-rus*). *See* TALIPES.

vas. A vessel, or duct of the body; as *vas deferens*, the duct of the testis.

vascular (*vas'-kū-lar*). Possessing many blood-vessels.

vascular system. System of blood-vessels.

vasectomy (*va-sek'-to-mi*). Removal of a part of the vas deferens.

vasoconstriction (*vā'-zō-kon-strik'-shon*). Contraction of blood-vessels.

vasodilatation (*vā'-zō-di-la-tā'-shon*). Dilatation of blood-vessels.

vasomotor (*vā-zō-mō'-tor*). Concerned with constriction of blood vessels. *V. nerves*. Sympathetic nerves which control the tone of smooth muscle in the walls of blood vessels.

vasopressin (*vā-zō-pres'-in*). Drug containing the pressor and antidiuretic principles of the posterior lobe of the pituitary gland. Given to control polyuria in diabetes insipidus and also to relieve distension after abdominal operations. Proprietary name Pitressin.

vasospasm (*vă'-zo-spasm*). Spasm of the blood-vessels.

vasovagal syndrome (*vā-zō-vā'-gal sin'-drōm*). Slowing of the heart rate with a feeling of nausea and grave distress. The attack may last a few minutes or an hour. The cause is unknown.

Vater's ampulla (*va'-ters ampoo'-la*). Small dilation in the terminal portion of the common bile duct where it empties into the duodenum.

vector (*vek'-tor*). A carrier. One who conveys the infection to another person.

vegetations (*ve-je-tā'-shons*). Concretion of small ducts on the diseased valves of the heart which occur in endocarditis.

vegetative (*ve'-je-tā-tiv*). Having the power of growth.

vein (*vān*). A vessel carrying the blood to the heart.

vena cava (*vē-na kă'-va*). The superior vena cava and the inferior vena cava are two large veins which return blood from the head and body and empty it into the right atrium of the heart.

venepuncture (*ve-nē-punk'-tūr*). Inserting a needle into a vein.

venereal (*ve-nē'-re-al*). Relating to sexual intercourse. *V. Diseases*. Infectious diseases transmitted during sexual intercourse, *e.g.* gonorrhoea, syphilis.

venereology (*ve-nār-ē-ol'-o-ji*). The study of venereal disease.

venesection (*vē-nē-sek'-shon*). Blood-letting. A vein is opened and blood drained off from it. Frequently performed in the past for almost any ailment. There are very few present-day indications for venesection.

venography (*ve-no'-gra-fi*). X-ray examination of veins.

venous (*vē'-nus*). Relating to the veins.

ventilation (*ven-ti-lā'-shon*). (1) Supply of fresh air. (2) Process of breathing.

ventral (*ven'-tral*). Relating to the belly. *V. root*. Anterior root, motor root. The nerve root containing the motor fibres.

ventricles (*ven-'tri-kls*). The two lower chambers of the heart are known as the right and left ventricles. The cavities in the brain also are known as ventricles.

ventriculography (*ven-tri-kūlog'-raf-i*). X-ray examination of the ventricles of the brain. Air or a radio-opaque dye is introduced into the ventricles, enabling their size and position to be observed.

ventrofixation (*ven'-tro-fiksā-shon*). The operation to suture an abdominal viscus to the anterior abdominal wall.

ventrosuspension (*ven-trō-sus-pen'-shon*). Another operation having the same object as ventrofixation, but fixing the round ligaments instead of the uterus to the abdominal wall.

venule (*ve'-nūl*). Small vein.

veratrum viride (*ve-rah'-trum vi'-ri-dā*). Green hellebore. It lowers blood pressure and slows the heart rate. Sometimes used in hypertension and toxaemia of pregnancy. Proprietary name, Veratrone.

vermicide (*ver'-mi-sīd*). Substance able to kill worms in the intestine.

vermiform appendix (*ver'-mi-form*). See APPENDIX VERMIFORMIS.

vermifuge (*ver-mi-fūj*). Substance used to dispel worms.

verminous (*ver'-min-us*). Infested with animal parasites.

vernix caseosa (*ver'-niks kā-sē-ō'-sah*). The sebaceous material which covers the skin of the fetus.

verruca (*ver'-ū'-ka*). A wart.

version (*ver'-shon*). The operation of altering the presentation of the fetus in the uterus so as to facilitate its delivery. *Cephalic version* is turning the fetus, so that the head presents, while *podalic version* brings about a breech presentation. *Bipolar version*, version by acting upon both poles of the fetus.

vertebrae (*ver'-te-brē*). The thirty-three small bones which form the backbone, or spinal column. See SKELETON, p. 320.

vertex (*ver'-teks*). The crown of the head.

vertigo (*ver-tī'-gō*). Giddiness.

vesica (*ves'-i-ka*). The bladder.

vesical (*ve-sī'-kal*). Relating to the bladder.

vesicant (*vēs'-i-kant*). A blistering agent.

vesicle (*vēs'-i-kl*). A blister. Blisters of greater diameter than 5 mm are termed bullae.

vesicovaginal (*ve-sī-kō-va-jī-nal*). Relating to the bladder and the vagina.

vesicular mole (*ve-sik'-ū-lar*). See MOLE.

vesicular breathing (*ve-sik'-ū-lar brē-thing*). The normal sound of inspiration heard on auscultation.

vesiculitis (*ve-si-kū-lī-tis*). Inflammation of seminal vesicles.

vestibular neuronitis (*ves-ti-bū-la nū-rō-nī-tis*). Disorder affecting the vestibular nerve which is characterized by extreme vertigo while hearing is unaffected. May result from streptomycin toxicity.

vestibule (*ves'-ti-būl*). (1) A small cavity of the ear into which the cochlea opens. (2) The space between the labia minora.

vestigial (*ves-tī'-ji-al*). Rudimentary. Bearing a trace of something now vanished or degenerate.

viable (*vī'-ab-l*). Capable of living. An obstetrical term implying that an unborn child is sufficiently developed to survive its birth.

Vibrio (*vi-brē-ō*). A genus of micro-organisms shaped like a bacillus but curved. One causes cholera.

vicarious (*vi-kā'-ri-us*). When one organ performs the work of another. *V. menstruation.* Menstruation from a passage other than the uterus.

villi (*vil-lī*) (sing., villus). Fine soft processes of living cells. *Intestinal v.* in the small intestines each contain a central vessel or lacteal, surrounded by a plexus of capillaries. *Chorionic v.* Processes arising from the chorion, the outer membrane of the developing ovum. Specialization of a mass of villi ultimately forms the placenta.

villous (*vil'-us*). Having the nature of villi, thus a villous tumour of the bladder is a growth consisting of long slender processes of cells.

Vincent's angina (*vin'-sents anji'-na*). Infection of the mucous epithelium of the mouth by a symbiotic (*see* SYMBIOSIS) association of a spirochaete Borrelia vincenti and a fusiform Gram-negative bacterium, Fusobacterium planti-vincenti.

vinegar (*vin'-e-gah*). A weak

solution of acetic acid formed by fermentation of wine and other alcoholic liquids.

vinum (*vē'-num*). Wine.

viomycin (*vī-ō-mī'-sin*). An antibiotic drug used in tuberculosis if the patient is resistant to streptomycin, etc.

viraemia (*vī-rē-mi-a*). Viruses present in the blood stream.

virilism (*vi'-ri-lism*). The appearance of masculine characteristics in the female.

virology (*vī-ro'-lo-ji*). The study of viruses and the diseases caused by them.

virulent (*vir'-ū-lent*). Violent, malignant.

virus (*vī'-rus*). Infecting agent that will pass through the finest filter known, *e.g.* the cause of mumps, anterior poliomyelitis and other infectious diseases.

viscera (*vis'-se-ra*). Plural of viscus.

visceroptosis (*vis-e-rop-tō-sis*). Prolapse of the abdominal viscera.

viscid (*vis'-kid*), **viscous** (*vis'-kus*). Sticky, thick, adhesive.

Viscopaste (*vis'-kō-pāst*). A proprietary zinc paste bandage.

viscus (*vis'-kus*). An internal organ; for example the heart, lung, or stomach.

vision (*vi-zhon*). The act or faculty of seeing. *Binocular vision*, use of both eyes without seeing double. *Central vision, direct vision,* that performed through the centre of the retina. *Double vision, diplopia,* a failure to fuse the images thrown upon the two retinae at the same time: two images are therefore seen and objects appear double. May be due to defect in muscles of the eye or an error of refraction. It is also a symptom of some nervous diseases, *e.g.* encephalitis lethargica. *Peripheral vision, indirect vision,* that performed by the peripheral or circumferential portion of the retina. *Stereoscopic vision,* that which gives perception of distance and solidity.

visual (*vi'-zū-al*). Pertaining to vision. *V. field.* The total area which can be seen at the same time without turning the head.

vital (*vi'-tal*). Pertaining to life. *V. capacity.* The amount of air that can be breathed out after a complete inspiration. *V. statistics.* Statistics of births, marriages, deaths and diseases in a population.

vitallium (*vi-ta'-li-um*). An alloy used in bone surgery for nails, screws, plates, etc.

vitamins (*vi'-ta-mins*). Chemical substances present in food, necessary for health and development. Those at present known are:

A. Anti-infective, fat soluble; found in animal fat such as butter, cream, milk, fish oil and derived from carotin, the colouring matter of carrots and tomatoes. Lack of A causes a lowered resistance to infection, night blindness and opacity of the cornea.

B complex (has different parts). Water soluble, found in whole-meal cereals, yeast, Marmite, liver, lean meat. B_1, or thiamine, anti-neuritic; prevents polyneuritis and beriberi, *q.v.*, B_2, or riboflavin. Deficiency causes a syndrome which includes visual disturbances. B_6, or pyridoxine: no deficiency symptoms are known, but the drug has been used in irradiation and pregnancy sickness. B_{12}, or cyanocobalamin, the specific anti-anaemia principle of liver. Nicotinic acid is also a constituent of the B complex.

C. Anti-scorbutic; found in rose hips, black currants, oranges, tomatoes, raw vegetables. Lack of C causes scurvy.

D. Anti-rachitic; found in animal fats and fish oils. The action of ultra-violet rays on certain fats, known as sterols, produces vitamin D. It is necessary for the metabolism of calcium. Lack of vitamin D causes rickets.

E. Anti-sterility, found in wheat germ oil, an ingredient of whole wheat. Lack of E causes sterility and insecurity of pregnancy.

K. The 'Koagulation Vitamin'. Fat soluble. Occurs in the green part of plants, particularly alfalfa grass, spinach, kale, carrot tops, and vegetable oils. It may be formed by bacterial action from food in the lower part of the intestine and absorbed. Bile salts in the intestine are necessary for absorption. Lack of vitamin K causes a deficiency of prothrombin in the blood, which is necessary for the clotting of blood. Prescribed in cases of obstructive jaundice.

vitelline (*vi'-te-lēn*). Pertaining to the vitellus, or yolk.

vitiate (*vi-shē-āt*). To make a substance less efficient.

vitiligo (*vit-il-ī'-go*). Disorder of pigment cells in which patches of depigmented skin arise, often in a symmetrical distribution.

vitreous chamber of the eye (*vi'-trē-us chăm'-ber*). The posterior five-sixths of the eyeball, that part behind the lens. It is filled with a clear jelly-like substance called the *vitreous humour*.

vitriol (*vit'-rē-ol*). Any crystalline sulphate. *Blue Vitriol*, copper sulphate or blue stone. Sometimes applied to granulation tissue on the eyelids. *Oil of V.* Sulphuric acid.

vivisection (*viv-i-sek'-shon*). Scientific examination of a living animal.

vocal cords (*vō'-kal kor'dz*). Two folds of mucous membrane in the larynx attached behind to the arytenoid cartilages, and in front to the back of the thyroid cartilage. Voice is produced by variation in position of these cords when acted on by small muscles of the larynx, and at the same time forcing through them an expiratory blast of air.

volatile (*vol'-a-tīl*). That which evaporates quickly.

volition (*vo-lish'-on*). The act or power of willing.

Volkmann's paralysis (*volk-munz*), V. **contracture**. A muscular paralysis caused by applying splints too tightly so that the blood supply is impaired. Most commonly seen in the forearm after fractures about the elbow joint.

Volkmann's spoon (*volk-munz*). A sharp spoon used for scraping a septic cavity.

VOLKMANN'S SPOON

volsellum (*vol'-sel-um*). *See* VULSELLUM.

volt (*vōlt*). A unit of electrical potential.

voluntary (*vol'-un-ta-ri*). Free. Regulated by choice and desire.

volvulus (*vol'-vū'-lus*). A twisting of a piece of intestine on its mesenteric attachment. Acute intestinal obstruction is the result.

vomer (*vō'-mer*). a bone of the septum of the nose.

vomit (*vo'-mit*). To eject the contents of the stomach through the mouth. *Projectile*

V. Forcible ejection of gastric contents without warning.

vomiting of pregnancy. The vomiting to which about two-thirds of pregnant women are subject at some time or other during the period of gestation. Occurs usually about the second, third and fourth months, and is commonest in the morning. In most cases no ill results follow, but occasionally the vomiting becomes so frequent and severe that a grave condition is produced, called the *Intractable,* or *Pernicious Vomiting of Pregnancy,* or *Hyperemesis Gravidarum.* Vomiting is also a symptom of toxaemia of pregnancy. *See* TOXAEMIA.

von Gierke's disease (*von gerkes di-sēz*). Glycogen storage disease. Recessively inherited defect in the metabolism of glycogen so that it cannot be used. The tissues become stuffed with glycogen while hypoglycaemia occurs.

von Recklinghausen's disease (*von rek'-ling-how-zenz*). Characterized by multiple tumours along cutaneous nerves of trunk and scalp, with areas of pigmentation. *See also* OSTEITIS FIBROSA.

vulnerable (*vul'-ne-rubl*). Susceptible.

vulsellum (*vul-sel'-um*), (plu. vulsella). Catch forceps with toothed blades. *See* above.

vulva *vul'-va*). The external organs of generation of the female.

teeth – enlarged view

VULSELLUM

vulvectomy (*vul-vek'-to-mi*). Excision of vulva.

vulvitis (*vul-vī'-tis*). Inflammation of the vulva.

vulvovaginal (*vul-vō-va-jī'-nal*). Pertaining to the vulva and the vagina.

vulvovaginitis (*vul-vō-va-ji-nī'-tis*). Inflammation of both the vulva and the vagina.

W

Waldeyer's ring (*vul-dā'-yers ring*). Circle of adenoid tissue in the pharynx formed by the faucial, lingual and pharyngeal tonsils.

Wallerian degeneration (*va-lār-i-an dē-je-ne-rā'-shon*). Degeneration of a nerve after it has been cut or severed.

wart (*wawt*). Small horny tumour from the skin. The *common wart* is due to a virus infection. A *plantar wart* is found on the sole of the foot. *Venereal warts* are common warts on the genitalia and not to be confused with flat condylomata of secondary syphilis.

washing soda (*wo'-shing sō'-dah*). Sodium carbonate.

Wassermann reaction (*vas'-er-man*). A blood test which shows whether the individual from whom the blood is taken is or is not the subject of active syphilis. Sometimes the cerebrospinal fluid is taken instead of blood. *See* KAHN TEST.

water-beds. Rubber mattress filled with warm water and used to prevent pressure sores.

water-borne (*waw'-ter-bawn*). Spread by water, such as certain diseases, *e.g.* typhoid fever.

water-brash. Regurgitation of stomach acid into the oesophagus.

water-hammer pulse. *See* CORRIGAN'S PULSE.

Waterhouse Friderichsen syndrome (*waw-te-hows fri-de-rik'-sen sin-drōm*). Syndrome resulting from bilateral adrenal haemorrhage accompanying the purpura of acute septicaemia, usually meningococcal.

watt (*wot*). The amount of power developed by an electrical current of one ampere having an electromotive force of one volt.

wave length. The distance between two adjacent crests of any wave motion.

weal (*wēl*). A white or pinkish elevation on the skin, as in urticaria.

wean (*wēn*). To cease feeding a baby at the breast.

Weber syndrome. Hemianopia

caused by posterior cerebral aneurysm.

Weil's disease (*vīls*). Epidemic spirochaetal jaundice. Disease caused by a Leptospira characterized by fever, headache, and pains in the limbs. Many patients develop jaundice and a purpuric rash.

Weil-Felix reaction (*vīl-fē'-liks rē-ak'-shon*). An agglutination reaction for typhus.

Welch's bacillus (*wel'-shes ba-si'-lus*). Clostridium perfringens, a spore-forming organism found in gas gangrene.

wen. *See* SEBACEOUS CYST.

Wernicke's encephalopathy (*ver-ni-kers en-ke-fa-lo-pa-thi*). Syndrome occurring in association with alcoholic polyneuritis, characterized by vertigo, nystagmus, ataxia and stupor. Considered to be due to thiamine deficiency.

Wertheim's operation (*vār'-tīms*). A radical operation for uterine cancer, whereby the uterus, tubes, ovaries, broad ligaments, pelvic lymph glands and cellular tissue around ureters are removed *en masse*.

wet-pack. *See* PACK.

Wharton's duct (*wor'-tonz*). The duct of the submaxillary gland.

Wharton's jelly. A special tissue of the umbilical cord.

wheal (*wēl*). Syn. weal.

Wheelhouse's operation. External (perineal) urethrotomy for stricture of the urethra.

whey (*whā*). The liquid left after milk has been clotted with rennin.

Whipple's disease (*wi-pels di-sēz*). Intestinal lipodystrophy. Disease of unknown cause. There is progressive deposition of mucoprotein material in the wall of the small intestine.

whipworm (*wip'-werm*). See TRICHOCEPHALUS.

Whitehead's varnish (*wīt-heds vah'-nish*). A protective covering sometimes used after a surgical procedure. The varnish contains iodoform, benzoin, storax, balsam of tolu and ether.

white cell (*wīt sel*). See BLOOD.

white leg (*wīt leg*). See PHLEGMASIA ALBA DOLENS.

whites (*wītz*). A popular term for leucorrhoea.

Whitfield's ointment (*wit'-fēldz oynt'-ment*). Contains salicylic and benzoic acids. Used for athlete's foot and ringworm.

whitlow (*wit'-lō*). Inflammation near a finger-nail, with suppuration. See ONYCHIA.

whooping cough (*hoop'-ing kof*). Pertussis, *q.v.*

Widal reaction (*vē'-dal*). A blood test for typhoid fever. Not available until patient has been ill for about ten days.

Willebrand's disease (*wi-lē-brans di-sēz*). Inherited defect of blood vessels and clotting mechanism.

willpower (*wil'-pow-er*). A voluntary effort which directs our actions and can overcome some primary impulse such as fear.

Wilm's tumour (*wilms tū'-mer*). A congenital tumour of the kidney which is malignant.

Wilson's disease (*wil'-sons di-sēz*). A rare metabolic disorder (hepatolenticular degeneration) in which copper accumulates in the liver and certain nuclei of the brain.

windpipe (*wind'-pīp*). The trachea.

Winslow's foramen (*winz'-lōz for-ā-men*). An aperture between the stomach and liver formed by folds of peritoneum. It forms a communication between the greater and lesser peritoneal cavities.

wintergreen, oil of. See METHYL SALICYLATE.

wisdom teeth (*wiz'-dom tēth*). The posterior molars. They erupt last, usually when a person is about 21 years old.

withdrawal (*with-draw'-al*). In psychology meaning to 'shrink into oneself'. A normal method of adjustment in a frightening situation. *W. symptoms.* Symptoms which appear when a drug, to which a person has become addicted, is withheld from him.

witch-hazel (*wich'-hāz'-el*). See HAMAMELIS.

womb (*woom*). The uterus, *q.v.*

wood-wool. An absorbent wool used for sterilized sponges, ice poultices, etc.

Wood's glass. Glass which contains nickel oxide. It causes fluorescence of certain objects and is used to detect ringworm, q.v.

woolsorter's disease (*wool'-sorterz*). See ANTHRAX.

word salad (*werd sal'-ad*). A jumble of disconnected words heard when certain schizophrenic patients speak.

worms (*werms*). Invertebrate animal. See ASCARIS, TAENIA, TRICHURIS and TRICHOCEPHALUS DISPAR.

Woulfe's bottle (*woolfs bot'-tel*). Bottle used to make a gas pass through a liquid in order to wash it.

wound (*woond*). Injury.

wrist (*rist*). The joint between the hand and the forearm. The carpus.

writer's cramp (*rī'-terz kramp*). Spasm of the hand and forearm brought on by efforts to write. Largely due to defective posture when writing.

wry-neck (*rī'-nek*). See TORTICOLLIS.

X

X chromosome (*eks krō-mō-sōm*). The sex chromosome which is paired in the homogametic sex. Unlike the Y chromosome, q.v., it carries many major genes.

xanthelasma (*zan-the-las'-ma*). A condition in which yellow patches or nodules occur on the skin, especially in the eyelids.

xanthine (*zan'-thin*). A nitrogenous substance produced in the body. Sometimes found in the urine.

xanthochromia (*zan-thō-krō-mi-a*). The distinctive yellow colour of cerebrospinal fluid following a subarachnoid haemorrhage. It is due to haemolysis of the blood in the subarachnoid space.

xanthoderma (*zan-thō-der'-ma*). Yellowness of the skin.

xanthoma (*zan-thō'-mah*). The same as xanthelasma, q.v.

xenopsylla cheopis (*zen-op-si'-la chē-ō'-pis*). A rat flea which can transmit plague and typhus.

xenopus test (*zen-'ō-pus test*). Test for pregnancy. The mother's urine is injected into the lymph sac of a female toad. If the woman is pregnant, the toad will pass ova, in from 24–48 hours.

xeroderma (*ze-rō-der'-ma*). A dry state of the skin.

xerophthalmia (*ze-rof-thal-mi-a*). Ulceration of the cornea occurring in vitamin A deficiency.

xerosis (*zer-ō'-sis*). Abnormal dryness, e.g. of the conjunctiva or the skin.

xerostomia (*ze-ro-stō'-mi-a*). Dryness of the mouth.

xiphoid process (*zif'-oyd prō-ses*). A sword-shaped cartilage attached to the breastbone. Also called the ensiform cartilage.

X-rays (*eks'-rāz*). Part of the electro-magnetic spectrum.

These rays are used (1) diagnostically, as in showing injury to bone, or the condition of hollow organs after they have been rendered opaque, and (2) therapeutically: (a) less penetrating rays are used for superficial skin lesions, such as warts or rodent ulcers; (b) deep X-ray therapy is used generally under a high voltage for the cure of cancer. See RÖNTGEN RAYS.

Xylene (*zī-lēn*). Xylol. Used as a solvent and also in microscopy.

Xylocaine (*zi'-lō-kān*). Lignocaine, q.v.

Characterized by fever, prostration, jaundice and gastrointestinal haemorrhage.

yellow mercuric oxide (*ye'-lō mer-kūr'-ik ok'-sīd*). An eye ointment sometimes used to treat styes and conjunctivitis.

Young's rule of dosage (*yungs rool of dōs'-āj*). To estimate dose for a child:

$$\frac{age}{age + 12}$$

e.g. child of six years

$$\frac{6}{6 + 12} = \frac{6}{18} = \frac{1}{3}$$

of the adult dose.

Y

Y chromosome (*wī krō-mō-sōm*). Sex chromosome found only in the heterogametic sex (male). It is shorter than the X chromosome and usually carries few major genes.

yaws (*yaws*). Framboesia. Tropical disease, resembling syphilis, caused by Treponema pertenue.

yeast (*yē'-st*). Unicellular fungi, Ascomycetes, which possess enzymes capable of converting sugars into ethanol with the release of carbon dioxide. Yeasts are also used as sources of protein and vitamins.

yellow fever (*ye'-lō fē-ver*). Virus-mediated disease transmitted by mosquitoes.

Z

zero (*zē'-rō*). The point on the scale of a thermometer at which the graduation begins, and which is marked with the numeral 0. The zero of the Centigrade and Réaumur thermometer is the melting-point of ice. That of the Fahrenheit is 32 degrees below the melting-point of ice.

Ziehl-Neelsen's stain (*zēl-nēl-sens stān*). Staining technique used to identify tubercle bacilli by their ability to retain the stain when treated with acid; hence acid-fast bacilli.

zinc (*zi'nk*). A metallic element. The chloride is used as a caustic and disinfectant, the sulphate as an emetic in cases of poisoning by atropine, opium, etc. Zinc oxide ointment is used for dressing sores.

zingiber (*zin'-ji-ber*). Ginger; given as a carminative.

Zollinger-Ellison syndrome (*zo-ling-er e-li-son sin-drōm*). Increased production of acid gastric juice in response to gastrin secreted by pancreatic neoplasm, resulting in peptic ulceration and inactivation of enzymes of small intestine which operate only in the alkaline range.

zona (*zō'-na*). Literally a girdle and applied to mean shingles. See HERPES. *Z. pellucida*. Membrane surrounding the ovum.

Zondek-Aschheim test (*zon-dek-ash'-hīm*). To diagnose pregnancy. The urine of a pregnant woman contains a counterpart of the luteinizing hormone of the pituitary gland. Where the diagnosis is uncertain, the urine is injected into immature mice. A few days later the mice are killed and if the generative organs of the mice have undergone the changes characteristic of puberty the woman is known to be pregnant.

zonula ciliaris (*zo-nū-la si-li-a-ris*). Suspensory ligament of lens of the eye.

zoogloea layer (*zō-ō-glē-a lā-er*). Colonies of bacteria in a jelly-like layer. Found on the top of a sand filter bed. This layer contains algae and protozoa and helps in water purification.

zoology (*zō-ol'-o-ji*). That part of biology which deals with the study of animal life.

zoosperm (*zō'-o-sperm*). Same as spermatozoon.

zoster (*zos'-ter*). Shingles. See HERPES.

zygoma (*zīg-ō'-ma*). The cheek-bone.

zygote (*zī-gōt*). The cell formed by combination of ovum with spermatozoon.

zymotic (*zī-mot'-ik*). A term which includes all epidemic, endemic and contagious diseases arising from germs.

APPENDIX I

BLOOD

The figures given below represent the approximate range of values for the constituents of the peripheral blood.

Red Cells

Haemoglobin	12 to 16 g per 100 ml
Red cells	4·5 to 6·0 million per cu. mm or mm³
Reticulocytes (newly formed red cells)	less than 1 per cent of total red cells
Mean cell volume (M.C.V.)	75 to 95 cu. μ is the average volume of a single red cell
Packed cell volume (P.C.V. or haematocrit)	35 to 55 per cent
Mean cell diameter (M.C.D.)	7·2μ
Mean corpuscular haemoglobin concentration (M.C.H.C.)	30 to 38 per cent

White Cells

Total white cells	5,000 to 10,000 per cu. mm or mm³
Neutrophils	60 to 70 per cent
Lymphocytes	25 to 35 per cent
Basophils	1 per cent
Eosinophils	1 to 4 per cent
Monocytes	4 to 8 per cent
Platelets (thrombocytes)	250,000 to 350,000 per cu. mm or mm³

Blood Chemistry

Urea	25 to 40 mg per 100 ml
Uric acid	3 to 6 mg per cent
Cholesterol	100 to 300 mg per cent
Bilirubin	0·1 to 1·0 mg per cent
Calcium	9 to 11 mg per cent

Blood Chemistry (*cont.*)

Phosphate	2·5 to 5·0 mg per cent
Bicarbonate	22 to 35 mEq/litre
Fasting blood sugar	80 to 120 mg per cent
Potassium	3·5 to 5·5 mEq/litre
Sodium	135 to 145 mEq/litre
Total Plasma Proteins	6·8 g per cent
Albumin	3·5 to 5·5 g per cent
Globulin	1·5 to 3·0 g per cent
Fibrinogen	0·2 to 0·4 g per cent

APPENDIX II

URINE TESTING

1. COLOUR.—Normal, straw to light amber.

(a) *Pale.* Low specific gravity urines are usually very pale.
   1. After drinking much fluid.
   2. In cold weather.
   3. Diabetes insipidus
   4. Chronic Bright's disease.
   5. Diabetes mellitus (high specific gravity).

(b) *High colour.* Concentrated urine.
   Concentration occurs:
   1. Febrile disease, *e.g.* pneumonia, rheumatic fever.
   2. Profuse vomiting.
   3. Profuse diarrhoea.
   4. Profuse sweating.
   5. Heart disease.

(c) *When coloured by blood it may be:*
   1. Bright red
   2. The colour of a } if blood is present in
      dark beer   large amounts.
   3. Brownish if there is only a small amount of blood.

(d) *When coloured by bile it may be:*
   Mahogany or greenish-brown, frothy.

2. QUANTITY.—During 24 hours the normal output of urine is about 50 oz. or 1500 ml.

3. SPECIFIC GRAVITY of water is taken as 1·0, formerly 1000.
   The specific gravity of urine depends on the amount of soluble solid matter, *e.g.* salts, urates, etc.
   Normal specific gravity varies from 1·010 to 1·025.
   Light-coloured urines, except in diabetes mellitus, as given in list under *colour*, are of low specific gravity and there is usually an increased amount of urine passed.
   Concentrated urines are of high specific gravity, and in diabetes mellitus may be 1·025 to 1·060.
   With concentrated urine the quantity is usually decreased.

4. REACTION.—Normal reaction slightly acid, due to acid phosphates:
    1. May be neutral.
    2. May become alkaline:
        (a) In cystitis.
        (b) After taking alkalis.
        (c) Specimen stale when tested.

5. SMELL.—Normal, sweet.
In diabetes mellitus—very sweet, like new-mown hay.
In cystitis—ammoniacal.

6. NAKED-EYE DEPOSITS.
    1. Urates.—Fawn, pink, or brick-red deposits occur in concentrated urines when the urine becomes cold.
    2. Uric acid.—Small red grains, like cayenne pepper.
    3. Mucus.—Light flocculent deposit.
    4. Pus.—Thick yellow or greenish-yellow.
    5. Blood.—Clots or brownish deposit.
    6. Phosphates.—Thick white deposit.

To Test a Specimen of Urine

1. Note the colour.

2. Note the specific gravity.

3. Note the reaction. This is tested with blue or red litmus paper.
    (a) Blue litmus turns red = acid reaction.
    (b) Red litmus turns blue = alkaline reaction.
    (c) Red and blue litmus do not change = neutral.

4. Note the smell.

5. Note the naked-eye deposits. Patients who are taking sulphonamide drugs should have their urine inspected for crystals which have a highly characteristic appearance.
    In many cases a bacteriological examination of the urine is required.

Tests for Albumin

    (a) Albustix Reagent Strips.
        Dip the test end of Albustix in the urine and remove immediately, comparing it with the colour scale. If albumin is present, the moistened end turns green or blue-green at once.

(b) *Heat.*
    1. Fill $\frac{2}{3}$ test tube with urine.
    2. If not acid, add 2 or 3 drops of acetic acid
    3. Heat the upper $\frac{1}{3}$ of the urine until it boils
    4. The part heated becomes white and opaque.
    5. Add 2 or 3 drops of acetic acid—
        (a) The deposit remains = albumin.
        (b) The deposit clears up = phosphates.
A cloudy urine which becomes clear on heating = urates.

(c) *Salicyl-sulphonic Acid.*
    Take 10 drops of urine in a test tube. If alkaline, add 3
drops of acetic acid. Add 1 drop of salicyl-sulphonic
acid 25%. If a cloud forms albumin is present.

(d) *Estimation of Quantity of Albumin by an Esbach's Albuminometer.*
Render the urine acid if not already so.
If the specific gravity is higher than 1·010 dilute with an equal
quantity of water.
Take a graduated Esbach's tube and put in urine up to the
mark U. Add Esbach's solution up to mark R. Cork tube and
mix by carefully inverting. Let it stand for twenty-four hours.
Read off the height of deposit in tube and record as parts per
thousand.
If the urine was diluted, the result must be multiplied by 2.

Tests for Blood

(a) *Tincture of Guaiacum and Ozonic Ether.*
    1. Stir the specimen.
    2. Pour about a drachm of urine into a test tube.
    3. Add 2 drops of tincture of guaiacum.
    4. Shake and mix.
    5. Add slowly a drachm of ozonic ether.
A blue ring appears at the junction of the fluids when blood is
present. (Fallacy: a similar result is obtained if a patient is taking
potassium iodide.)

(b) *Occultest Reagent Tablets.*
    1. Place one drop of well-mixed uncentrifuged urine
       in the centre of the test paper.
    2. Put one Occultest tablet in the centre of the moist
       area.
    3. Place two drops of water on the tablet.
The result is negative if there is no blue colour on the test paper
after two minutes. If the result is positive, a diffuse area of blue

colour appears on the test paper around the tablet within two minutes.

Tests for Sugar

(a) *Clinitest Reagent Tablets.*

    1. Place five drops of urine in a test tube. Rinse the dropper and add ten drops of water.

    2. Drop in a Clinitest tablet and watch the reaction.

    3. Fifteen seconds after boiling has ceased, shake the tube gently and compare with the colour chart.

The result is negative if the solution turns blue. It is positive if it turns any other colour. Results are recorded as $\frac{1}{4}$%, $\frac{1}{2}$%, $\frac{3}{4}$%, 1%, 2% or over 2%. If the fluid, even fleetingly, passes through orange to dark greenish-brown, this is recorded as "over 2%".

(b) *Clinistix Reagent Strips.*

    Dip the test end of Clinistix in the urine and remove.

There is glucose in the urine if the moistened end turns blue (usually within one minute).

(c) *Benedict's Test.*

    1. Take 5 ml of Benedict's solution and to this add 8 drops of urine with a pipette.

    2. Boil for three minutes.

If sugar is present the colour will change. Greenish-yellow denotes a trace of sugar; yellow: some sugar; and orange-brown: much sugar.

Tests for Acetone

(a) *Acetest Reagent Tablets.*

    Place one tablet on a clean white surface and add one drop of urine on tablet.

If the tablet turns mauve it indicates the presence of diacetic acid and acetone in the urine.

(b) *Rothera's Test.*

    1. To half a test tube full of urine add ammonium sulphate crystals until the liquid is saturated.

    2. Dissolve two or three nitro-prusside crystals in 8 ml of water and add four drops of this to the urine.

    3. Shake well.

    4. Add ten drops of strong ammonia.

There will be a purple colour in 15 minutes if acetone or diacetic acid is present.

Tests for Bilirubin

(a) *Ictotest Reagent Tablets.*

Place five drops of urine on the test mat and put one Ictotest tablet in the middle of the moist area. Then put two drops of water on the tablet.

If the mat round the tablet turns bluish-purple, bilirubin is present.

(b) *Iodine Test.*

To 5 ml of urine add a few drops of tincture of iodine which has been diluted with equal parts of water.

A green ring will form where the two liquids join if bilirubin is present.

Test for Pus

Liquor Potassae.

1. Take two test tubes and fill one a quarter full with liquor potassae and the other a quarter full with urine.
2. Mix the two together by pouring the contents of one tube into the other several times.

If the mixture becomes thick and ropey this indicates the presence of pus. If present, pus cells can be seen with the microscope after the urine has been centrifuged.

Test for Chlorides

Fantus' Quantitative Test.

A nurse may have to ascertain the presence or absence of chlorides in urine before saline is given intravenously.

1. Measure 10 drops urine into test tube with a pipette. Rinse pipette.
2. Add 1 drop potassium chromate 20% sol. Rinse pipette.
3. Add silver nitrate 2·9 sol. drop by drop until the solution turns brown. The number of drops of silver nitrate solution required to do this equals the number of grams of sodium chloride per litre of urine.

N.B. The same pipette must be used throughout.

APPENDIX III

POISONS: Antidotes and Treatment

In a case of suspected poisoning:

1. Send for medical aid, and if possible state in writing the type of poison taken.
2. Prevent any more poison being taken.
3. Give artificial respiration if necessary.
4. If the patient is conscious and is not convulsing and there is no evidence that a corrosive acid or alkali has been taken then vomiting should be induced either by tickling the back of the throat with your index finger, or giving a strong solution of salt and water (one tablespoon of salt to a pint of water).
5. Do not give anything by mouth if the patient is convulsing, unconscious or semi-conscious.
6. Any poison on the skin should be washed away with water.
7. Preserve any urine, vomit, faeces, sputum.
8. Keep any bottles or box which may have contained the poison.
9. Treat the patient for shock. Lie him down and cover him with a blanket.

POISON	SYMPTOMS	TREATMENT
Strong Acid	Immediate intense burning pain from mouth to stomach. Ulcerated mouth. Vomiting shreds of mucous membrane and altered blood. Dyspnoea due to oedema of the glottis. Shock.	Do not use a stomach tube or an emetic. Give an alkali immediately: ideally lime water, but soap solution in an emergency. Next give milk or olive oil. Strong analgesics to relieve pain. Tracheostomy. Intravenous fluids to combat shock.
Strong Alkali and Ammonia	As with acid poisoning but less severe if a weak solution has been taken.	Give dilute acid such as acetic acid, vinegar or lemon juice. Otherwise treat as for acid poisoning.
Antihistamine	Initial drowsiness and lassitude. Followed by confusion, coma and convulsions.	Gastric lavage with sodium bicarbonate solution. Oxygen, artificial respiration and amphetamine if the respiration is depressed. Convulsions are controlled by paraldehyde.
Arsenic (see also p. 387)	*Acute:* Burning abdominal pain. Severe vomiting and diarrhoea,	Gastric lavage with copious amounts of water. Dimercaprol (B.A.L.).

POISON	SYMPTOMS	TREATMENT
Arsenic—contd.	leading to dehydration and shock. Muscle cramps. *Chronic:* Mild gastroenteritis. Dry cough with a husky voice. Grey skin pigmentation and hyperkeratosis. Jaundice. Peripheral neuritis. Anaemia.	Analgesics. Intravenous fluid to counter dehydration. Remove source, otherwise symptomatic.
Aspirin (salicylates)	Initially, nausea and tinnitus (ringing in the ears), followed by deafness, confusion, restlessness, then coma. Profuse sweating leading to dehydration. 'Air hunger.' Haematemesis.	Gastric lavage with water. Intravenous sodium chloride and bicarbonate to counter acidosis and dehydration. Nikethamide if respiration is depressed.
Barbiturates	Initial drowsiness and vertigo. There may be hallucinations, followed by coma, which becomes profound with absent reflexes, respiratory depression and fall in blood pressure. Erythematous rashes occasionally occur.	Gastric lavage with copious amounts of water. Oxygen and artificial respiration.

POISON	SYMPTOMS	TREATMENT
Belladonna (atropine)	Dry mouth, flushed skin, pupils dilated. Rapid pulse and respirations. Restlessness, excitement. Convulsions and later paralysis and coma.	Gastric lavage with very dilute potassium permanganate. Oxygen and artificial respiration may be required. Convulsions controlled by short-acting barbiturates.
Coal Gas (carbon monoxide)	Headache, nausea and giddiness, followed by coma and convulsions. Cherry-pink discoloration of skin and mucosae	Artificial respiration. Oxygen with 5 % carbon dioxide. Warmth. Respiratory stimulants
Chloral Hydrate	Initial drowsiness passing into deep coma with respiratory depression. Low blood pressure and a sub-normal temperature.	Gastric lavage. Stimulants. Oxygen and artificial respiration.
Cyanides	Very rapid unconsciousness followed by convulsions, then flaccid paralysis. Respirations at first rapid then slow. Strong smell of bitter almonds.	Immediate inhalation of amyl nitrite, and artificial respiration. Intravenous injection of sodium nitrite 3%, followed by sodium thiosulphate 50%, then niketha-mide. Gastric lavage with dilute potassium permanganate solution. Repeat the injections in one hour.

POISON	SYMPTOMS	TREATMENT
Ferrous sulphate (tablets containing iron)	Vomiting, diarrhoea and haematemesis. Drowsiness. Shock. 2–4 days later, after apparent recovery, sudden collapse may occur.	Gastric lavage. Give bismuth carbonate 4 hourly by mouth. Vitamin B mixture and tocopherol.
Lead	*Acute:* Vomiting. Intestinal colic. Shock and collapse. *Chronic:* Tiredness. Constipation. Anaemia. Blue line on gums. Weakness and palsies. Acute bouts of colic and vomiting. Convulsions and mania.	Gastric lavage with dilute sodium sulphate solution, then demulcents such as milk and albumin. Sodium calcium edetate intravenously. Symptomatic. Remove from exposure. 10% calcium gluconate intravenously for colic. Control convulsions with intravenous barbiturates.
Mercury (*see also* p. 390)	*Acute:* Severe abdominal pain. Vomiting. Diarrhoea. Shock. Anuria. *Chronic:* Gingivitis.	Gastric lavage, followed by egg white. Dimercaprol. Morphine. Warmth. Remove from further exposure.

POISON	SYMPTOMS	TREATMENT
Mercury—*contd.*	Blue line on gums. Tremor. Anaemia. Psychosis.	Symptomatic treatment.
Morphine (codeine, heroin, pethidine)	Euphoria with increasing drowsiness, then profound sleep followed by deep coma. Respirations slow and feeble. Pulse slow. Cyanosis. Pupils: pin-point.	Intravenous nalorphine hydrobromide. Oxygen, artificial respiration. Gastric lavage with dilute potassium permanganate. Stimulants if necessary.
Phenol (lysol)	Immediate burning pain from mouth to stomach. Lips white and hardened. Vomiting. Collapse. Delirium and coma.	Gastric lavage with magnesium or sodium sulphate. Demulcents such as milk or olive oil. Oxygen and artificial respiration, if necessary.
Strychnine	Convulsions. Sweating. Muscular rigidity. Respiratory paralysis.	Thiopentone sodium intravenously or other short-acting barbiturate. Muscle relaxant such as tubocurarine. Gastric lavage with potassium permanganate or tannic acid solution. Oxygen and artificial respiration may be necessary.

POISON	SYMPTOMS	TREATMENT
Turpentine	Smell of turpentine in breath. Headache, giddiness, drowsiness and sometimes delirium. Respirations slow. Pulse thready. Skin blue and clammy.	Gastric lavage. Demulcent drinks, such as milk and olive oil. Saline purge. Morphia for pain.
D.N.O.C. or other derivatives of dinitrophenol, used as weed killer.	Increased metabolic rate. Whites of the eyes may become yellow before symptoms arise. Sweating, fatigue, insomnia. Respiration increased in rate and depth. Tachycardia. Temperature raised.	No specific antidote available. Keep the patient at rest, and give a barbiturate intramuscularly; saline intravenously. Oxygen.

APPENDIX IV

SOME COMMON DRUGS

listed in alphabetical order

Proprietary names commence with a capital letter
B.P. signifies British Pharmacopoeia
B.P.C. signifies British Pharmacopoeia Codex

acetazolamide (B.P.)	Diamox	Diuretic and used to control intra-ocular pressure
acetomenaphthone (B.P.)	Prokayvit	Used to treat low prothrombin level
A.C.T.H.	corticotrophin (B.P.)	Hormone of anterior lobe of pituitary
Achromycin	tetracycline hydrochloride (B.P.)	Antibiotic often used to treat mixed infections
Actidil	triprolidine hydrochloride	Antihistamine
Actifed	triprolidine hydrochloride with pseudoephedrine	Treatment of nasal and respiratory congestion
Adalin	carbromal (B.P.)	Mild hypnotic
Adcortyl	triamcinolone (B.P.C.)	Corticosteroid drug
Aerotrol	isoprenaline hydrochloride	Bronchodilator
Albucid	sulphacetamide sodium (B.P.)	Bacteriostatic action
Aldactone-A	spironolactone (B.P.)	Increases excretion of sodium and reduces excretion of potassium
Aldocorten	aldosterone	Given in Addison's disease
Aldomet	methyldopa (B.P.)	Used to lower blood pressure
aldosterone	Aldocorten, Electrocortin	Given in Addison's disease
Aleudrin	isoprenaline sulphate (B.P.)	Bronchodilator
Alkeran	melphalan	Cytotoxic drug
Aludrox	aluminium hydroxide	Antacid

Alupent	orciprenaline sulphate	Antispasmodic
amethopterin	methotrexate	Cytotoxic drug
amidone hydrochloride	methadone hydrochloride, Physeptone	Analgesic which resembles morphine
aminopterin		Cytotoxic drug
amiphenazole hydrochloride (B.P.C.)	Daptazole	An analeptic. It reduces respiratory depression
amitriptyline hydrochloride (B.P.)	Laroxyl, Saroten, Triptafen-DA Tablets, Tryptizol	Antidepressant and tranquilizer
amoxil	amoxycillin trihydrate	Antibiotic
amphetamine sulphate (B.P.)	Benzedrine	Stimulates central nervous system
ampicillin (B.P.)	Penbritin	Wide-spectrum antibiotic
amylobarbitone sodium (B.P.)	Sodium Amytal	Hypnotic, usually acting within half an hour and lasting up to 6 hours
Amytal	amylobarbitone (B.P.)	Hypnotic and sedative
Angised	glyceryl trinitrate	Relaxes involuntary muscle. A vasodilator
Anovlar 21	norethisterone acetate (ethinyl oestradiol dichlorophen (B.P.)	Oral contraceptive
Anthiphen		Anthelmintic used in tapeworm infection
Anthisan	mepyramine maleate (B.P.)	Antihistamine
aprotinin	Trasylol	Used in the treatment of haemorrhage
Aprinox	bendrofluazide (B.P.)	Diuretic
Aquamox	quinethazone	Diuretic
Aralen	chloroquine phosphate (B.P.)	Antimalarial drug
Aramine	metaraminol tartrate (B.P.)	A vasoconstrictor drug
Arfonad	trimetaphan camsylate (B.P.)	A hypotensive drug

Artane	benzhexol hydrochloride (B.P.)	Used to treat paralysis agitans
Asilone	dimethicone sorbitol and aluminium hydroxide	Antacid
A.T. 10	dihydrotachysterol	Raises calcium level in the blood
Atromid S	clofibrate	Reduces serum cholesterol levels
atropine methonitrate (B.P.)	Eumydrin	Antispasmodic action. Given in pyloric stenosis
Avloclor	chloroquine phosphate (B.P.)	Antimalarial drug
Avlosulfon	dapsone (B.P.)	Drug used to treat leprosy
Avomine	promethazine theoclate (B.P.)	Antihistamine drug often used as antiemetic
azapropazone		Analgesic, anti-inflammatory
B.A.L.	dimercaprol (B.P.)	Antidote to poisoning by arsenic, mercury, etc.
bemegride (B.P.)	Megimide	Restorative drug used in barbiturate poisoning
Benadryl	diphenhydramine hydrochloride (B.P.)	Antihistamine drug
bendrofluazide (B.P.)	Aprinox, Centyl, Neo-NaClex	Diuretic
Benemid	probenecid (B.P.)	Used to treat gout
benzathine penicillin (B.P.)	Dibencil, Penidural	Antibiotic
Benzedrine	amphetamine sulphate (B.P.)	Stimulates central nervous system
benzhexol hydrochloride (B.P.)	Artane, Pipanol	Used to treat paralysis agitans
benzylpenicillin (B.P.)	There are numerous proprietary preparations	Antibiotic

bethanidine sulphate	Esbatal	Hypotensive drug
bisacodyl	Dulcolax	Laxative
Brevidil M	suxamethonium bromide (B.P.)	A muscle relaxant
Brevital Sodium	methohexitone sodium	A short-acting barbiturate
Brietal Sodium	methohexitone sodium	A short-acting barbiturate
Brocadopa	levodopa	Used in parkinsonism
Brocillin	propicillin potassium	Antibiotic
Broxil	phenethicillin potassium (B.P.)	Antibiotic
busulphan (B.P.)	Myleran	Cytotoxic drug
Butazolidin	phenylbutazone (B.P.)	Used to allay pain in rheumatoid arthritis, etc.
butobarbitone (B.P.)	Soneryl	Hypnotic, usually acting within half an hour and lasting up to 6 hours
Cafergot	ergotamine tartrate and caffeine	Treatment of migraine
carbachol (B.P.)		Used in post-operative urinary retention
carbimazole (B.P.)	Neo-Mercazole	Used in thyrotoxicosis
carbromal (B.P.)	Adalin	Mild hypnotic
Celbenin	methicillin sodium (B.P.)	Antibiotic
Centyl	bendrofluazide	Diuretic
cephalexin	Ceporex	Antibiotic
cephaloridine	Ceporin	Antibiotic
cephradine	Velosef	Antibiotic
Ceporex	cephalexin	Antibiotic
Ceporin	cephaloridine	Antibiotic
chlorambucil (B.P.)	Leukeran	Cytotoxic drug
chloramphenicol (B.P.)	Chloromycetin	Antibiotic used especially in typhoid fever
chlordiazepoxide hydrochloride (B.P.)	Librium	Mild tranquillizing drug

Chloromycetin	chloramphenicol	Antibiotic used especially in typhoid fever
chloroquine phosphate (B.P.)	Aralen, Avloclor, Resochin	Antimalarial drug
chloroquine sulphate (B.P.)	Nivaquine	Antimalarial drug
chlorothiazide (B.P.)	Saluric	A diuretic
chlorpheniramine maleate (B.P.)	Piriton	Antihistamine
chlorpromazine hydrochloride (B.P.)	Largactil	A tranquillizing drug
chlorpropamide (B.P.)	Diabinese	Oral drug used to treat mild diabetes mellitus
Choledyl	choline theophyllinate (B.P.)	Bronchodilator and mild diuretic
choline theophyllinate (B.P.)	Choledyl	Bronchodilator and mild diuretic
clofibrate	Atromid S	Reduces serum cholesterol levels
cloxacillin sodium (B.P.)	Orbenin	Antibiotic esp. used for penicillin-resistant organisms
Cortef	hydrocortisone (B.P.)	Steroid drug
Cortelan	cortisone acetate (B.P.)	Steroid drug
corticotrophin (B.P.)	ACTH, Cortrophin	Hormone of anterior lobe of pituitary
cortisone acetate (B.P.)	Cortelan, Cortistab, Cortisyl	Steroid drug
Cortistab	cortisone acetate (B.P.)	Steroid drug
Cortisyl	cortisone acetate (B.P.)	Steroid drug
Cortrophin	corticotrophin (B.P.)	Hormone of anterior lobe of pituitary
Coumadin Sodium (U.S.A.)	Warfarin Sodium (B.P.)	Anticoagulant drug

Cremodiazine	sulphadiazine (B.P.)	Sulphonamide drug
Crystapen V	phenoxymethylpenicillin (B.P.)	Antibiotic
cyanocobalamin (B.P.)	Cytamen, vitamin B$_{12}$ (B.P.)	Used to treat pernicious and other anaemias
cyclizine hydrochloride (B.P.)	Marzine	An antiemetic
cyclobarbitone (B.P.)	Phanodorm	Hypnotic, usually acting in 15 minutes and lasting up to 3 hours
Cyclogyl	cyclopentolate hydrochloride	A mydriatic drug
cyclopenthiazide	Navidrex	Diuretic
cyclopentolate hydrochloride	Cyclogyl, Mydrilate	A mydriatic drug
cyclophosphamide (B.P.)	Cytoxan (U.S.A.) Endoxana	Cytotoxic drug
Cytamen	cyanocobalamin (B.P.)	Used to treat pernicious and other anaemias
Dalmane	flurazepam hydrochloride	Hypnotic
dapsone (B.P.)	Avlosulfon	Drug used to treat leprosy
Daptazole	amiphenazole hydrochloride (B.P.C.)	An analeptic. It reduces respiratory depression
DeCortisyl	prednisone (B.P.C.)	Steroid drug
Degranol	mannomustine hydrochloride (B.P.C.)	Cytotoxic drug
Delta-Cortef	prednisolone (B.P.)	Steroid drug
Deltacortone	prednisone (B.P.)	Steroid drug
Delta-Stab	prednisolone (B.P.)	Steroid drug
desoxymethasone	Esperson	Topical corticosteroid
dexamphetamine sulphate	Dexedrine	Stimulates central nervous system and decreases appetite

Dexedrine	dexamphetamine	Stimulates central nervous system and decreases appetite
dextran	Dextraven, Intradex	Given intravenously to restore blood volume
Dextraven	dextran	Given intravenously to restore blood volume
dextromoramide tartrate (B.P.)	Palfium	An analgesic
D.F. 118	dihydrocodeine acid tartrate	An analgesic
D.F.P.	dyflos (B.P.C.)	Drug, with miotic action, used to treat glaucoma
Diabinese	chlorpropamide (B.P.)	Oral drug used to treat mild diabetes mellitus
diamorphine hydro- chloride (B.P.)	heroin	Analgesic
Diamox	acetazolamide (B.P.)	Diuretic and used to control intraocular pressure
Dianabol	methandienone (B.P.)	Anabolic steroid
diazepam	Valium	Tranquillizer
Dibencil	benzathine penicillin (B.P.)	Antibiotic
Dibenyline	phenoxybenzamine hydro- chloride (B.P.)	Vasodilator
Dibotin	phenformin hydrochloride	Oral drug used to treat diabetes mellitus
dichloralphenazone (B.P.)	Welldorm	Hypnotic and sedative
dichlorophen	Anthiphen	Anthelmintic used in tapeworm infection
diclofenac	Voltarol	Anti-inflammatory
diethazine hydro- chloride (B.P.)	Diparcol	Drug used to reduce rigidity in parkinsonism
digoxin (B.P.)	Lanoxin	Slows heart rate and increases cardiac output

dihydrocodeine acid tartrate	D.F. 118	An analgesic
dihydrotachysterol Dilaudid	A.T. 10 hydromorphone hydrochloride	Raises calcium level in the blood Analgesic more potent than morphine but action of shorter duration
dimercaprol (B.P.)	B.A.L.	Antidote to poisoning by arsenic, mercury, etc.
dimenhydrinate (B.P.) Dindevan Diparcol	Dramamine phenindione (B.P.) diethazine hydro- chloride (B.P.)	Antihistamine which is an antiemetic Anticoagulant drug Drug used to relieve rigidity in parkinsonism
diphenhydramine hydro- chloride (B.P.)	Benadryl	Antihistamine drug
diphenoxylate hydrochloride	Lomotil	Used to control diarrhoea
Disprin	aspirin soluble and calcium carbonate	Analgesic drug
Distalgesic	dextropropoxyphene hydrochloride and paracetamol	Analgesic drug
Doriden	glutethimide (B.P.)	Hypnotic usually acting within 20 minutes and lasting up to 6 hours
Dramamine Dromoran	dimenhydrinate (B.P.) levorphanol tartrate (B.P.)	Antihistamine which is an antiemetic Analgesic drug
Dulcolax Durabolin Durenate	bisacodyl nandrolone sulphamethoxydiazine (B.P.)	Laxative Steroid drug Used in urinary infections, etc.
dyflos (B.P.C.)	D.F.P.	Drug with miotic action used to treat glaucoma

edrophonium chloride (B.P.)	Tensilon	Used in diagnosis of myasthenia gravis
Electrocortin	aldosterone	Given in Addison's disease
Eltroxin	L-thyroxine	Treatment of hypothyroidism
Endoxana	cyclophosphamide (B.P.)	Cytotoxic drug
Entacyl	piperazine adipate (B.P.)	Anthelmintic used against roundworms and threadworms
Epanutin	phenytoin sodium (B.P.)	Anticonvulsant drug
Equanil	meprobamate (B.P.)	A tranquillizing drug
Eraldin	practolol	Treatment of angina and cardiac arrhythmias
ergometrine maleate (B.P.)	Ergotrate, Syntometrine	Causes contraction of uterine muscle. Given in post-partum haemorrhage
ergotamine tartrate (B.P.)	Femergin	Used in migraine
	ergometrine maleate (B.P.)	Contracts uterine muscle
Ergotrate	erythromycin (B.P.)	Antibiotic
Erythrocin	Erythrocin, Ilotycin	Antibiotic
erythromycin	Ilosone	Antibiotic
erythromycin estolate	bethanidine sulphate	Hypotensive drug
Esbatal	desoxymethasone	Topical corticosteroid
Esperson	Zactane, Zactipar	Analgesic drug
ethoheptazine	Tromexan	Anticoagulant drug
ethyl biscoumacetate (B.P.C.)		
ethyloestrenol	Orabolin	Anabolic steroid
Eumydrin	atropine methonitrate (B.P.)	Antispasmodic action. Given to infants with pyloric stenosis
Fefol	exsiccated ferrous sulphate	Iron-containing drug
Femergin	ergotamine tartrate (B.P.)	Used in migraine
Fentazin	perphenazine (B.P.)	Tranquillizing drug

Feospan Spansule	exsiccated ferrous sulphate	Iron-containing drug
Ferlucon	ferrous gluconate (B.P.)	Iron-containing drug
Ferromyn	ferrous succinate	Iron-containing drug
ferrous gluconate (B.P.)	Ferlucon	Iron-containing drug
ferrous succinate	Ferromyn	Iron-containing drug
ferrous sulphate (B.P.)	Fersolate	Iron-containing drug
Fersolate	ferrous sulphate	Iron-containing drug
Flagyl	metronidazole (B.P.)	Used to treat *Trichomonas vaginalis* infections
Flaxedil	gallamine triethiodide (B.P.)	A muscle relaxant
Florinef	fludrocortisone	Steroid drug
fludrocortisone	Florinef, Fludrocortone	Steroid drug
Fludrocortone	fludrocortisone	Steroid drug
fluphenazine hydrochloride and nortriptyline hydrochloride	Motival	Antidepressant
flurazepam hydrochloride	Dalmane	Hypnotic
folic acid	vitamin B group	
Fortral	pentazocine	Analgesic
Franol	ephedrine hydrochloride (phenobarbitone (theophylline	Bronchial dilator
frusemide	Lasix	Diuretic
Fucidin	fusidic acid	Antibiotic
Fulcin	griseofulvin (B.P.)	Antibiotic used in fungus infections
Furacin	nitrofurazone (B.P.C.)	Antibacterial drug
Furadantin	nitrofurantoin	Urinary antiseptic
fusidic acid	Fucidin	Antibiotic

gallamine triethiodide (B.P.)	Flaxedil	Muscle relaxant
gamma benzene hexachloride (B.P.)	Lorexane, Quellada	Antiparasitic
Gantrisin	sulphafurazole (B.P.)	Urinary antiseptic, etc.
Gelusil	magnesium trisilicate (B.P.) aluminium hydroxide	Adsorbent and antacid drug
Glucophage	metformin	Oral drug given in diabetes mellitus
glutethimide (B.P.)	Doriden	Hypnotic usually acting within 20 minutes and lasting up to 6 hours
glyceryl trinitrate (B.P.)	Angised	Relaxes involuntary muscle. A vasodilator
griseofulvin (B.P.)	Fulcin, Grisovin	Antibiotic used in fungus infections
Grisovin	griseofulvin (B.P.)	Antibiotic used in fungus infections
guanethidine sulphate (B.P.)	Ismelin	Hypotensive drug
heparin		Anticoagulant drug usually given intravenously
Heptalgin	phenadoxone hydrochloride (B.P.)	Analgesic
heroin hydrochloride	diamorphine hydrochloride (B.P.)	Analgesic more potent than morphine but its action of shorter duration
hexachlorophane (B.P.)	Phisohex	Antiseptic
Hydrenox	hydroflumethiazide (B.P.)	A diuretic
hydrochlorothiazide (B.P.)	Hydrosaluric, Salupres	A diuretic
hydrocortisone acetate (B.P.)	Cortef, Hydrocortistab, HydroCortisyl	Corticosteroid drug
Hydrocortistab	hydrocortisone acetate (B.P.)	Corticosteroid drug
HydroCortisyl	hydrocortisone acetate (B.P.)	Corticosteroid drug

hydroflumethiazide (B.P.)	Hydrenox, NaClex	Diuretic
hydromorphone hydrochloride	Dilaudid	Analgesic, more potent than morphine but action of shorter duration
Hydrosaluric	hydrochlorothiazide	Diuretic
hyoscine hydrobromide (B.P.)	scopolamine hydrobromide	Hypnotic, antispasmodic and mydriatic
Ilosone	erythromycin estolate	Antibiotic
Ilotycin	erythromycin (B.P.)	Antibiotic
imipramine hydrochloride (B.P.)	Tofranil	Antidepressant
Inderal	propranolol hydrochloride	Blocking agent acting on adrenergic beta receptors. Reduces response of heart to exercise
Indocid	indomethacin	Analgesic and anti-inflammatory drug
INH	isoniazid (B.P.)	Antituberculous drug
Insulin		Given in diabetes. There is a delayed action
globin zinc insulin injection		Given in diabetes but action of longer duration than that of globin zinc insulin
isophane insulin injection		Insulin is slowly absorbed throughout the day
protamine zinc insulin injection		Rapid in action
insulin, soluble		
insulin zinc suspensions (B.P.)	Insulin Lente, Insulin Semilente, Insulin Ultralente	These forms of insulin are frequently given to diabetics
Intal	sodium cromoglycate	Treatment of asthma
Intradex	dextran	Plasma substitute used to restore blood volume
iproniazid phosphate	Marsilid	Antidepressant drug. It is a monoamine oxidase inhibitor

Ismelin	guanethidine sulphate (B.P.)	Hypotensive drug
isocarboxazid (B.P.C.)	Marplan	Antidepressant drug. It is a monoamine oxidase inhibitor
Isolevin	isoprenaline hydrogen tartrate	Bronchodilator
isoniazid (B.P.)	INH	Antituberculous drug
isoprenaline sulphate (B.P.)	Aleudrin, Neodrenal, Neo-Epinine, Norisodrine	A bronchodilator
isoprenaline hydrochloride	Aerotrol, Isovon, Saventrine, Suscardia	A bronchodilator
isoprenaline hydrogen tartrate	Isolevin	A bronchodilator
Isovon	isoprenaline hydrochloride	A bronchodilator
L-dopa	levodopa, Brocadopa, Larodopa	Used in parkinsonism
Lanoxin	digoxin (B.P.)	Used in atrial fibrillation
Largactil	chlorpromazine hydrochloride (B.P.)	Sedative and tranquillizer
Larodopa	L-dopa	Used in parkinsonism
Laroxyl	amitriptyline hydrochloride (B.P.)	Antidepressant and tranquilizer
Lasix	frusemide	Diuretic
Ledercort	triamcinolone (B.P.C.)	Corticosteroid drug
Lethidrone	nalorphine hydrobromide (B.P.)	Antidote to morphine
Leukeran	chlorambucil	Cytotoxic drug
levallorphan tartrate (B.P.)	Lorfan	Respiratory stimulant
levodopa	L-dopa, Brocadopa, Larodopa	Used in parkinsonism

Levophed	noradrenaline acid tartrate (B.P.)	Produces peripheral vasoconstriction
levorphanol tartrate (B.P.)	Dromoran	Analgesic
Librium	chlordiazepoxide hydrochloride (B.P.)	Tranquilizing drug
lignocaine hydrochloride (B.P.)	Lignostab, Xylocaine, Xylotox	Local anaesthetic
Lignostab	lignocaine hydrochloride (B.P.)	Local anaesthetic
liothyronine	Tertroxin	Drug used in thyroid deficiency
Lomotil	diphenoxylate hydrochloride	Used to control diarrhoea
Lorexane	gamma benzene hexachloride (B.P.)	Antiparasitic. Used in pediculosis
Lorfan	levallorphan tartrate (B.P.)	Respiratory stimulant
L.S.D.	lysergide	Drug used in psychotherapy
lucanthone hydrochloride (B.P.)	Nilodin	Used in treatment of schistosomiasis
Luminal	phenobarbitone (B.P.)	Sedative and hypnotic. Usually acting an hour after being taken and lasting from 6 to 10 hours
lysergide	L.S.D.	Drug used in psychotherapy
magnesium hydroxide (B.P.C.)		Antacid and mild laxative
magnesium trisilicate (B.P.)		Antacid and adsorbent
Mandrax	methaqualone and diphenhydramine hydrochloride	Hypnotic drug
mannomustine hydrochloride (B.P.C.)	Degranol	Cytotoxic drug
Marevan	Warfarin Sodium (B.P.)	Anticoagulant drug

Marplan	isocarboxazid (B.P.C.)	Antidepressant drug, a monoamine oxidase inhibitor
Marsilid	iproniazid phosphate	Antidepressant drug. It is a monoamine oxidase inhibitor
Marzine	cyclizine hydrochloride (B.P.)	An antiemetic
medazepam	Nobrium	Tranquillizer
Megimide	bemegride (B.P.)	Restorative drug used in barbiturate poisoning
melphalan	Alkeran	Cytotoxic drug
menadiol sodium diphosphate	Synkavit	A vitamin K analogue
meprobamate (B.P.)	Equanil, Miltown	A tranquillizing drug
mepyramine maleate (B.P.)	Anthisan	Antihistamine
mercaptopurine (B.P.)	Puri-Nethol, 6-Mercaptopurine	Cytotoxic drug
Mestinon	pyridostigmine bromide (B.P.)	Used in treatment of myasthenia gravis
metaraminol tartrate	Aramine	A vasoconstrictor drug
metformin	Glucophage	Oral drug given in diabetes mellitus
methadone hydrochloride	amidone hydrochloride, Physeptone	Analgesic which resembles morphine
methandienone (B.P.)	Dianabol	Anabolic steroid
methaqualone hydrochloride	Mandrax	Hypnotic drug
methicillin sodium (B.P.)	Celbenin	Antibiotic
methohexitone sodium	Brevital Sodium, Brietal Sodium	A short-acting barbiturate
methotrexate	amethopterin	Cytotoxic drug
methoxamine hydrochloride (B.P.C.)	Vasoxine	A vasoconstrictor drug

methyldopa (B.P.)	Aldomet	Used to lower blood pressure
methylpentynol (B.P.C.), methyl phentynol hydrochloride	Oblivon, Somnesin	Short-acting hypnotic
	Ritalin	Antidepressant drug
metronidazole (B.P.)	Flagyl	Used to treat *Trichomonas vaginalis* infection
Migril	ergotamine tartrate, caffeine and cyclizine hydrochloride	Treatment of migraine
Miltown	meprobamate (B.P.)	A tranquillizing drug
Mogadon	nitrazepam	Hypnotic drug with fairly rapid action
morphine		Analgesic and sedative
Motival	fluphenazine hydrochloride and nortriptyline hydrochloride	Antidepressant
Mycostatin (U.S.A.)	nystatin	Antibiotic
Mydrilate	cyclopentolate hydrochloride, Cyclogyl	A mydriatic drug
Myleran	busulphan (B.P.)	Cytotoxic drug
Mysoline	primidone	Treatment of epilepsy
NaClex	hydroflumethiazide (B.P.)	Diuretic
nalidixic acid	Negram	Antibiotic
nalorphine hydrobromide (B.P.)	Lethidrone	Antidote to morphine
naloxone hydrochloride	Narcan	Narcotic antagonist
nandrolone	Durabolin	Steroid drug
Narcan	naloxone hydrochloride	Narcotic antagonist
Nardil	phenelzine sulphate	Antidepressant drug, a monoamine oxidase inhibitor

Navidrex	cyclopenthiazide	Diuretic
Negram	nalidixic acid	Antibiotic
Nembutal	pentobarbitone sodium (B.P.)	Hypnotic usually acting within 15 minutes and lasting for up to 3 hours
Neodrenal	isoprenaline sulphate (B.P.)	A bronchodilator
Neo-Epinine	isoprenaline sulphate (B.P.)	A bronchodilator
Neo-Mercazole	carbimazole (B.P.)	Used in thyrotoxicosis
Neomin	neomycin sulphate (B.P.)	Antibiotic used in skin infections, etc.
neomycin sulphate (B.P.)	Neomin	Antibiotic used in skin infections, etc.
Neo-Naclex	bendrofluazide	Diuretic
neostigmine methyl-sulphate (B.P.)	Prostigmin	A miotic. Increases intestinal tone. Used in myasthenia gravis
nicotinamide (B.P.)		Used to treat pellagra
Nilevar	norethandrolone (B.P.)	Anabolic steroid
Nilodin	lucanthone hydrochloride (B.P.)	Used in treatment of schistosomiasis
nitrazepam	Mogadon	Hypnotic drug with fairly rapid action
nitrofurantoin	Furadantin	Urinary antiseptic
nitrofurazone (B.P.C.)	Furacin	Antibacterial drug
Nivaquine	chloroquine sulphate (B.P.)	Antimalarial drug
Nobrium	medazepam	Tranquillizer
noradrenaline acid tartrate (B.P.)	Levophed	Produces peripheral vasoconstriction
norethandrolone (B.P.)	Nilevar	Anabolic steroid
norethisterone (B.P.)	Primolut N	Steroid drug
Norisodrine	isoprenaline sulphate (B.P.)	A bronchodilator
novobiocin sodium (B.P.)	Streptonivicin	Antibiotic sometimes used for patients sensitized to penicillin
Nystan	nystatin (U.S.A.), Nystan	Antibiotic used in treatment of moniliasis
nystatin (B.P.)	Mycostatin	Antibiotic used in treatment of moniliasis

Oblivon	methylpentynol (B.P.C.)	Hypnotic with short action
oestradiol benzoate (B.P.)		Oestrogenic hormone
Omnopon	papaveretum (B.P.C.)	Analgesic
Orabolin	ethyloestrenol	Anabolic steroid
Orbenin	cloxacillin sodium (B.P.)	Antibiotic esp. used for penicillin-resistant organisms
orciprenaline sulphate	Alupent	Antispasmodic
oxytetracycline	Terramycin	Antibiotic
Palfium	dextromoramide tartrate (B.P.)	An analgesic
Panadol	paracetamol (B.P.)	Analgesic and antipyretic
papaveretum (B.P.C.)	Omnopon	Analgesic
paracetamol (B.P.)	Panadol, Tabalgin	Analgesic and antipyretic
PAS	para-aminosalicylic acid	Used in treatment of tuberculosis
Penbritin	ampicillin (B.P.)	Wide-spectrum antibiotic
Penicillin V	phenoxymethylpenicillin (B.P.)	Antibiotic
Penidural	benzathine penicillin (B.P.)	Antibiotic
Penspek	phenbenicillin potassium (B.P.)	Antibiotic
pentazocine	Fortral	Analgesic
pentobarbitone sodium (B.P.)	Nembutal	Hypnotic drug usually acting within 15 minutes and lasting up to 3 hours
perphenazine (B.P.)	Fentazin	Tranquillizing drug
Pethidine hydrochloride (B.P.)		Analgesic
Phanodorm	cyclobarbitone (B.P.)	Hypnotic usually acting in 15 minutes and lasting up to 3 hours
phenadoxone hydro-chloride (B.P.)	Heptalgin	An analgesic
phenbenicillin potassium	Penspek	Antibiotic

phenelzine sulphate	Nardil	Antidepressant drug, a monoamine oxidase inhibitor
Phenergan	promethazine hydrochloride (B.P.)	Antihistamine drug
phenethicillin potassium (B.P.)	Broxil	Antibiotic
phenformin hydrochloride	Dibotin	Oral drug used to treat diabetes mellitus
phenindione (B.P.)	Dindevan	Anticoagulant
phenobarbitone (B.P.)	Luminal	Sedative and hypnotic. Usually acting an hour after being taken and lasting from 6 to 10 hours
phenoxybenzamine hydrochloride (B.P.)	Dibenyline	Vasodilator
phenoxymethylpenicillin (B.P.)	Crystapen V, Penicillin V	Antibiotic
phenylbutazone (B.P.)	Butazolidin	Used to allay pain in rheumatoid arthritis, etc.
phenytoin sodium (B.P.)	Epanutin	Anticonvulsant drug
Phisohex	hexachlorophane (B.P.)	Antiseptic
phthalylsulphathiazole	Sulfathalidine	Used in gastrointestinal infections
Physeptone	amidone hydrochloride	Analgesic which resembles morphine
Pipanol	benzhexol hydrochloride (B.P.)	Used to treat paralysis agitans
piperazine adipate (B.P.)	Entacyl	Anthelmintic used against roundworms and threadworms
piridoxilate		Treatment of angina
Piriton	chlorpheniramine maleate (B.P.)	Antihistamine drug
Pitressin	vasopressin	Used in diabetes insipidus

practolol	Eraldin	Treatment of angina and cardiac arrhythmias
prednisolone (B.P.)	Delta-Cortef, Delta-Stab	Steroid drug
prednisone (B.P.)	DeCortisyl, Deltacortone	Steroid drug
Primolut N	norethisterone (B.P.)	Steroid drug
Priscol	tolazoline hydrochloride (B.P.)	Used in treatment of peripheral vascular disorders
Pro-Banthine	propantheline bromide (B.P.)	Used in treatment of gastric ulcer
probenecid (B.P.)	Benemid	Used to treat gout
procainamide hydrochloride	Pronestyl	Used in treatment of arrhythmias, etc.
prochlorperazine maleate (B.P.)	Stemetil	Tranquillizing drug
Prokayvit	acetomenaphthone (B.P.)	Used to treat low prothrombin level
promazine hydrochloride (B.P.)	Sparine	Tranquilizer
promethazine hydrochloride (B.P.)	Phenergan	Antihistamine drug
promethazine theoclate (B.P.)	Avomine	Antihistamine drug often used as anti-emetic
Pronestyl	procainamide hydrochloride	Used in treatment of arrhythmias, etc.
propantheline bromide (B.P.)	Pro-Banthine	Used in treatment of gastric ulcer
propicillin potassium	Brocillin, Ultrapen	Antibiotic
propranolol hydrochloride	Inderal	Blocking agent acting on adrenergic beta receptors. Reduces response of heart to exercise
Prostigmin	neostigmine methylsulphate (B.P.)	A miotic. Increases intestinal tone. Used in myasthenia gravis

Puri-Nethol	mercaptopurine (B.P.)	Cytotoxic drug
pyridostigmine bromide (B.P.)	Mestinon	Used in treatment of myasthenia gravis
pyridoxine hydrochloride	vitamin B₆	
Quellada	gamma benzene hexachloride	Used in treatment of nausea
quinalbarbitone sodium (B.P.)	Seconal Sodium	Antiscabetic
		Hypnotic acting within 15 minutes and action lasting up to 3 hours
quinethazone	Aquamox	Diuretic
Rastinon	tolbutamide	Oral drug used in diabetes mellitus
reserpine	Serpasil	Antihypertensive drug
Resochin	chloroquine phosphate (B.P.)	Antimalarial drug
Ritalin	methyl phenidate hydro-chloride	Antidepressant drug
Rynacrom	sodium cromoglycate	Treatment of allergic rhinitis
Salazopyrin	sulphasalazine	Sulphonamide drug
salbutamol	Ventolin	Antispasmodic
Salupres	hydrochlorothiazide	Diuretic
Saluric	chlorothiazide (B.P.)	Diuretic
Saroten	amitriptyline hydro-chloride (B.P.)	Antidepressant and tranquilliser
Saventrine	isoprenaline hydrochloride (B.P.)	A bronchodilator
Scoline	suxamethonium chloride	Muscle relaxant
scopolamine hydro-bromide	hyoscine hydrobromide (B.P.)	Hypnotic, antispasmodic and mydriatic
Seconal Sodium	quinalbarbitone sodium (B.P.)	Hypnotic acting within 15 minutes and action lasting up to 3 hours
Serpasil	reserpine	Antihypertensive drug

Sodium Amytal	amylobarbitone sodium (B.P.)	Hypnotic, usually acting within half an hour and lasting up to 6 hours
sodium cromoglycate	Intal, Rynacrom	Treatment of asthma and allergic rhinitis
solapsone (B.P.)	solasulfone, Sulphetrone solapsone (B.P.)	Used in treatment of leprosy
solasulfone		Used in treatment of leprosy
Solupen	benzylpenicillin	Antibiotic
Somnesin	methylpentynol (B.P.C.)	Short-acting hypnotic
Soneryl	butobarbitone (B.P.)	Hypnotic usually acting within half an hour and lasting up to 6 hours
Sparine	promazine hydro-chloride (B.P.)	Tranquillizer
spironolactone (B.P.)	Aldactone-A	Increases excretion of sodium and reduces excretion of potassium
Stelazine	trifluoperazine hydro-chloride (B.P.)	Tranquillizing drug
Stemetil	prochlorperazine maleate (B.P.)	Tranquilling drug
streptomycin sulphate (B.P.)		Used in the treatment of tuberculosis
Streptonivicin	novobiocin sodium (B.P.)	Antibiotic sometimes used for patients sensitized to penicillin
succinylsulphathiazole (B.P.)	Sulfasuxidine	Used in infections of gastrointestinal tract
Sulfasuxidine	succinylsulphathiazole (B.P.)	Used in infections of gastrointestinal tract
Sulfathalidine	phthalylsulphathiazole (B.P.)	Used in infections of gastrointestinal tract
sulphacetamide sodium (B.P.)	Albucid	Bacteriostatic action
sulphadiazine (B.P.)	Cremodiazine	Sulphonamide drug

sulphadimidine (B.P.)	Sulphamezathine	Sulphonamide drug sometimes given in urinary infections
sulphafurazole (B.P.)	Gantrisin	Sulphonamide drug useful in urinary tract infection
Sulphamezathine	sulphadimidine (B.P.)	Sulphonamide drug sometimes given in urinary infections
sulphamethizole (B.P.)	Urolucosil	Sulphonamide drug, may be used in urinary tract infections
sulphamethoxydiazine (B.P.)	Durenate	Long-acting sulphonamide drug
sulphasalazine	Salazopyrin	Sulphonamide drug
Sulphetrone	solapsone (B.P.)	Drug used to treat leprosy
Suscardia	isoprenaline hydrochloride	A bronchodilator
suxamethonium bromide (B.P.)	Brevidil M	A muscle relaxant
suxamethonium chloride	Scoline	Muscle relaxant
Synkavit	menadiol sodium diphosphate	A vitamin K analogue
Tabalgin	paracetamol (B.P.)	An analgesic
Tensilon	edrophonium chloride (B.P.)	Used in diagnosis of myasthenia gravis
Terramycin	oxytetracycline	Antibiotic
Tertroxin	liothyronine	Drug used in thyroid deficiency
testosterone (B.P.)		Androgenic drug
tetracycline hydrochloride (B.P.)	Achromycin, Tetracyn	Used to treat many infections
thyroxine sodium (B.P.)		Used to treat thyroid deficiency
Tofranil	imipramine hydrochloride (B.P.)	Antidepressant
tolazoline hydrochloride (B.P.)	Priscol	Used in treatment of peripheral vascular disorders

tolbutamide	Rastinon	Oral drug used in diabetes mellitus
Trasicor	oxprenolol hydrochloride	Treatment of angina and cardiac arrhythmias
Trasylol	aprotinin	Used in the treatment of haemorrhage
tretamine (B.P.C.)		Cytotoxic drug
triamcinolone (B.P.C.)	Adcortyl, Ledercort	Corticosteroid drug
trifluoperazine hydrochloride (B.P.)	Stelazine	Tranquilizing drug
trimeprazine tartrate (B.P.C.)	Vallergan	Sedative and has properties of anti-histamine drug
trimetaphan camsylate (B.P.)	Arfonad	A hypotensive drug
triprolidine hydrochloride	Actidil	Antihistamine
triprolidine hydrochloride with pseudoephedrine	Actifed	Treatment of nasal and respiratory congestion
Triptafen-DA Tablets	amitriptyline hydrochloride (B.P.)	Antidepressant and tranquilizer
Tromexan	ethyl biscoumacetate (B.P.C.)	Anticoagulant drug
Tryptizol	amitriptyline hydrochloride (B.P.)	Antidepressant and tranquilizer
Ultrapen	propicillin potassium	Antibiotic
Urolucosil	sulphamethizole (B.P.)	Sulphonamide drug, may be used in urinary tract infections
Valium	diazepam	Tranquilizer
Vallergan	trimeprazine tartrate (B.P.C.)	Sedative and has properties of anti-histamine drug
vasopressin	Pitressin	Used in diabetes insipidus
Vasoxine	methoxamine hydrochloride (B.P.C.)	A vasoconstrictor drug

Velosef	cephradine	Antibiotic
Ventolin	salbutamol	Antispasmodic
vitamin B_{12}	cyanocobalamin	Used to treat pernicious and other anaemias
Voltarol	diclofenac	Anti-inflammatory
Warfarin Sodium (B.P.)	Coumadin Sodium (U.S.A.), Marevan (B.P.)	Anticoagulant drug
Welldorm	dichloralphenazone (B.P.)	Hypnotic and sedative
Xylocaine	lignocaine hydrochloride (B.P.)	Local anaesthetic
Xylotox	lignocaine hydrochloride (B.P.)	Local anaesthetic
Zactane	ethoheptazine	Analgesic
Zactipar	ethoheptazine	Analgesic

APPENDIX V

DIETS IN HEALTH AND IN ILLNESS

Dietetic Requirements

The amount and kind of food each individual requires depends on his age and sex, the climate of his country and the sort of work he does, or the life he leads. A man lying in bed needs only 1,700 Calories to fulfil his body's requirements, whereas a man doing extremely heavy work may need 5,000 Calories—nearly three times as much.

Diets are made up of: proteins.
carbohydrates.
fats.
water.
vitamins.
minerals, such as calcium, iron and iodine.

1 gram of protein yields: 4 Calories.
1 gram of carbohydrate yields: 4 Calories.
1 gram of fat yields: 9 Calories.

Calories are the amount of heat needed to raise 1,000 grams of water one degree Centigrade. The Calorie is used as a unit of measurement in dietetics.

Every diet must contain some protein and the tables show the amount of Calories and the weight of protein in grams required by various groups of people. (One ounce is roughly equivalent to 30 grams.)

Total Calorie Requirements in Various Conditions of Life
(NB. The proportion of protein required should be noted.)

	Age	Calories	Grams of Protein
Children	0–1	1000	37
	2–6	1500	56
	7–10	2000	74
	11–14	2750	102
Woman	15–19	2500	93
Man	15–19	3500	130

Requirements of a Woman during pregnancy and lactation.

Stage	Calories
First half of pregnancy.	2500
Second half of pregnancy.	2750
During lactation.	3000

Calorie requirements of a *Man* and *Woman*

In bed.	1750	1500
Sedentary work.	2250	2000
Light work.	2750	2250
Medium work.	3000	2500
Heavy work.	3500	3000
Very heavy work.	4250	3750
Extremely heavy work.	5000	—

Composition of Some Common Foodstuffs per Ounce

	Calories	Protein grams	Fat grams	Carbohydrate grams
Bread	73	2·2	0·2	15·5
Potato	21	0·6	—	4·6
Sugar	108	—	—	26·9
Butter	211	0·1	23·4	—
Cheese	117	7·1	9·8	—
Egg	45	3·5	3·3	0·3
Milk	17	0·9	1·0	1·2
Bacon	128	3·1	12·8	—
Beef	89	4·2	8·0	—
Apple	12	0·1	—	3·0
Orange	10	0·2	—	2·2

Diet in Disease

Many diseases are caused by errors in diet. In other cases patients are unable to utilize certain foods and so the treatment is largely dietetic.

The diet is ordered by the physician and the nurse must keep strictly to the physician's orders.

The following specimen diets carry out all the general principles involved and are widely used.

Light Diet

This should consist of easily digested foods, attractively served, so that they stimulate the patient's appetite. Highly seasoned and fatty foods should be avoided.

Avoid rich soups, highly seasoned meats such as sausages, fat meat such as pork, and fried foods.

Do not give fried egg or cheese dishes.

Avoid fried vegetables and gas-producing vegetables such as onions, radishes, green peppers, cucumbers, raw cabbage, dried beans and peas. Raw apples and pears, grapes and melon are all gas-producing and may not be well tolerated.

Avoid pastry and rich puddings and cakes, new bread, fried bread and rye bread.

Do not give effervescent drinks or alcohol.

Low Residue Diet

(For ulcerative colitis, steatorrhoea, and in acute conditions such as enteric fever and dysentery.)

Avoid all pips, and skins of fruit (whether raw, cooked or in jams, and currants, raisins and lemon peel in cakes), nuts and all unripe fruit. Fruit juice may be taken. Currants, raisins and figs are particularly undesirable, and all fruit is better stewed than raw. Red currant, apple and other fruit jellies allowed, but no ordinary jams.

Avoid all raw vegetables, whether taken alone (celery, watercress), or in pickles or salad; green vegetables must be passed through a sieve and mixed with butter in the form of a purée. Porridge is only allowed if made with the finest oatmeal.

Avoid alcohol, vinegar, pepper, mustard, curry, chutney, new bread or tough meat.

Reducing Diet

In general, avoid starchy foods, such as bread, cakes, potatoes, etc.; avoid sugary foods and fatty foods.

The diet may contain adequate quantities of lean meat, poultry, lean fish and plenty of green-leaf vegetables and fruit.

N.B. Beer is to be avoided as it contains starch, and fish such as salmon, turbot, herrings, mackerel and sardines are classed as 'fat' fish and are not recommended.

Diet for Constipation

Full diet with the following additions:

Wholemeal bread.

Porridge, made with coarse oatmeal; oatcake.

Vegetables twice a day, especially green vegetables, onions, carrots, parsnips, turnips, tomatoes, watercress and lettuce.

Fruit three times a day, raw or cooked, especially fresh plums and greengages, raspberries, currants, gooseberries, strawberries and figs, pears, apples, oranges and grapes, dried figs, raisins and dates.

Ten stewed prunes for breakfast every morning.

Jam and marmalade with bread and puddings.

Glass of cold water on waking and on going to bed.

Low Purine Diet

(For gout.)

It is not generally agreed that the contents of the food have much effect upon gout, but if a low purine diet is advised *avoid entirely*:

> Salmon, halibut, plaice.
> Liver, sweetbread, kidney, roe, brain.
> Coffee, Alcohol.

Take sparingly:

> Cod, chicken, mutton, veal, beef. Porridge.
> Potatoes, onions, turnips, carrots, parsnips.
> French beans, spinach, asparagus.
> Dates, figs, rhubarb. Tea and cocoa.

Cholesterol-free Diet

(For arteriosclerosis, especially coronary disease.)

Avoid yolk of eggs in any form, including cakes and sweets made with eggs.

> Avoid cream, cheese.
>   ,,   kidney, liver, sweetbread, brain.
>   ,,   duck and goose.
>   ,,   the fat of meat, pork, suet, sausages.

Take as little butter as possible.

Fat-free Diet

(For liver and gallbladder disease and steatorrhoea.)

Butter should be replaced by honey or golden syrup. No cheese. No nuts, chocolate or cocoa.

Eggs are best avoided, but may not cause nausea if cooked in puddings and cakes.

Lean meat is allowed: all fat should be carefully separated by the patient.

Fat meat, ham, bacon and pork to be avoided. No suet. No sausages, liver, kidneys or offal. No fish or meat pastes.

Haddock, cod, whiting, turbot, brill and plaice are allowed, but no other fish.

The patient should have skimmed milk.

Diabetic Diets

In treating diabetes, the patient's intake of carbohydrates may be restricted or he may be ordered a diet with an ordinary amount of carbohydrate and adequate insulin to cover it. In a fat diabetic patient, a diet containing only 1,300 Calories may be ordered; whereas, with a thin diabetic patient, or with a patient who does manual labour, a full diet may be required with sufficient insulin covering it.

Diabetic Diet with 180 grams of carbohydrate

*grams of
carbohydrate*

Breakfast
    Egg, bacon, ham or fish
    2 oz. bread or equivalent (*see* p. 423) 30
    *Milk
    Butter or margarine
    Diabetic marmalade if desired
    Coffee or tea

Mid-morning
    *Milk
    Coffee or tea
    2 semi-sweet biscuits 10

Lunch
    Meat, fish, cheese or eggs
    Green vegetables or salad as desired
    Small portion of root vegetables
    7 oz. potato (*i.e.* 2 medium potatoes) 30
or 3 oz. potato and 3 tablespoons unsweetened milk
      pudding
    Fruit (raw or stewed without sugar) 10

Tea
    *Milk
    1 oz. bread or equivalent................................. 15
    Butter or margarine
    Diabetic jam if desired

Supper
    Meat, fish, cheese or eggs
    Green vegetables or salad as desired
    Small portion of root vegetables
    3 oz. potato (*i.e.* 1 medium potato) 15
    2 oz. bread or equivalent................................. 30
    Butter or margarine
    Fruit (raw or stewed without sugar) 10
    *Milk

Bedtime
    *Milk. *Milk taken during the day must not exceed
          30 g C.H.O. *i.e.* 1 pint 30
                                   180

Diabetic Diet with 300 grams of carbohydrate

*grams of
carbohydrate*

Breakfast
    Egg, bacon, ham or fish
    4 oz. bread or equivalent (*see* p. 423) 60
    *Milk
    Butter or margarine
    Fruit (raw or stewed without sugar) 10
    Coffee or tea

Mid-morning
    *Milk
    Coffee or tea
    3 semi-sweet biscuits 15

Lunch
    Meat, fish, cheese or eggs
    Green vegetables or salad as desired
    Small portion of root vegetables
    6 oz. potato (*i.e.* 2 medium potatoes) 30
  or 3 oz. potato and 3 tablespoons unsweetened milk
      pudding
    Fruit (raw or stewed without sugar) 10

Tea
    *Milk
    3 oz. bread or equivalent................................. 45
    Butter or margarine
    Diabetic jam if desired

Supper
    Meat, fish, cheese or eggs
    Green vegetables or salad as desired
    Small portion of root vegetables
    3 oz. potato (*i.e.* 1 medium potato) 15
    3 oz. bread or equivalent................................. 45
    Butter or margarine
    Fruit (raw or stewed without sugar) 10
    *Milk

Bedtime
    1 oz. bread or equivalent................................. 15
    Butter or margarine
    *Milk *Milk allowance = 45 g C.H.O. *i.e.* 1½ pints
       a day 45
                                             ————
                                           300

Equivalents for use in Diabetic Diets

Bread: The equivalent to 1 oz. of bread (*i.e.* 15 grams of carbohydrate) is found in the following:

    2 Ryvita or Vita-Weat
    3 Cream Crackers or Water Biscuits
    3 semi-sweet biscuits
    ¾ cupful Cornflakes or other breakfast cereal
    3 tablespoons porridge
    1 medium-sized potato (3 oz.)
    2 tablespoons boiled rice, spaghetti or macaroni
    ½ pint of milk.

Drinks: The following are equivalent to 20 grams of carbohydrate.

    {1 glassful milk (7 oz.) and
    {2 teaspoons Horlicks, Ovaltine or Bournvita.
    {⅔ cupful fresh orange juice (4 oz.) and
    {2 lumps or 2 teaspoonfuls of sugar.
    {Diabetic fruit squash and
    {4 lumps or 4 teaspoons of sugar.
    {½ cup milk (3 oz.) in tea or coffee and
    {1 oz. bread (or equivalent).

Fruit: The following portions of fruit are equivalent to 10 grams of carbohydrate.

Apple, dessert	1 small
Apple, stewed	1½ cups
Apricots, dried	6 halves
Apricots, fresh	2 medium
Banana	1 small
Cherries	10 large
Dates	2
Figs, dried	1 small
Figs, fresh	2 large
Gooseberries	6 large
Grapefruit	1 medium
Grapes	12
Greengages	4 medium
Melon	1 slice, 2 in. thick
Orange	1 small
Orange juice	⅔ cup
Peach	1 medium
Pear	1 medium
Pineapple, fresh	1 slice, 1 in. thick
Plums, dessert	2 large

Plums, stewed	3 medium
Prunes	6 small
Raspberries	1 cup
Strawberries	1 cup
Tangerine	1 large

Foods to be avoided in a diabetic diet.

The following foods contain a high percentage of carbohydrate, and are therefore to be avoided by the diabetic: sugar, sweets and chocolate; jam, marmalade, honey or syrup; puddings, cakes and pastries; biscuits (except as equivalents to bread); thickened soups, sauces and gravies; sweetened fruit drinks and minerals.

Foods allowed at will in a diabetic diet.

The following foods may be taken as desired by the diabetic: Coffee, tea or soda water; clear broth, Bovril, Oxo or Marmite, and the following vegetables:

artichokes	chicory	lettuce	radishes
asparagus	cucumber	mustard & cress	rhubarb
broccoli	endive	marrow	runner beans
Brussels sprouts	French beans	mushrooms	sauerkraut
cabbage	kale	onions	spinach
cauliflower	leeks	parsley	swedes
celery	lemons	pepper, green	tomatoes
			watercress

Distribution of carbohydrate in the diet according to the amount of insulin taken by the patient

If no insulin is being taken by the patient, the amount of carbohydrate should be distributed evenly over breakfast, lunch, tea and supper. If protamine zinc and soluble insulin is given, $\frac{1}{3}$ of the total carbohydrate should be given at breakfast, $\frac{1}{3}$ divided between lunch and tea and $\frac{1}{3}$ at supper. With globin insulin, $\frac{1}{6}$ carbohydrate should be given at breakfast, $\frac{2}{6}$ at lunch, and $\frac{2}{6}$ at supper time. When lente insulin is being taken, $\frac{1}{4}$ carbohydrate at breakfast, $\frac{1}{4}$ at lunch, $\frac{1}{4}$ at tea, and $\frac{1}{4}$ at supper and $\frac{1}{20}$ at bedtime. With Isophane insulin, $\frac{1}{5}$ carbohydrate should be given at breakfast, $\frac{3}{10}$ at lunch, $\frac{1}{5}$ at tea time, $\frac{1}{5}$ at supper, and about $\frac{1}{20}$ at bedtime.

Diet for Patients with Gastric Ulcer

Stage I

All patients have to be given the appropriate medicines, such as magnesium trisilicate, aluminium hydroxide or other alkaline powder, and tinct. belladonna or propantheline before meals, and milk ad. lib.

Patients should avoid soups made with meat stock, meat, fish and poultry, cheese, fried eggs; vegetables, raw fruit, brown and wholemeal bread, cereals and biscuits except plain ones.

Avoid alcohol, strong tea or coffee, Oxo, Bovril, condiments and seasonings.

Specimen menu giving approximately 2,000 Calories:

Breakfast
    Strained porridge
    Milk
    Soft egg (boiled, poached or scrambled)
    White bread toasted
    Jelly jam, honey or jelly marmalade
    Milk drink or very milky tea with sugar

Mid-morning
    Egg flip
    Buttered Cream Crackers

Lunch
    Strained cream soup
    Melba toast or Cream Crackers
    Milk pudding or puréed fruit
    Milk drink or very milky tea with sugar

Tea
    Toast and butter
    Jelly jam
    Milky tea with sugar

Supper
    Egg custard
    Plain cereal pudding or jelly
    Milk drink or very milky tea with sugar

Bedtime
    Milk drink
    Plain biscuits

The patient should have milk ad. lib. and the appropriate medicines.

Avoid soups made with meat stock, highly seasoned meat such as sausages, tinned meat and fish; re-cooked food, pork and bacon; strong cheese, fried eggs, fried vegetables and gas-forming vegetables such as onions, green peppers, dried peas and beans; raw vegetables. All cooked vegetables should be sieved.

Avoid fresh fruit except bananas and any cooked fruit with seeds, or skins; avoid dried fruit. Do not give pastry, rich puddings or cakes; brown and wholemeal bread, biscuits and cereals.

Avoid strong tea, coffee, Oxo and Bovril, and alcohol. Avoid seasoning and condiments.

Specimen menu giving approximately 2,100 Calories.

Breakfast
    Cereal (as allowed)
    Milk
    Soft egg, plain fish or ham (not fried)
    White toast or bread
    Butter or margarine
    Jelly jam or marmalade jelly
    Weak tea or coffee with sugar and milk

Mid-morning
    Milk or milky drink
    Plain biscuits

Lunch
    Lean meat, fish or poultry (as allowed)
    Potato (not roast or fried)
    Vegetables (as allowed)
    Fruit or milk pudding (as allowed)
    Tea or coffee with sugar and milk

Tea
    White bread
    Butter or margarine
    Jelly or Marmite
    Weak tea with sugar and milk

Supper

Meat, fish, cheese or egg dish (as allowed)
Potato
Vegetables   ⎫
Fruit or pudding ⎬ as at lunch
            ⎭
White bread
Butter or margarine
Weak tea with sugar and milk

Bedtime

Milk or milky drink
Toast and butter or plain biscuits.

POST-PEPTIC ULCER REGIME

Avoid alcohol. Avoid effervescing drinks and coffee.

Avoid all pips and skins of fruit (whether raw, cooked or in jam, and currants, raisins and lemon peel in puddings and cake), nuts and all unripe fruit. For example, an orange may be sucked but not eaten. Currants, raisins and figs are particularly undesirable.

Avoid all raw vegetables, whether taken alone (celery, watercress), or in pickles or salad; green vegetables must be passed through a sieve and mixed with butter in the form of a purée. Porridge is only allowed if made with the finest oatmeal.

Avoid vinegar, lemon juice, sour fruit, spinach, pepper, mustard, curry, chutney, excess of salt, new bread, tough meat.

Take plenty of butter and a tablespoonful of olive oil before each meal.

Eat slowly and chew very thoroughly. An adequate time should be allowed for meals, and rest for at least a quarter of an hour before and after meals. Meals must be punctual.

Don't smoke excessively. No smoking at all if any indigestion.

For six months: A meal or feed should be taken at intervals of not more than two hours from waking till retiring, and again if awake during the night. The feed should consist of a glass of the following mixture, which should be prepared each morning: a quart of milk, and 120 grains of sodium citrate in 1 oz. of water.

After six months of complete freedom: A feed should be taken in the middle of the morning, on going to bed, and again if awake during the night, in addition to the ordinary meals.

A teaspoonful of the 'alkaline powder' should be taken an hour after meals and also directly the slightest indigestion or heartburn is felt.

The bowels should be kept regular by means of magnesia emulsion taken two or three times a day, and, if necessary, liquid paraffin, but no other aperients should be taken.

The teeth should be attended to by the dentist regularly every six months.

No drugs should be taken in pill or tablet form.

If there is the slightest return of symptoms, the patient should go to bed on a strict diet, and consult his doctor, not waiting for the symptoms to become serious.

High Protein, Low Fat Diet

(For cirrhosis of liver, steatorrhoea, certain cases of nephritis, carcinoma.)

Lean meat, fish, eggs, Cheddar cheese.
White bread, Cornflakes, boiled potatoes, cauliflower, peas.
Small occasional helpings of jam and marmalade.
Baked custards and milk puddings made from skimmed milk.
2 pt. daily of fortified milk consisting of:
    2 pt. skimmed milk
    2 oz. Sprulac
    2 oz. Casilan
    1 oz. lactose.

Low Sodium Diet

Avoid adding salt to food at meal times, and only very small quantities may be used in cooking.

The following food should be avoided: Soups made from ham or salt meat; Oxo, Bovril; tinned and preserved meats; smoked and dried products such as ham and bacon; salt fish and offal (though heart and liver may be taken).

The patient should also avoid cheese; beetroot, celery and spinach; puddings made with baking powder or soda; and anything made with self-raising flour.

He should not take meat sauces, pickles, condiments, salad cream or mayonnaise.

Gluten-free Diet

(This diet is used chiefly to treat coeliac disease and in steatorrhoea. Rye and wheat gluten has to be avoided and special bread, cakes and biscuits are given made of wheat starch.)

Breakfast
    Oatmeal porridge, Cornflakes or other suitable cereals
        (with milk and sugar)
    Egg, bacon, ham, kipper or haddock
    Wheat starch bread, toasted if desired
    Butter, honey or marmalade
    Tea or coffee

Mid-morning
> Tea, coffee or milk
> Oatcakes or wheat starch biscuits if desired

Lunch
> Meat, poultry, or steamed, baked or grilled fish
> Potatoes
> Cooked vegetables or salad
> Sago, rice, tapioca, egg custard, blancmange, **junket**, jelly
> or fruit
> Tea, coffee or fruit juice

Tea
> Wheat starch bread
> Butter
> Jam, honey, syrup or tomatoes
> Oatcakes or wheat starch cakes or biscuits
> Tea or coffee

Supper
> Meat, fish, cheese or eggs
> Potatoes or wheat starch bread and butter
> Cooked vegetables or salad if desired
> Pudding or fruit as at lunch

Bedtime
> Tea, milk or coffee.

APPENDIX VI

FIRST AID

Artificial Respiration

(a) **Mouth to Mouth Method.** This is the most efficient first aid method of giving artificial respiration and the procedure is as follows:

1. Lay the patient flat on his back, if possible on a table, or on ground higher than that on which the rescuer stands.
2. See that the mouth is cleared of any obstruction.
3. Place some soft article, such as a coat, under the patient's shoulders so that his head falls well back.
4. Stand or kneel opposite to the patient's head.
5. Put one hand on the crown of the patient's head and press gently so that the head is fully extended. Put the other hand on the patient's jaw so that it is drawn well forward. (See Fig. 1.)

AREA COVERED BY RESCUER'S MOUTH

AIRWAY CLEAR

Fig. I

6. The rescuer breathes in deeply and then places his
   mouth over the patient's mouth whilst pinching the
   patient's nose to block the nasal orifice. The rescuer
   breathes out strongly into the patient's lungs (See Fig.
   II). If the patient is a child or baby the rescuer should
   breathe delicately.

Fig. II

7. The patient expires passively and the rescuer takes another deep breath and repeats the cycle every 3 to 5 seconds. The jaw must be kept drawn well forward (see Fig. III) so that the patient's airway is always kept patent.

Fig. III

A special tube or airway, if available in the emergency, can be used so that the rescuer is not in direct contact with the patient's mouth.

A manikin should be used to teach this method of artificial respiration.

(*b*) **Schäfer's Method.**—Lay the patient on his face, loosen tight clothing, turn his head to one side, and carry the arms forward so that one rests on each side of the head. Kneel astride the patient, facing his head. Place your hands flat over the lower

Artificial Respiration (Schäfer's method, I)

Artificial Respiration (Schäfer's method, II)

part of the back, one on each side, with the thumbs near the spine. Lean forward keeping the arms stiff, and press steadily and firmly to drive the air out of the patient's lungs. Keeping your hands in position, relax the pressure and fall back towards the heels. Air will now enter the lungs. Repeat movements 15–18 times a minute.

(c) **Holger Nielsen Method.**—Place the patient on his face and give a slap in the middle of the back to jerk the tongue forward.

Position of Operator

Place one knee with the inner side in line with the patient's cheek six to twelve inches from the top of the patient's head.

Place the other foot with the heel in line with the patient's elbow.

Place the hands on the patient's back with the palms resting on the shoulder blades, the thumbs on the spine and the fingers pointing to the patient's feet. (Figs. A and B.)

Fig. A

Fig. B

Movement (1)

Keeping the arms straight rock gently forward until the arms are vertical, using no special force. The movement takes 2½ seconds counting 'One, two, three'. This pressure causes expiration. (Figs. C and D.)

FIG. C

FIG. D

Movement (2)

The operator now rocks back counting 'four' and slides his hands past the patient's shoulders until they can grip his upper arms near the elbows. He raises and pulls on the arms for a period of 2½ seconds counting 'Five, six, seven.'

This movement causes inspiration. The arms should remain straight for the whole period. (Figs. E and F.)

FIG. E

FIG. F

Counting 'Eight' the operator lowers the patient's arms to the ground and replaces his hands in the original position.

The whole operation should be rhythmic in character and should be continued until breathing re-commences.

When the patient begins to show signs of breathing the operator should continue with Movement 2 only, raising and lowering the arms alternately counting, 1, 2, 3 ($2\frac{1}{2}$ seconds) for Inspiration and 4, 5, 6 ($2\frac{1}{2}$ seconds) for Expiration. This will now give a rate of 12 times per minute. (Figs. G and H.)

FIG. G

FIG. H

Children

For children down to the age of 5 years the pressure on the shoulder blades should be considerably reduced and applied with the finger tips only. The rates should be 12 times per minute. (Figs. I and J.)

Fig. I

Fig. J

Below 5 years of age the arms should be laid by the sides and a support placed under the child's head, or with the head supported by a helper, grasp the shoulders with the fingers underneath and the thumbs on top. Lift the shoulders steadily with the fingers to expand the chest: lower the shoulders and with the thumbs press gently on the shoulder-blades. (Figs. K and L.)

The rate should be 2 seconds Inspiration and 2 seconds Expiration or 15 times per minute.

This method may be done with the patient on a table and the operator standing.

FIG. K

FIG. L

Bites

Dog.—Encourage the wound to bleed by pressing around it, and bathe with warm antiseptic lotion. Apply 3 per cent. solution of tincture of iodine, and cover with the inner surface of a clean pocket handkerchief. If the dog appeared to be savage a tourniquet should be applied as soon as possible proximal to the wound. The patient should be taken to a doctor, and the name and address of the owner of the dog should be ascertained.

Snake.—Tie a tourniquet around the limb, proximal to the wound. Squeeze the wound and encourage bleeding. If the wound does not bleed, open it with a penknife or needle that has been previously sterilized in a match flame. If potassium permanganate crystals are available, rub a few into the wound. Apply a dressing and take the patient to see a doctor as soon as possible.

Bee Sting.—If the sting is visible, squeeze it out, or remove it with the point of a needle that has been previously sterilized in a match flame. Apply a compress of saturated solution of sodium bicarbonate, or a wet 'blue-bag'. The compress should be changed every two hours until the inflammation has subsided.

Burns and Scalds

If the patient is seen in flames, cover him with some thick garment to put out the flames, and lay him flat. Send for the doctor. Keep the patient quiet, apply warmth and give a stimulating drink. Keep the head low. Remove burnt clothing, cutting away where necessary, and apply a compress of soda bicarbonate lotion or normal saline.

Coal Gas Poisoning

Enter the room and open the window as soon as possible. Turn off the gas. Drag the patient out of the room into the fresh air, and send for a doctor. Loosen all tight clothing and perform artificial respiration until the doctor arrives. When respiration is established apply warmth, and give stimulants if necessary.

Convulsions, Epilepsy, etc.

Draw the patient to a place of safety. Put something hard between the teeth to prevent him biting his tongue. Loosen tight clothing. Control the movements but do not try to stop them. Make the following observations to report to the doctor: Evidence of any warning; where the twitching began; duration and severity; loss of consciousness; any damage to the tongue;

incontinence; colour of the patient; size and equality of the pupils; termination of the fit; smell of the breath; condition after the fit.

Infants.—Keep the child warm. As sedatives will be needed, lose no time in sending for the doctor.

Drowning

If other people are available send for the doctor, and hot-water bottles, blankets, a hot drink and a conveyance. Loosen tight clothing and clear the mouth of water, weeds, etc. Perform artificial respiration until the doctor arrives. If recovery takes place, remove wet clothing, apply friction and warm dry clothes. Give a hot drink.

Electric Shock

Disconnect the patient from the current by turning off the switch. If this is not possible the nurse must move the patient, protecting herself first either by standing on wood or rubber or by placing rubber or thick, dry woollen material, such as a coat, between her hands and the patient. The doctor should be sent for, clothing loosened and artificial respiration applied. Treat for shock by warmth and stimulants. Any burns should be covered with clean linen.

Foreign Bodies

(*a*) *Eye.*—Prevent the patient from rubbing the eye. Examine the lower lid first. If the foreign body is not seen, pull the upper lid over the lower one and the lashes of the lower lid will often remove it from the upper. To examine the upper lid, tell the patient to look down and evert it over a match stick. The foreign body can be removed with a camel-hair brush or a small piece of blotting paper cut to a point. If the irritant is a liquid, the patient should put his face into a bowl of water and open and shut the eyes several times. Liquid paraffin or castor oil should be dropped into the eye afterwards, and a pad and bandage applied. If there is any difficulty, the patient should be taken to a doctor.

(*b*) *Ear.*—Insects. Lay the patient down on the unaffected ear. Fill up the meatus with oil, and the insect will float to the top. In the case of other small objects such as a pencil, straw, beads or peas, if they can be seen and grasped they are pulled out; if not, the patient must be taken to a doctor. The condition is often made worse by trying unsuccessfully to remove the foreign body. Water will only make the foreign body swell and so increase the difficulty.

(*c*) *Nose.*—Children may put shoe buttons, peas, beads into the nose. Blowing the nose or inducing the patient to sneeze may help. A better result may be obtained by blocking the unaffected nostril and then directing the patient to blow. If this is not successful, take the child to a doctor.

(*d*) *Trachea.*—Loosen clothing, bend patient forwards and thump back. This may dislodge the foreign body. If a child, hold him upside down and slap sharply between the shoulders. If this is unsuccessful, pass a finger as far down the throat as possible. This may remove the object or cause the patient to retch and cough which may dislodge it. If these measures fail, a doctor must be obtained immediately. If the patient stops breathing and is completely asphyxiated, the nurse would be justified in attempting a tracheotomy if medical aid is not available.

Fractures

Send for some means of transport. A stretcher will be necessary for certain cases. Except in the case of small bones the fracture should be immobilized before the patient is moved. Improvised splints of pieces of wood may be used, but if an ambulance is obtainable splints will be brought. The joint above, and the joint below the injury should be immobilized. If the skin is broken the wound must be covered as soon as possible. Haemorrhage requires immediate treatment.

Treat the patient for shock by keeping the head low, giving a hot drink, applying warmth; arrange as comfortably as possible for transport.

Haemorrhage

May be internal or external, and come from arteries, veins, or capillaries.

1. Send for the doctor.
2. Cover the wound with clean linen and apply pressure.
3. If not arrested, in the case of arterial bleeding apply pressure above the wound: (*a*) digital compression on the nearest spot where the artery crosses a bone, (*b*) tourniquet as a last resort.

N.B. Wool or some other material should be placed between the tourniquet and the skin. It should not be left on for longer than twenty minutes. It is dangerous to apply a tourniquet to the arm as damage to the superficial nerves may cause paralysis.

4. Elevate the bleeding point.
5. Application of hot lotion (115° F), or ice will aid clotting.
6. Treat for shock.

In the case of venous haemorrhage apply pressure below the wound.

Bleeding from a tooth socket.—1. Sit the patient up. 2. Remove any clots. 3. Pack the socket with a strip of styptic gauze. 4. Make the patient bite on a pad and apply a jaw bandage. If the patient has no teeth, the nurse should apply pressure to the bleeding part. The pressure may have to be maintained for as long as twenty minutes.

Bleeding from the nose.—1. Put the patient in the recumbent position with the head raised and thrown back. 2. Remove clots from the back of the mouth. 3. Apply cold or iced water over the nose and to the sides of the neck.

Poisons

See Appendix III, p. 385 *et seq.*

Sunstroke

The patient should be removed to the shade and have cold water applied to the head and nape of the neck. He should be put into a cool, darkened room with a current of moving air. The iced compresses to the head and neck should be renewed frequently. The clothing should be regulated according to the patient's temperature. If there is hyperpyrexia, pending the doctor's arrival the nurse may perform a tepid sponge.

APPENDIX VII

THEATRE INSTRUMENTS

It must be understood that lists of instruments for different operations vary with different surgeons and circumstances, but the following have been found generally satisfactory:

General Set (Plate I)

15 Lane's tissue forceps (I, 1).
 9 Spencer Wells' artery forceps (I, 2).
 9 Mayo Ochsner's forceps (I, 3).
 4 toothed dissecting forceps (I, 4).
 2 non-toothed dissecting forceps (I, 5).
 2 retractors (I, 6).
 2 sponge-holding forceps (I, 7).
 4 towel clips (I, 8).
 1 small probe (I, 9). ⎫
 1 long   „   ⎪
 1 grooved director (I, 10). ⎪
 1 blunt dissector (I, 11). ⎪
 1 raspatory (I, 12) ⎬ 9 extras.
 1 sharp spoon (I, 13). ⎪
 1 aneurysm needle (I, 14). ⎪
 1 needle holder (I, 15). ⎪
 1 suture holder (I, 16). ⎭
 1 pair curved scissors (I, 17).
 2 pairs straight scissors (I, 18).
 2 scalpels (I, 19).

Plate I

Bone Set (Plate II)

9 skin clips (II, 1).
2 lion bone-holding forceps (II, 2).
2 small lion   „   „
1 large straight bone cutting forceps (II, 3).
1   „   curved   „   „   „   (II, 4).
1 small straight   „   „   „
1   „   curved   „   „   „
2 pairs necrosis forceps (II, 5).
1 pair sequestrum   „   (II, 6).
1 awl (II, 7).
1 grooved awl (II, 8).
1 mallet (II, 9)
Langenbeck retractors (II, 10).
1 pair sinus forceps (II, 11).
2 rugines (II, 12).
1 pair bone levers or spikes (II, 13).
1 pair medium bone levers (grooved) (II, 14).
1 pair small bone levers (or more according to operation).
1 file (II, 15).
1 mechanical drill and drill points (II, 16).

Plate II

Bone Sharps (Plate IIIA)

1 large saw (III, 1).
1 small saw.
Chisels of varying sizes (III, 2).
Osteotomes   ,,   ,,   (III, 3).
Gouges   ,,   ,,   (III, 4).
Drill points ,,   ,,   (II, 16).

Bone Plating Set (Plate IIIB)

General Set and Bone Set, plus—
2 plate holding forceps (III, 5).
2 plate benders (III, 6).
2 screw holding forceps (III, 7).
2 screwdrivers (III, 8).
Plates (III, 9) and screws (III, 10).

Extra Laparotomy Instruments (Plate IIIC)

General Set, plus—
1 malleable probe (III, 11).
1 pliable   ,,   (III, 12).
1 malleable spoon or scoop (III, 13).
1 gall-stone forceps (Desjardin's) (III, 14).
} 4 gall bladder extras.
2 Moynihan's pedicle forceps (III, 15).
2 straight compression forceps (III, 16).
2 abdominal retractors (III, 17).
2 pairs curved intestinal clamps (III, 18).
2 curved compression forceps (III, 19).

Plate III

A
1
2
3
(chisel)
4

B
5
6
7
8
9
10

C
11
12
14
13
15
16
17
18
19

Gastrectomy and Resection of Gut (Plate IVA)

General Set, plus—
2 abdominal retractors (III, 17).
1 self-retaining retractor (IV, 1).
2 straight compression forceps (III, 16).
2 curved   „   „   (III, 19).
2 Moynihan's pedicle forceps (III, 15).
1 double intestinal clamp (IV, 2).
2 large straight intestinal clamps (IV, 3).
2 small   „   „
2 curved intestinal clamps (III, 18).
4 Judd's or Allis's basting forceps (IV, 4).
1 large Payr's clamp (IV, 5).
1 small   „   „

Colostomy (Plate IVB)

General Set, plus—
Abdominal retractors (III, 17).
2 small intestinal clamps (III, 18).
Paul's tube (IV, 6) and colostomy rod (IV, 7).

Empyema (Plate IVC).

General Set, plus—
Rugine (II, 12).
2 rib raspatories (IV, 8).
Rib cutting forceps (II, 3, 4).
Rib shears (IV, 9).
Necrosis forceps (II, 5).

Herniotomy (Plate IVD).

General Set, plus—
Hernia needle (IV, 10).

Haemorrhoids (Plate IVE)

General Set, plus—
Proctoscope (IV, 11).
4 haemorrhoid clamps (IV, 12).

Amputation (Plate IVF)

General Set, plus—
Extra artery forceps (I, 2).
Bone set (II).
Bone sharps (IIIA).
Flat retractor (IV, 13).
Amputation knife (IV, 14).

Plate IV

Tonsillectomy (Plate V)

1 towel clip (I, 8).
4 tongue depressors (V, 1).
1 Davis gag (V, 1).
Suspension apparatus for gag (V, 2).
2 tonsil guillotines (V, 3).
2 Doyen's gags (V, 4).
2 Mayo Ochsner's artery forceps (I, 3).
1 tracheotomy dilator (V, 5).
2 tonsil snares (V, 6).
1 tonsil dissector (V, 7).
2 adenoid curettes (V, 8).
2 pairs toothed dissecting forceps (I, 4).
2 curved tonsil forceps (V, 9).
1 toothed   ,,   ,,   (V, 10).
4 straight artery forceps (I, 2).
4 curved   ,,   ,,

Plate V

Plate VI

Some special instruments for gynaecological work: Plate VI

Vaginal speculae, Auvard's (VI, 1).
    „   „   Sims' (VI, 2).
    „   „   Fergusson's (VI, 3).
Pessaries (VI, 5).
Uterine sound (VI, 6).
Playfair's probe (VI, 7).
Ovum forceps (VI, 8).
Vulsellum forceps (VI, 9).
Intra-uterine douche nozzle (VI, 10).
Dilators for cervix (VI, 11).
Intra-uterine flushing curette (VI, 12).

Some special instruments for ophthalmic work: (Plate VIIA)

Retractor (VII, 1).
Undine (VII, 2).
Ophthalmoscope (VII, 3).
Graefe's knife (VII, 4).
Keratome (VII, 5).
Beer's knife (VII, 6).
Iris scissors (VII, 7).
Elliott's trephine (VII, 8).
Iris forceps (VII, 9).
Roller forceps for trachoma (VII, 10).

Operative Treatment of Fractures (Plate VIIB)

Steinmann's pin, introducer, stirrup (VII, 11).
Apparatus for the insertion of Kirschner's wire (VII, 12).
A Böhler's iron (VII, 13).
A Smith-Petersen nail (VII, 14).
(This plate is much reduced from the actual size).

Plate VII

APPENDIX VIII

STERILIZATION

Catgut.—Most of the catgut is supplied sterile in hermetically sealed glass tubes. The tubes are placed in carbolic acid 5 per cent or in 'sterilizing solution' for $\frac{1}{2}$ hour. The following are two methods by which catgut can be sterilized:

(1) Immerse in iodine 1 per cent in spirit for 7 days, transfer to iodine 0·75 per cent in spirit ready for use.

Or,

(2) Steep in iodine 1 per cent for 7 days. Wash daily in biniodide 1-500 for 3 days until clear. Store in biniodide 1-500.

Horsehair } Boil 20 minutes.
Silkworm or salmon gut } Store in carbolic 5 per cent.

Silk and thread.—Boil for 40 minutes, store in carbolic 5 per cent.

Synthetic materials, *e.g.* Gossamer silk and Nylon. Boil for 20 minutes, store in biniodide or perchloride of mercury 1 in 1000 in spirit or water.

All except catgut can also be sterilized in the autoclave 20 lb. pressure for $\frac{1}{2}$ hour.

Rubber tubing, etc.—Boil for 10 minutes, store in formalin 1 in 250, or autoclave 5 lb. pressure for $\frac{1}{2}$ hour.

Gum elastic catheters.—After thorough cleansing, wipe with sterile olive oil, store in paraform jars for 24 hours before use.

Silver and glass catheters.—Boil for 20 minutes.

Gloves.—Boil for 10 minutes, put in boracic lotion. If required dry, boil for 3 minutes, dry on sterile towel, pack in drums—autoclave, 5 lb. pressure for 30 minutes. Boracic powder should be sterilized separately and made up into small packages to be dusted on the hands.

Dressings.—Autoclave at 20 lb. pressure for 30 minutes.

Instruments.—(1) Autoclave 20 lb. pressure for 30 minutes.

Or,

(2) Boil for 5 to 20 minutes in the case of clean instruments, 20 minutes for contaminated instruments.

Scissors and scalpels.—(1) 'Sterilizing Solution' for 30 minutes. (2) Wrapped in lint and boiled as above.

Sharp instruments for bones.—(1) Arranged on lint on a sterilizer tray and boiled as above. (2) Autoclaved.

Needles.—After use, immerse in 2 per cent Lysol, dry and clean with monkey soap or emery paper (fine). Store in sterilizing solution containing a few grains of soda bicarbonate. Alternatively may be boiled or autoclaved as instruments.

Sterilizing Solution.

Borax 1·5 %
Formalin 2·5 % } in water
Phenol 0·4 %

In most cases a Central Sterile Supply Department provides sterile equipment for theatre and ward use. However, emergencies may arise and the above methods may have to be used.

Feeding bottles and teats may be sterilized by boiling for 5 minutes, or they may be rendered sterile by immersing them in a 1–80 solution of 1 % electrolytic sodium hypochlorite (Milton) for at least 1½ hours.

Drinking water may be rendered sterile in an emergency by first filtering it and then adding one teaspoonful of 1 % electrolytic sodium hypochlorite to every gallon of water. It must be left for 5 minutes before drinking.

APPENDIX IX

ABBREVIATIONS OF SOME DEGREES, DIPLOMAS AND OTHER TITLES

A.I.M.S.W.	Associate of the Institute of Medical Social Workers
A.M.S.	Army Medical Services
A.R.R.C.	Associate of the Royal Red Cross
A.R.S.H.	Associate of the Royal Society of Health
B.A.	Bachelor of Arts
B.Ch., B.S.	Bachelor of Surgery
B.Ch.D., B.D.S.	Bachelor of Dental Surgery
B.M.	Bachelor of Medicine
B.Sc.	Bachelor of Science
C.M., Ch.M.	Mastery in Surgery
D.A.	Diploma in Anaesthetics
Dip.Bact.	Diploma in Bacteriology
D.C.H.	Diploma in Child Health
D.C.P.	Diploma in Clinical Pathology
D.D.S.	Doctor of Dental Surgery
D.M.	Doctor of Medicine
D.M.D.	Doctor of Dental Medicine
D.M.R.	Diploma in Medical Radiology
D.M.S.	Director of Medical Services
D.N.	Diploma in Nursing
D.O.	Diploma in Ophthalmology
D.Obst.R.C.O.G.	Diploma in Obstetrics of the Royal College of Obstetricians and Gynaecologists
D.P.H.	Diploma in Public Health
D.P.M.	Diploma in Psychological Medicine
D.Sc.	Doctor of Science
D.T.H.	Diploma in Tropical Hygiene
D.T.M.	Diploma in Tropical Medicine
F.Ch.S.	Fellow of the Society of Chiropodists
F.F.A.R.C.S.	Fellow of the Faculty of Anaesthetists of the Royal College of Surgeons
F.F.R.	Fellow of the Faculty of Radiologists
F.P.S.	Fellow of the Pharmaceutical Society
F.R.C.O.G.	Fellow of the Royal College of Obstetricians and Gynaecologists
F.R.C.P.	Fellow of the Royal College of Physicians

F.R.C.P.E.	Fellow of the Royal College of Physicians of Edinburgh
F.R.C.P.I.	Fellow of the Royal College of Physicians of Ireland
F.R.C.S.	Fellow of the Royal College of Surgeons
F.R.C.S.E.	Fellow of the Royal College of Surgeons of Edinburgh
F.R.C.S.I.	Fellow of the Royal College of Surgeons of Ireland
F.R.F.P.S.G.	Fellow of the Royal Faculty of Physicians and Surgeons, Glasgow
F.R.S.	Fellow of the Royal Society
F.R.S.E.	Fellow of the Royal Society of Edinburgh
H.V.	Health Visitor
L.A.H.	Licentiate of Apothecaries' Hall, Dublin
L.D.S.	Licentiate in Dental Surgery
L.D.Sc.	Licentiate in Dental Science
L.M.S.S.A.	Licentiate in Medicine and Surgery, Society of Apothecaries, London
L.R.C.P.	Licentiate of the Royal College of Physicians
L.R.C.P.E.	Licentiate of the Royal College of Physicians of Edinburgh
L.R.C.S.I.	Licentiate of the Royal College of Surgeons of Ireland
L.R.F.P.S.G.	Licentiate of the Royal Faculty of Physicians and Surgeons, Glasgow
L.S.A.	Licentiate of the Society of Apothecaries, London
L.S.Sc.	Licentiate in Sanitary Science
M.A.	Master of Arts
M.A.O.	Master of Obstetrics
M.B.	Bachelor of Medicine
M.C., M.S., M.Ch.	Master of Surgery
M.Ch.D., M.D.S.	Master of Dental Surgery
M.Ch.S.	Member of the Society of Chiropodists
M.C.S.P.	Member of the Chartered Society of Physiotherapy
M.D.	Doctor of Medicine
M.O.H.	Medical Officer of Health
M.P.S.	Member of the Pharmaceutical Society
M.R.C.O.G.	Member of the Royal College of Obstetricians and Gynaecologists
M.R.C.P.	Member of the Royal College of Physicians
M.R.C.S.	Member of the Royal College of Surgeons
M.S.	Master of Surgery
M.S.A.	Member of the Society of Apothecaries

M.S.R.(D).	Member of the Society of Radiographers (Diagnostic)
M.S.R.(T).	Member of the Society of Radiographers (Therapy)
M.T.D.	Midwife Teacher's Diploma
P.M.O.	Principal Medical Officer
P.M.R.A.F.N.S.	Princess Mary's Royal Air Force Nursing Service
Ph.C.	Pharmaceutical Chemist
Q.A.R.A.N.C.	Queen Alexandra's Royal Army Nursing Corps
Q.A.R.N.N.S.	Queen Alexandra's Royal Naval Nursing Service
Q.H.N.S.	Honorary Nursing Sister to the Queen
Q.H.P.	Honorary Physician to the Queen
Q.H.S.	Honorary Surgeon to the Queen
R.A.M.C.	Royal Army Medical Corps
R.G.N.	Registered General Nurse (Scotland)
R.M.N.	Registered Mental Nurse
R.M.O.	Regimental Medical Officer (military); Resident Medical Officer (institutional)
R.N.	Registered Nurse (America)
R.N.M.D.	Registered Nurse for Mental Defectives
R.N.M.S.	Registered Nurse for the Mentally Sub-normal
R.R.C.	Royal Red Cross
R.S.C.N.	Registered Sick Children's Nurse
Sc.D.	Doctor of Science
S.C.M.	State Certified Midwife
S.E.N.	State Enrolled Nurse
S.M.O.	Senior Medical Officer
S.R.N.	State Registered Nurse

MULTISTIX*

Reagent Strips

The most comprehensive clinical profile ever offered by reagent strip urinalysis. Seven important areas of information on a single strip — in just 60 seconds.

Urobilinogen
Read 60 seconds after wetting

Blood
Read 30 seconds after wetting

Bilirubin
Read 20 seconds after wetting

Ketones
Read 15 seconds after wetting

Glucose
Read 10 seconds after wetting

Protein
Read next

pH
Read immediately

Further information is available from:

 Ames Company, Division of Miles Laboratories Limited, P.O. Box No. 37, Stoke Court, Stoke Poges, Slough, SL2 4LY
CHEMICAL AND BIOLOGICAL INFORMATION SYSTEMS SERVING MEDICINE AND INDUSTRY

 *TRADEMARK